DR. BRALY'S FOOD ALLERGY AND NUTRITION REVOLUTION

DR. BRALY'S FOOD ALLERGY AND NUTRITION REVOLUTION

For Permanent Weight Loss and a Longer, Healthier Life

James Braly, M.D.
Laura Torbet

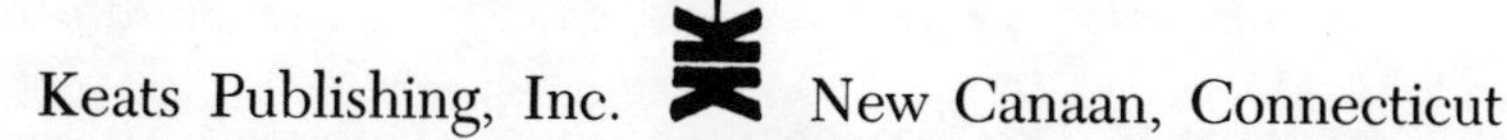
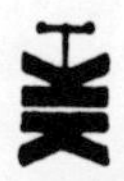

Keats Publishing, Inc. New Canaan, Connecticut

Dr. Braly's Food Allergy & Nutrition Revolution is not intended as medical advice. Its intent is solely informational and educational. Please consult a health professional should the need for one be indicated.

DR. BRALY'S FOOD ALLERGY & NUTRITION REVOLUTION

Library of Congress Cataloging-in-Publication Data

Braly, James.
[Optimum health program]
Dr. Braly's food allergy and nutrition revolution / James Braly.
p. cm.
Originally published: Dr. Braly's optimum health program. New York Times Books, 1985.
Includes bibliographical references and index.
ISBN 0-87983-590-7 : $17.95
1. Food allergy—Diet therapy. I. Title. II. Title: Doctor Braly's food allergy and nutrition revolution. III. Title: Food allergy and nutrition revolution.
RC588.D53B73 1992
616.97'50654—dc20 92-27994
CIP

Printed in the United States of America

Published by Keats Publishing, Inc.
27 Pine Street, P. O. Box 876
New Canaan, Connecticut 06840-0876

15 14 13

TO MY THREE-YEAR-OLD SON, ZACHARY:
Thank you, my son, for bringing
more joy into my life than I thought possible!

Acknowledgments

I want to thank Nathan Keats for his vote of confidence by inviting me to have this book reprinted. A special thanks to Doug Horton, my friend and associate, who made it his personal project to get the book out again into the hands of the public. Dr. Jonathan Wright and Dr. Alan Gaby have kept my "fire in the belly" aglow with their three-day "Nutritional Therapies for the 1990's" medical seminars (highly recommended to anyone interested in *practical and scientific* nutritional education). Thanks, also, to Michael Murray, N.D., who has done a masterful job of introducing me to the science of botanical medicine.

And a deeply felt thanks to my colleague, Lendon Smith, M.D., for his kind words in the foreword and his always inspiring work and writings in nutritional medicine.

Contents

Foreword
xv

Introduction
xix

PART I: The Promise of Optimum Health

1: A New Approach to Weight Loss and Good Health
3
What Exactly Do You Do on the Optimum Health Program? . . . Food May Be a Hazard to Your Health . . . Things Are Looking Up . . . Why the Optimum Health Program? . . . There Is No Such Thing as a Free Lunch

2: Me, Modern Medicine, and the Optimum Health Program
14
Old Medicine and New . . . What's in Store for Medicine? . . . There's Hope . . . Medicine at Optimum Health Labs

3: Thirteen Commonsense Truths About Good Health
25

PART II: How the System Works: Allergy, Digestion, and the Immune System

4: The Allergy Epidemic
37
What Are the Facts? . . . Food Allergy: A Widely Ignored and Misunderstood Illness . . . The Symptoms of Food Allergy . . . Why We Have Allergies

5: The Allergy/Addiction Syndrome and the Dilemma of Diagnosis
54

The Delayed Response: Eat Now, Suffer Later . . . The Progression from Allergy to Addiction . . . Addiction and the Dieter's Dilemma . . . The Difficulties of Testing for Allergies

6: Digestion and the Immune System
63

Tracking the Gastrointestinal Tract . . . The Immune System: The Great Defender . . . How Food-Allergy Reaction Works . . . It All Starts with Malnutrition . . . Getting Well Again

PART III: All About Supplementation

7: Supplementation: Your Nutritional Safety Net
77

Why Do You Need Supplements? . . . How Much Supplementation Do We Need? . . . Guidelines for Your Personal Supplementation Program

8: Vitamins
91

The Name and Numbers Game . . . Fat-Soluble/Water-Soluble . . . Vitamin A—Retinol . . . Beta Carotene—Provitamin A . . . The B Complex . . . Vitamin B1—Thiamine . . . Vitamin B2—Riboflavin . . . Vitamin B3—Niacin . . . Vitamin B5—Pantothenic Acid . . . Vitamin B6—Pyridoxine . . . Vitamin B 12—Cobalamin . . . Folic Acid . . . Biotin . . . PABA, or Para-aminobenzoic Acid . . . Choline . . . Inositol . . . Vitamin C . . . Vitamin E—Tocopherol

9: Minerals
118

Iron . . . Calcium . . . Magnesium . . . Zinc . . . Selenium

10: Amino Acids
126

Dietary and Supplementary Sources of Amino Acids . . . Guidelines for Amino-Acid Supplementation . . . Tryptophan . . . DL-Phenylalanine . . . Arginine and Ornithine . . . L-Carnitine . . . L-Lysine . . . L-Glutamine

11: Essential Fatty Acids:
The Missing Piece of the Nutrition Puzzle
137

Understanding the Essential Fats . . . Stalking the Essential Fats . . . The Prostaglandin Connection . . . How Essential Fatty Acids Grow Up to Become Prostaglandins . . . The Remarkable Health Benefits of Essential Fatty Acids . . . Essential-Fatty-Acid Therapy on the Optimum Health Program

Vitamin Tables
158

Mineral Tables
174

Amino-Acid Tables
186

Essential-Fatty-Acid Tables
193

PART IV:
The Optimum Health Program

12: Permanent Weight Loss—
A Natural By-Product of the Optimum Health Program
197

Losing Weight: The Wrong Way . . . Losing Weight: The Right Way . . . Therapy for Optimum Weight . . . The Optimum Health Weight-Loss Program

13: Getting Started on the Optimum Health Program:
First of All, How's Your Health?
215

Finding Out About You

14: Testing for Food Allergies: Finally, the FICA!
221

The Old Way . . . The New Way . . . FICA: The Breakthrough . . . The Candidiasis Complication . . . Methods of Self-Testing for Food Allergy

15: How to Eat: Thirteen Basic Nutrition Guidelines
234

16: The Rotation Diet: Backbone of the Optimum Health Program
248

What Makes the Rotation Diet So Sensible and Effective for Everyone? . . . Can Allergies Be Eliminated Through Rotation Only? . . . Planning Your Own Rotation Diet . . . Tips for Following the Rotation Diet . . . Keeping a Food and Symptom Journal . . . How to Take Your Supplements . . . Coping with Withdrawal . . . Digestive Support . . . Reintroducing Allergic Foods . . . You've Done It

17: Cooking, Shopping, and Coping on the Optimum Health Program
268

Shopping . . . Substitutes for Allergic Foods . . . A Few Cooking Tips . . . Dining Out on Your Diet . . . Recipes

18: Exercise: Nutrition's Partner
277

The Health Benefits of Exercise . . . Aerobic Conditioning: The Most Effective Exercise . . . Evaluating Personal Risk Factors of Exercise . . . Your Personal Exercise Program . . . Tips and Cautions

19: Notes to Parents: Optimum Health for Children
291

Getting a Head Start: Prepregnancy, Pregnancy, and Infancy . . . The Problem with Cow's Milk . . . How to Bring Up Healthy Children . . . Menu Suggestions . . . Is Your Child Allergic? . . . Allergy-Related Childhood Diseases

PART V: Therapeutic Applications for the Optimum Health Program

20: Getting Well on the Optimum Health Program
311

How to Use Part V . . .

Discussion and Protocols:

Addiction . . . Anti-Aging . . . Arthritis . . . Asthma . . . Atopic Allergies . . . Blood-Sugar Disorders . . . Brain Allergies . . . Candidiasis . . . Cardiovascular Disease (Including Hypertension) . . . Constipation . . . Depression . . . Diabetes Mellitus . . . Diarrhea . . . Digestive Disorders . . . Eczema . . . Gallbladder Problems . . . Gluten Sensitivity . . . Headache . . . Herpes Simplex. . . Hives . . . Hypoglycemia . . . Hypotension . . . Hypothyroidism . . . Insomnia . . . Iron Deficiency and Iron-Deficiency Anemia . . . Irritable Bowel Syndrome . . . Kidney Stones . . . Leg Cramps . . . Multiple Sclerosis . . . Osteoporosis . . . Pain . . . Premenstrual Syndrome (PMS). . . Stress Management . . . Tinnitus . . . Ulcers . . . Uric Acid (Elevated) . . . Viral Infection

Afterword:
A Healthy Future?
418

Appendices

Glossary
423

Mail-Order Food Sources
431

Sources of Common Allergens
432

Substitutes and Alternatives to Allergic Foods
441

Fiber Foods: Sources of Nongrain Dietary Fiber
452

Sugar Alternatives
454

Recipes
456

Rotation Diet Planning Form
486

Diet Diary Form
487

Bibliography
488

Index
495

Foreword

Ten years ago I realized that food sensitivities were responsible for hyperactivity and Jekyll-and-Hyde behavior in children. Therefore, I joined the American College of Allergists for some encouragement and validation. At a national meeting I discovered that a splinter group had formed. This subgroup was trying to get some recognition for their belief that food sensitivities *did* exist, but were often not recognized by the standard or orthodox allergist because the patients' food allergies were not revealed by the standard scratch test on the skin nor were they revealed by the RAST (a blood test for the allergic tendency).

At one of the subgroup's meetings where I was invited to speak, the members were encouraging each other to become comfortable in the knowledge that foods *could* be responsible for bedwetting, stomachaches, headaches, colic, arthritis, muscle aches, and, in short, just about any symptom the body was capable of producing—even obesity. Here are two quotes I learned at this meeting. They were well worth the $70 membership fee: "Food sensitivities cannot do everything, but they can do anything." Here is the other as a corollary to the first: "Eighty percent of those people with food sensitivities have hypoglycemia."

I was encouraged by these intelligent doctors who were trying to explain scientifically something that they had seen clinically. Symptoms and signs that are definitely related to food ingestion can be explained by blood tests and specimen analysis; it is more than just a series of anecdotes. One investigator showed proof that the bladder wall will swell like a giant hive and prevent the victim from holding enough urine to stay dry all night. Many diseases are due to the body's reaction to ingested foods, chemicals, and pollutants. The body is trying to tell the owner that something is wrong.

Thus reassured that I was on the right track, I returned to my practice to do the detective work of finding the offending food, preservative, or environmental poison that was irritating this particular patient. We used to tell patients, when we did not know what was causing their symptoms or disease, "We have investigated your case extensively, but we can find nothing in the examination or the blood tests that gives us a clue of the cause. Do you have a stressful life, job or marriage?" Everyone has something in their life that is a stressor. Get rid of that, and everything will be back to normal. Now we have a few more conditions to explain symptoms before we march the patient off to the psychiatrist.

When I investigated hyperactive children, I found that many of them were "wild and crazy" because they were sensitive to dairy products. In some the connection was easy to spot because they were pale, had dark circles under their eyes, and made snorting, throat-clearing noises as if they had some rubber bands hanging down their throats. The past history revealed colic as a baby, ear infections as a toddler, sometimes asthma as a complication of colds, and then the symptoms moved to bedwetting or nosebleeds. Headaches, constipation, sinus trouble, irritability and episodic violent behavior were often present, but we had to remember to ask about them.

The next step was to obtain patient compliance. We had to stop the food that triggered the symptoms. Sounds easy, but that food was usually the one that the patient craved, and, as we found out, the one to which the patient was addicted. This helped to explain why the victim *had* to have the food at regular intervals or he would develop some nasty withdrawal symptoms. Apparently the food was causing the blood sugar to rise, and then plummet—as the allergists explained at the meeting. This low-blood sugar attack would set up the foraging reaction to ingest that food again. (And, as Dr. Braly points out, "We eat a food to which we are addicted, not to feel good, but in order *not* to feel bad.")

Our job as doctors is to educate the patient about the lifestyle changes that are necessary to achieve optimum health. We have to explain the reasons for the sickness, and then support the patient's weak ego and flagging immune system until the symptoms are gone and the patient's renewed vigor takes over. The patient must heal himself; the doctor is only available to provide insight and support until healthy homeostasis is established.

I began to see the connection between sensitivities and diseases. Genetics played a role. Stressors were always there to blame. Depression often lurked in the background of these people, but it was difficult to establish whether the depression acted as a stressor and produced the symptoms, or the depression was the result of the food or chemical sensitivity. But it was an enjoyable challenge to use the food sensitivity or chemical overload as the working diagnosis and try to get the patient to feel well again, no matter what the cause.

I used vitamin shots, intramuscularly or intravenously, because I had read that food sensitivities will damage the intestinal lining cells to the point that these cells could not digest and absorb the foods and vitamins and minerals the patient was swallowing. After a few shots to "prime the pump," these victims could take the foods and supplements orally without symptoms. The patients became less sensitive to the offenders as the cells were able to break the foods down into their non-allergenic simple sugars, fats and amino acids. Still, this did not work for everyone.

We had people get their protein from mixed amino acids if we felt they were sensitive to soy, milk, pork, chicken and beef. It was expensive and inconvenient, but it worked on those who were desperate.

I had patients fast for four days, and that helped some, but compliance was a problem. We used the rotation diet, in which the patient did not eat the same thing every day. Eating wheat or dairy only every four days was helpful, but hard to follow. (What do you do with last night's leftover meat loaf?)

These patients with their variable symptoms of fatigue, irritability, depression, insomnia, frequent infections, anxiety, obesity, and "being sick and tired of being sick and tired" needed our help. However, this group of symptoms were covered in medical school only as a motivation to write out a prescription for Valium. There were no good tests to give away the condition. It is often called chronic fatigue syndrome now. Virus? Sensitivity? Yeast infection? Parasites? Emotional? But why are there so many of these conditions and questions now? It is almost an epidemic. Something has happened to the health of the people in our country.

Most of us doctors who care about our patients and are willing to believe them, and who do not feel they are crocks or hypochondriacs, will keep searching for better diagnostic and therapeutic answers. I would like to propose that the basic underlying condition that allows people to be chronically sick, have autoimmune diseases, and all the vague symptoms mentioned above, is that the immune system has failed. Our impoverished, overcooked food, the polluted air, the crowded conditions, our lack of exercise, all add up together to hurt the buffering capacity of our bodies so there is no reserve to handle stress, and the viruses and germs that are in us and on us invade and set up housekeeping. The disease that follows is an opportunity, if you will, to stop and figure out what is wrong with one's lifestyle.

If a person is alive, it means that most of the enzymes are working, but if one feels punk, it means that the building blocks are not available, or the acid/base balance is off enough to prevent the minerals and vitamins—if they even are present—to serve their function because they are not soluble. Farmers know this about the soil. If it is acid, they throw on some lime, which is alkaline. But too much will prevent some other minerals which are present in normal amounts to be unavailable to the plants because of the solubility factor.

Chemistry rules apply to the soil, to the plants and to man. There is no escaping them, just as we know that gravity works, and ice is cold. Universal truisms are there to bring us up short when we have strayed from the way we are supposed to live. You cannot fool Mother Nature.

You cannot fool Dr. Braly, either. He has examined all these aspects of what is holding us together and his book has it all. It is a bible of healthy living, and should be used as a textbook in schools. Parents should read aloud to their children from this book.

The Braly Bible is a must. Thanks, Dr. Braly, for making my work easier.

—Lendon H. Smith, M.D.
Portland, Oregon

Introduction

The Victory Is Ours!

A favorite story of mine involves the 1986 survey in which the FDA (the seemingly well-intentioned but badly misdirected federal regulatory agency) contacted the Harris Poll people to conduct a nationwide survey to investigate America's changing attitude towards so-called holistic or alternative (nondrug, nonsurgical, nonpsychiatric) medicine. Much to their surprise and embarrassment, I strongly suspect, the poll's landmark conclusions were:

> The health consumer (that is, you) is smart, educated, often successful in his or her career, an individual resolute, regardless of propaganda to the contrary, in getting the best health care available. More to the point, the higher your education, the higher your income, the more likely you are to seek unorthodox, nonmainstream, "holistic" health care!

Although you do not totally reject the commonplace medicine of prescription drugs, psychiatric and surgical intervention, you have become more keenly aware of science-based, frequently more effective, and consistently less toxic alternatives (that is, the contents of this book).

This particular Harris Poll survey (largely ignored by the medical establishment, of course) is, from an historical perspective, extremely encouraging. I'm convinced it portends incredibly exciting opportunities for America's health care delivery system. *When the educated class of a country or culture, even though in the minority, has been won over to a new way of thinking, whether in the field of politics, economics, morality or medicine, human destiny, at that very point in time, has been immutably set and predetermined. Our battle with entrenched medicine has been won!*

Others may claim the victory, public announcements of the outcome may be delayed (or never admitted), events may get worse before they get better, and others less deserving may receive the accolades for our victory, but the much maligned and regulated "alternative" health care provider, the young physician of tomorrow, and especially you, the health care consumer, have won!

THE NEW MEDICINE

In the relatively short time span since my book was first published and released (1985), some mind-boggling research has occurred, giving us a somewhat privileged glimpse at what this hard-earned victory will mean to you and future generations. As an excellent example, an impressive body of research now exists strongly suggesting that with the general acceptance of nutritional medicine by the medical community we should quickly see a significant reduction in deaths from surgery, a substantial reduction in surgical complications, and startling cuts in the cost of surgical care. A 1990 article published in the peer reviewed *Journal of Enteral and Parenteral Nutrition* reports that when the investigators compared two randomly selected groups of American patients scheduled for elective (nonemergency) surgery, *the group that showed a clear sign of malnutrition*—namely, low serum albumin, the commonly ordered blood test used to measure general protein nutritional status—*in this study represented over 30% of all patients.*

This group, it was found, *could expect to spend twice the time in the hospital (10 days versus five days), pay twice as much to the hospitals and doctors ($16,000 versus $8,000), have 250% more complications from surgery (infections, slow healing, abnormal blood clotting, etc.)* **and die six times more frequently than their better nourished counterparts!**

Therefore, nutritionally sophisticated doctors will insist (like many of my colleagues and I have been insisting for years) that none of their patients will be allowed to have elective surgery until all common measurements of nutritional status are well within the normal limits. (Should you feel the importance of serum albumin/protein status has been overstated, I would be remiss if I didn't share with you the recent published reports that a *high normal* serum albumin level [4.8mg/dl or higher] may not only protect you from the complications and runaway expenses of surgery, but is also associated with a 300% or more *reduction* in the incidence of premature deaths from all common causes. How one pushes his serum albumin up to this level involves—you guessed it—optimizing your overall nutritional status.)

NO MORE NUTRITIONALLY ILLITERATE DOCTORS

Traditional medicine embracing clinical nutrition will mean that young physicians graduating from medical schools will no longer be unaware or ignorant about nutrition and botanical/herbal medicine. As a consequence they will be less dangerous to their patients. To phrase it more bluntly, medical knowledge without nutritional awareness but with a compulsive inclination to use and abuse prescription drugs and surgery, may in fact be quite dangerous to your health.

The late Dr. Mendelsohn, author of *Confessions of a Medical Heretic*, popularized the disturbing reports of *decreased* patient deaths during the absence of medical care; that is while physicians were out on strike. The Canadian doctors' strike in the late 1960's, the Los Angeles-USC doctors' strike in the early 1970's, the subsequent physicians' strike in Colombia, South America, and the two separate Israeli physicians' labor strikes some 25 years apart were all associated with *reductions* in patient mortality during the strike period, ranging from 15% to 50%. *Depressingly, the longer the physicians' labor strike, the larger the reduction in the patient death rate.* (As I'm writing this introductory chapter [January, 1992] I'm informed that we now have yet another opportunity to test this disturbing hypothesis. The Israeli physicians are again threatening to go on a prolonged labor strike against the State and the State-owned hospital system. *If the allopathic-doctors-are-dangerous-to-your-health hypothesis is correct, we should again see people living who would have died if the prescribing- and surgery-crazed doctors were there to treat them.)*

The graduating American physician of the 1980's, at a time of breathtaking advances in nutrition and herbal medicine, averaged well under 30 hours of required medical school education in clinical nutrition over the entire four years of medical school, with little-to-no exposure to the dizzying number of medical conditions caused or complicated by delayed/hidden food allergies. (Below I have included an abbreviated, updated list of the more common conditions I see in my practice.) Plus, they receive absolutely no instructions in the promising area of scientific botanical/herbal medicine. What knowledge was taught came only from sterile books and impersonalized lecture halls with no patients around. To make matters much worse, most all of the book and lecture learning came during the first year of medical school. No clinical nutrition was applied to patients during the hands-on, patient-oriented third and fourth years of school. (As most seasoned teachers know, the best way, if not the only predictably effective way, to learn complicated material is to apply it *daily*.) Most of the medical student's nutritional education was lost forever by the time of graduation.

This kind of educational insanity, I predict, will gradually come to an end. Instead, the young physicians of tomorrow will be schooled in scientifically-based alternative medicine all four years of medical school. There will be a special emphasis on *applied* clinical nutrition and botanical/herbal medicine during the critically important clinical years of medical school. The physicians of tomorrow will have a more balanced and comprehensive education, including the equivalent of a post-graduate degree in clinical nutrition and herbology. It will represent literally hundreds and hundreds of hours of study and practical application. Thirty hours over four years of medical education should and will be replaced by thirty hours a semester.

I personally read and research my specialties—clinical nutrition, food allergy, and herbology—*at least 40 to 50 hours a month and have for over 12 years. Yet I still have great, seemingly hopeless difficulty staying abreast of all the new discoveries and advances in naturopathic medicine.* Six years ago I wrote that new knowledge in clinical nutrition and allergy was doubling every three years or so. Today, I'm convinced the speed of new discoveries is accelerating!

AN UPDATE ON FOOD ALLERGY

Theron Randolph, M.D., an extraordinary physician, original thinker and relentless researcher, wrote over the years about the ubiquitous nature of "hidden" or delayed-onset food allergy. He made famous the quote, "Food allergy is the most commonly undiagnosed illness in medicine today." And you know what? He was right! What doctors today ascribe to neuroses, hypochondriasis or normal ailments of everyday living are often caused or aggravated by delayed-onset food allergies.

A few years ago, *USA Today* had a sizeable story dealing with a new book by a Harvard Medical School professor, in which the focus appeared to be the long list of common symptoms and ailments that patients *needlessly* present to their already overworked physicians, symptoms that were really "normal," minor everyday symptoms (normal and minor only to the physician, of course) that the patient really should learn to live with. The list of symptoms and "minor" ailments reads like a list of common, everyday *food allergy symptoms: nasal stuffiness, coughing, aches and pains, stiffness, headaches, sleep problems, fatigue, gas, fluid retention, overweight, etc.* According to research, the professor said, the would-be patients should *expect* about 80 such episodes per year, and they should learn that these symptoms mean "nothing" and not to worry about or seek medical consultation for them. *Too many Americans are encouraged to be hypochondriacs,* the professor said, and the public and doctors alike should be warned against overindulgence and overconcern.

This is a perfect illustration of the continuing problem, still evident in medical school, that if traditional medicine has no solution to a medical problem, the patient is to blame, and then labelled as neurotic and a hypochondriac (i.e., time-consuming and therefore troublemaking for the physician). As a result, medical students are instructed that they should expect at least 50% or more of their patient visits to be for such typical psychologically-induced complaints.

I've personally been laboratory testing and treating literally thousands of food-allergic, undernourished patients for over a decade now, *and am continuously impressed by the number of medical conditions that include food allergy as an underlying cause or exacerbating agent.* Here is an updated list from the first edition of *common diseases* with food allergy as a prominent cause or aggravating factor. They include (but are not limited to) the following:

Rheumatoid arthritis, juvenile rheumatoid arthritis, joint stiffness, muscle and joint pain, perhaps some cases of osteoarthritis and low back pain
Epilepsy, when accompanied by recurrent headaches and/or abdominal symptoms and/or hyperactivity
Migraines and cluster headaches, perhaps so-called "tension headaches" as well
Attention deficit disorder/hyperactivity/hyperkinesis
Anxiety and panic attacks
Addiction
Asthma
Chronic bronchitis
Nonseasonal rhinitis
Sinusitis
Middle ear infection
Eczema
Hives
Dermatitis herpetiformis (gluten allergy)
Exercise-caused anaphylaxis and hives
Chronic fatigue syndrome
Duodenal ulcers

Inflammatory bowel disease
Glaucoma
Weight gain, obesity
Fluid retention/edema
Kidney inflammation, kidney failure

No longer can the skeptics in medicine reject out-of-hand the notion that food allergy is a very, very common problem. They may honestly disagree with the estimates of its overall etiological prevalence. (For example, I have no problem with a challenge to estimates that over 80% of patients with rheumatoid arthritis, migraines, asthma and epilepsy suffer from delayed food allergies.) However, if the skeptics have stayed abreast of the supportive scientific literature, they can no longer *rationally* defend their frequently repeated argument that food allergies are rare in adults and limited to the airways, digestive tract and skin. These same doctors may also disagree with the alternative methods being used today to diagnose food allergy. *The skeptical medical community, however, can no longer objectively refuse to acknowledge and accept the desperate need of an accurate means of diagnosing food allergy in their own practices. Food allergy is just too common to ignore any longer!*

The new physicians, well-trained in allergy and immunology, will actively search for food allergy and chemical sensitivity in their patients, and they will frequently find it, just as I have. Not only will they encourage the customary food allergen avoidance and elimination diets, *but more importantly these allergy educated physicians will look for the many underlying nutritional and lifestyle* causes *of food allergy.* Being teachers, they will routinely teach their patients the importance of complete abstinence from alcohol and nonsteroidal anti-inflammatory drugs (aspirin substitutes). They will look for the underlying nutritional deficiencies that might contribute to allergic reactions (zinc, magnesium, bioflavonoid, tannin, Vitamin C and Vitamin A deficiencies, etc.), and they will not hesitate to introduce highly effective anti-allergy, anti-inflammatory, *nonprescription herbal remedies* to reverse and control allergic symptoms.

Two of my favorite anti-allergy herbs in capsule form include *capsaicin* (also found in cayenne pepper) and *quercetin bioflavonoid* (a natural substance found in high concentrations in yellow and red onions) in synergistic combination with Vitamin C. Besides being potent anti-inflammatory agents, both act to stabilize those devilishly unstable, allergy-related immune cells called mast cells and basophils. The effect of the combination of these two herbs in the treatment of food allergy is often close to miraculous. The new breed of doctor, having been taught this in medical school, will make frequent use of such herbs and perhaps others of even greater efficacy, then take time to teach you where to buy and use them intelligently.

(This is, of course, assuming the government still allows you that precious freedom of choice. There are persistent rumblings from Washington's anti-libertarian special interest groups—those ever-present political activists that feel you, the consumer, are inherently stupid and unable to make intelligent decisions on your own—warning us that herbs, as well as amino acids, may soon become highly restricted, regulated, and perhaps even prescription items. Recalling my previous assertion that the "victory is ours," the situation may become worse before it gets better. This is one area that looks the most discouraging at this time.)

Being an outspoken advocate of self-reliance and self-responsibility, the new doctors' conscious goal and guiding principle will be to teach you how to regain control of your allergies without the need of a physician.

BY POPULAR DEMAND—NEW RESEARCH FINDINGS, MY TOP 10 PICKS:

I've been frequently asked when lecturing what new research of the last five years I personally find most promising and exciting. Although admittedly subjective, here's my "Top 10:"

1) Synthetic growth hormone injections given to elderly men three times weekly over a period of six months or so resulted in near universal reports of significantly more youthful-looking skin, increased muscle tone with far less body fat—and the participants reported they felt 20 years younger. Are we getting close to conquering the aging process?

   What I find particularly intriguing here is that we now know how to increase growth hormone release through nutritional supplementation (arginine, ornithine, niacin, phosphatidylcholine, etc.). Expensive and potentially toxic synthetic growth hormone injections also have nutritional alternatives.
2) Dr. Eggers, noted English neurologist and researcher, had published in the journal *Pediatrics* his study on the causal relationship between food allergy and epilepsy.

   His study included 100 epileptics, representing all five

common forms of epilepsy. He concluded that 80% of all epileptic patients studied could and did elicit epileptic seizures by eating food allergens! Meanwhile, at least two prominent medical publications—one in the U.S. and one in England—have refused to publish this astounding and controversial bit of research.

3) Dr. Terrence Leighton, professor of immunology at University of California at Berkeley, reported to me during a phone call recently that, of all the plant-derived nutrients with proven anti-cancer benefits he and his staff of scientists had studied over the last few years, by far the most potent anti-tumor effects could be found in the bioflavonoid quercetin. (Recall that quercetin with bromelain is one of my favorite anti-food allergy herbs, one that I have been using with allergic patients for over eight years now.) When I asked him if human studies had been conducted with quercetin, he admitted that these had not been done. However, he shared with me a study just completed in Europe in which human cancer cells were injected into the abdomens of laboratory animals with subsequent metastasis or spreading throughout the body of the animals. With injection of quercetin, the cancer went into complete remission!
4) With the use of such amino acids as DL-phenylalanine, tyrosine, glutamine, and L-tryptophan, vitamins such as Vitamin C, B6 and niacin, and herbs such as valerian, Korean ginseng, cayenne pepper, and green oat straw, addictive behavior can be strongly curtailed. In one study of recovering alcoholics such nutritional therapy resulted in a reduction of six-month alcohol relapses from the normal 52% to 13% and an overall increase in alcohol- and drug-free days by over 700%—without the customary (and generally ineffectual) psychological counseling and group therapies to explain this remarkable improvement. I was so taken aback by this new research that I have decided to make this the subject of my next book.
5) The conclusion I've reached from research of the obesity and overweight scientific literature published over the last five to ten years is that being overweight is rarely the result of overeating, or lack of will power. In fact, there is no published well-controlled scientific study that clearly demonstrates that fat people eat more calories than normally thin or lean people. I have personally retrieved and read seven articles that conclude fat people on the average eat 300 to 400 *fewer* calories daily than thin people. It's a brand new ball game! (Most all the research going on today is focusing on metabolism and thermogenesis, not human psychology and human discipline. About time, don't you think?)
6) The January, 1991 issue of *American Journal of Clinical Nutrition* presented evidence that low normal blood levels of

"lipid standardized" Vitamin E were better predictors of an impending heart attack than high cholesterol, high blood pressure or smoking cigarettes! Reported in the January 13, 1992 issue of *USA Today*, the American Heart Association convention, held in Galveston, Texas, gave lots of attention to vitamins and coronary heart disease. They concluded that blood levels of such important antioxidant vitamins as Vitamin C, E and beta-carotene play an extremely important role in the prevention of LDL cholesterol (the "bad" cholesterol) oxidation, thereby suspected of preventing atherosclerosis and heart attacks! (But even with this evidence and the extraordinarily safe history of these three common vitamins, the authors could not bring themselves to advocate supplementation with antioxidant vitamins for the prevention of heart attacks. Amazing!)

7) Introduced into the U.S. by Doctor's Best, Inc. of San Clemente, California, the ancient Ayurvedic herb Guggul (brand name Guggulow) was reborn. After 2500 years of use in the lowering of body fats, treatment of obesity and "clearing the channels of the body," 20th-century science finally got around to studying its effects on serum cholesterol. The conclusion was that on average guggul lowered the total cholesterol by 27%, triglycerides by over 30% and amazingly increase the good HDL cholesterol by over 35%—the single best natural therapy I have seen for elevated cholesterol in over 20 years of medical practice. And many overweight people report a weight loss of one-half to one pound each week without reducing calories!

Please keep in mind that the Pritikin-style low-fat, high complex carbohydrate diet has serious shortcomings, the most obvious—and too often ignored—is the tendency for the good HDL cholesterol to come plummeting down right alongside the bad cholesterols. In addition the *extremely low total and HDL cholesterol* that accompany an across-the-board low-fat diet are reported to be associated with increased risks of other common deadly diseases—namely, cancer, strokes and sudden death. A tragic example of this unreported phenomenon involves Nathan Pritikin who experienced the recurrence of leukemia before his unfortunate death—*with a total cholesterol under 125 mg/dl.* The scientific literature records an increased risk of cancer as total cholesterols fall below 160 mg/dl or lower.

8) Kabi Pharmacia of Sweden and their immunodiagnostic division have just introduced into the U.S. new allergy testing laboratory technology that surpasses any immunoassay protocol I have researched. I was so impressed by the precision and accuracy of their new IgE CAP fluorescent immunoassay that I have just added it to the existing technology we have

been using to diagnose food allergy. For those of you who are interested, at the present time the state of the art for the laboratory diagnosis of immediate and delayed food allergy—type I, II and III allergic reactions—includes: the IgE CAP (type I), IgG RAST (type II) and IgG food immune complex assay (type III). At the time of this writing, Immuno-Nutritional Clinical Laboratory (INCL) in North Hollywood, California is the only nonresearch clinical laboratory offering this combination. The tools for diagnosing food allergy are getting better.

9) In 1991 I attended a two-and-a-half day seminar in Santa Monica, California at which over 25 papers were presented by the scientific community on one essential nutrient only—magnesium! I left the seminar with my mouth open, completely dazzled by the new knowledge I had gained. Some pearls of wisdom include: There are two distinct kinds of hypertensive patients who are responsive to nutritional supplementation. The magnesium-responsive high blood pressure is one in which the patient is not salt sensitive and has an elevated or high normal blood level of the kidney hormone, renin. Give these hypertensive individuals magnesium supplements and their blood pressure will come down. The other group includes those individuals who are salt sensitive (about 20% of all hypertensive patients) and have normal or low normal levels of blood renin. Give these people calcium supplements and their blood pressure will come down.

If the attending physicians at your nearby hospital were to simply place one gram of magnesium sulfate into the IV bottle upon admission of any heart attack victim, begin and continue running magnesium-supplemented intravenous fluid into these patients during their stay in the coronary care unit of the hospital, they could reduce the death rate the first 30 days after a heart attack (by far the most dangerous time following a heart attack) by two thirds. Most recurring kidney stones are composed of calcium oxalate. Published research papers now argue that simply supplementing with therapeutic doses of both magnesium and vitamin B6, practically speaking, bring these excruciatingly painful kidney stone attacks to a complete stop.

10) Rheumatoid and juvenile rheumatoid arthritis are now accepted throughout the international scientific research community as clinical consequences of food allergy. Five years ago such talk was heresy. Today, the only serious debate that remains involves the answer to the question, "Just how frequently does food allergy cause or aggravate rheumatoid or juvenile rheumatoid arthritis?" Is the frequency well under 10% (the position of many rheumatologists) or well over 70% (still my position)? The significance of this debate

is reflected by the *Lancet* article several years back that exposed the dangers of prolonged anti-rheumatoid arthritis prescription drug therapies. Although such patients did seem to do better the first five to ten years on a drug regimen, they did worse (and died at an average age of 56) thereafter. The summary of their prospective 20-year study was that rheumatologists cannot claim that their prescribed drugs reverse or even retard the natural history of this disabling disease.

1994 UPDATE

Dear Reader:

It's been over seven years since I first wrote *Dr. Braly's Optimum Health Program,* and almost one year since it was revised and reprinted in paperback as *Dr. Braly's Food Allergy and Nutrition Revolution*—well over 30,000 copies ago!

Since then, there have been many favorable changes in both the public's and the health professionals' acceptance of the growing science and clinical practice of food allergy and nutrition. These favorable changes have added support to the often-repeated truism that food allergy is the most commonly undiagnosed medical condition in the United States today.

In addition to the growing acceptance of clinical nutrition and food allergy, several exciting events have very recently transpired personally affecting me. After much thought I decided to consolidate my laboratory, INCL, with the Fort Lauderdale, Florida–based laboratory, Immuno Laboratories, Inc. and at the same time proudly accept the position of medical director for the merged company.

As you may have already noted in my book, my former laboratory, INCL, provided specialized food allergy testing to doctors and thousands of patients through a blood test process known as the IgG RAST and the additional test we called the FICA.

My choice to unite INCL with Immuno Laboratories was based in large part upon my knowledge and approval of their "Immuno 1 Bloodprint" (an improved counterpart to INCL's IgG RAST—i.e., a more automated, superior in quality control and faster laboratory assay for the detection of IgG antibody to allergic foods). After investigation, I had to conclude that Immuno Laboratories' food allergy testing and services were the most clinically useful ones available today and that I have chosen the best organization to join forces with.

The subject of food allergy and clinical nutrition understandably will continue to provoke heated ideological and scientific debate for years to come. With all the controversy, claims and counterclaims being thrown about, I commend you as an individual for your courage and wisdom in seeking health through knowledge. You made a smart decision! I sincerely wish to thank you for choosing my book as one of your many avenues of reaching that all-important goal.

For more information about food allergy testing, please contact Immuno Laboratories Client Services, 1-800-231-9197.

Yours in the very *best* of health,

—James Braly, M.D.

This book is not intended as a substitute for the medical advice of physicians. The reader should regularly consult his doctor in matters relating to health and particularly in respect to symptoms that may require diagnosis or medical attention.

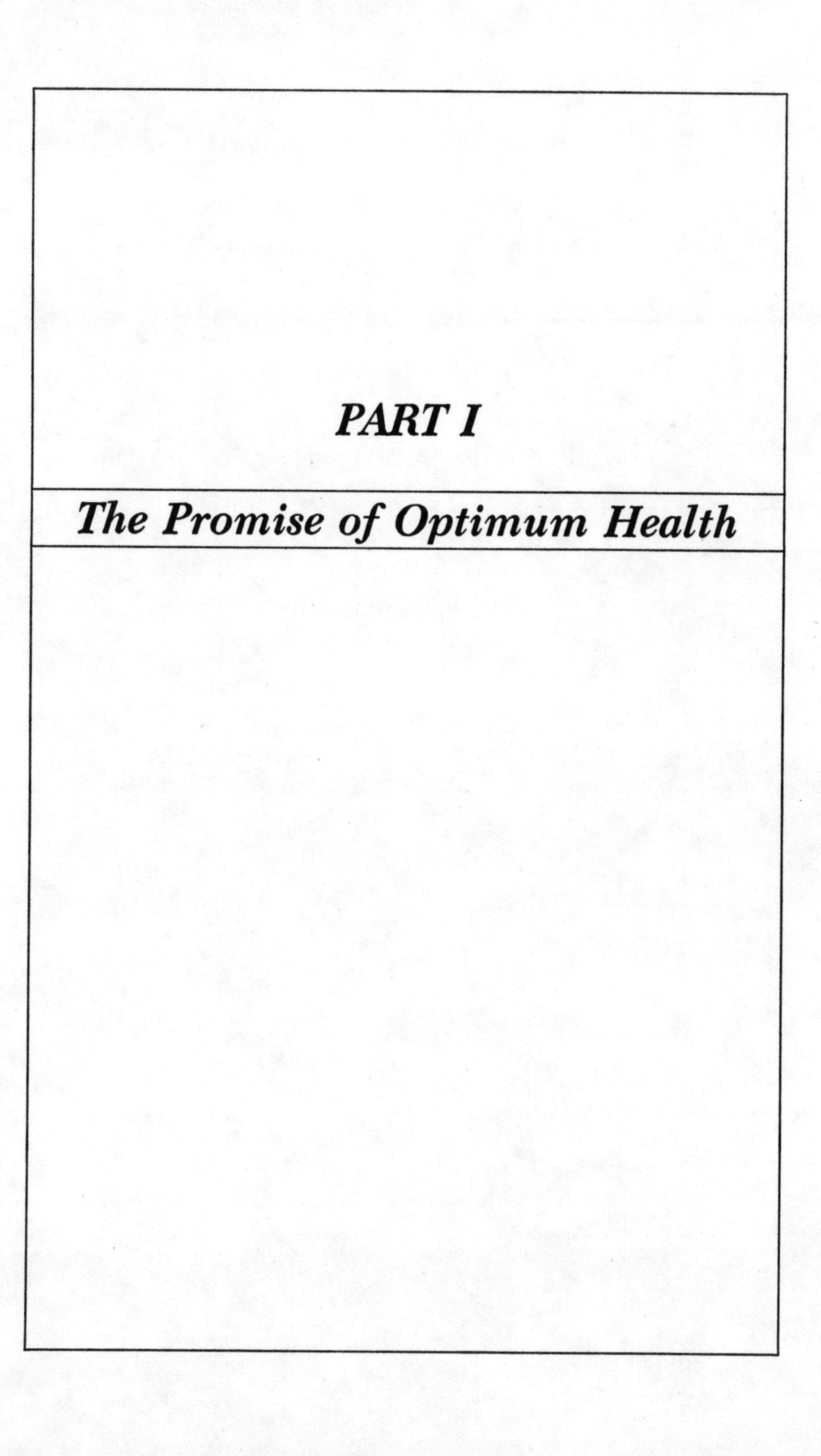

PART I

The Promise of Optimum Health

1

A New Approach to Weight Loss and Good Health

If you follow the program outlined in this book, you will almost certainly lose weight, without feeling hungry and without counting calories. You will function better physically and mentally. Nagging, chronic symptoms you may have gotten used to—pain, fatigue, indigestion, puffy eyes, muscle aches, a runny nose, insomnia, skin rashes, depression, irritability—will lessen or disappear. Substantial relief can be expected from allergies and even from serious ailments such as migraine, rheumatoid arthritis, premenstrual syndrome, high blood pressure, alcoholism, and adult-onset diabetes mellitus. You will likely lead a longer and healthier life.

Such claims may sound exaggerated, even outrageous, but I assure you they are well-founded. I am a physician specializing in nutrition, immunology, and allergy. The Optimum Health Program is the result of my own quest to overcome physical, mental, and emotional problems, some of which had remained untreated and undiagnosed since childhood.

In Chapter 2, I'll tell you more of my own story and about Optimum Health Labs, where the Optimum Health Program originated and where it continues to evolve. For now, let me whet your appetite with some case histories.

People who have been on the Optimum Health Program.

- Talk show host Merv Griffin came in with a lifetime history of overweight, having been diagnosed as hypoglycemic. Though he'd been following the traditional hypoglycemic diet of frequent high-protein meals, he felt increasingly vulnerable to symptoms. His tests revealed that he was allergic to numerous foods. After two or three days of withdrawal symptoms on our diet, he felt exceptionally energetic and healthy. Without trying and without counting calories, he lost 35 pounds in less than three months, a feat he had been unable to accomplish on dozens of calorie-restrictive diets.
- We treated an eight-year-old child with a history of frequent

psychomotor seizures. In over two years on the program, the child had only two minor seizures, both the result of eating foods he should have avoided.

- A forty-five-year-old woman came to us with a fifteen-year history of totally immobilizing migraine headaches—two or three a week, each lasting from two to ten hours. Her headaches were gone completely after two weeks on the program, and she has remained completely pain-free.
- Every form of diagnostic test and therapy had failed for a fifty-year-old lawyer who came to us with a five-year history of constant, unremitting muscle spasms in his back. Before he was referred to our clinic, he had tried surgery, acupuncture, prescription painkillers, alcohol and narcotics, and had even contemplated suicide. After seven days on the Optimum Health Program, he was totally pain-free.
- When actor James Coburn came in, he had to be helped in and out of his chair by the friend who brought him. Recurring bouts of rheumatoid arthritis (which runs in his family) had gotten so bad in the last six months that he could barely move without help. He had recently gone on a fifteen-day juice fast, which partially relieved his symptoms, but they had returned when he went back to normal foods. So, suspecting something in his diet, he came to us. He experienced a 90 percent improvement within two weeks and has remained basically pain-free over the last four years.
- We treated a thirty-year-old unemployed welfare recipient, who was unable to work because of recurring episodes of hallucinations and paranoid feelings. He went on a diet, eliminating not only allergic foods, but also pastries, sweets, alcohol, and all processed foods. Aggressive vitamin, mineral, and essential-fatty-acid supplementation was included in his program. The psychosis was brought under control, and he is now employed.
- A housewife of sixty lost 33 pounds in three months. When she came to us, she weighed 205 pounds, had a blood sugar reading of 319, a triglyceride level of 229, and her blood pressure was a dangerously high 180/98. In the first two weeks she lost 14 pounds, and her blood pressure dropped to 148/80.
- Actor Joel Lewin came to the clinic at 227 pounds (he's 5 feet 11 inches tall). Three months later he weighed 170 pounds and reported that his concentration was also much improved, his energy level was more consistent, and he was sleeping better.
- A sixty-one-year-old man entered the program with the following complaints: hypertension, arthritis, overweight, and back pain. In three months, he lost 38 pounds, his blood pressure dropped, and his arthritis improved substantially. Only

the back pain remained, and that may be related to structural alignment.

- Singer Engelbert Humperdinck lost 30 pounds in three months on the Optimum Health Program.

Athletes who have followed the program also report improvement in their performance as a result of the allergy-free diet and special nutrition and supplementation programs we've developed for them:

- Ultramarathoner Dave Prokop reported in *Runners World* that "the diet provided me with one of the most remarkable experiences of my life. In two weeks I lost about 14 pounds, getting my weight down to 148 from 162 (the lowest it had been since college), even though I was eating fairly large meals and my training mileage was actually decreased." He also reported increased energy and endurance, and he overcame his water-retention problem.
- Cyclist John Marino was diagnosed as having thirty-eight allergies. On the diet, he broke his Los Angeles-to-New York record by completing the ride in twelve days, three hours, and forty-one minutes. To set the record he rode twenty hours a day, and he reported that he had a very high energy level during the ride, without the ups and downs he usually felt and without the achy, sore legs he always assumed were inevitable on those long rides.
- Triathlete and physician Dr. Ferdie Massimino came to us to try to lose the weight he couldn't seem to shake (in spite of his grueling workout schedule). After being on the program, he won the championship for his age group (over thirty) at the internationally acclaimed 140-mile Ironman Triathlon in Hawaii and won first place in the United States national championship in the Ironman Triathlon three weeks later. He had lost 25 pounds while consuming 3,700 calories a day.
- While on our program, thirty-seven-year-old John Powell threw the longest discus throw of his illustrious career, the world record throw for 1984, and the third longest throw of all time. Although he was losing weight, his strength was at a lifetime high.

These are true stories, and they are not the result of miracle cures. At OHL we are used to seeing people get better, often after years of suffering and searching for answers. These results were not achieved through crash diets or wonder drugs—it's more typical for our patients to give up or reduce their medications. They were following the Optimum Health Program, a commonsense, multidisciplinary approach to good health that consolidates recent scientific findings in allergy and nutrition research as well as in other related fields—nutritional biochemistry, orthomolecular medicine, clinical ecology, sports medicine, immunology, etc.

WHAT EXACTLY DO YOU DO ON THE OPTIMUM HEALTH PROGRAM?

1. Find out if you have allergies and identify them. At OHL we believe that allergies, especially to food, are almost universal and that they contribute to, or are the underlying cause of, many symptoms and diseases, as well as overweight. People are often skeptical when they hear so much emphasis placed on food allergies, for they often have preconceived and outdated ideas on the subject, because, as we will see, allergies tend to be "masked" or covered up by the way we eat; because it takes a long time for damage to accumulate and cause serious trouble; and (since allergies masquerade as other conditions) because they are generally misunderstood, misdiagnosed, and ignored, even by physicians. But their effects are far-reaching. Chapters 4 and 5 discuss in detail the nature of allergy, the difficulty of diagnosing allergies, and the methods of treatment. Chapter 14 is the how-to chapter that tells you all about how to be tested—or to test yourself—for allergies.

2. Eliminate all allergic food from your diet for three months. Most people are allergic to an average of five to fifteen or more foods; furthermore, many of those foods (as we'll explain) are likely to be staples in one's diet. So this first stage of the Optimum Health Program may involve considerable change in the way you eat. During these ninety days, your body will desensitize itself to most of your allergic foods. At the same time your digestive tract and immune system, which may be profoundly affected by food allergy, have a chance to repair themselves. After ninety days, you will be able to go back to eating nearly all your allergic foods (only 5 percent of the usual range of five-to-fifteen allergic foods are likely to be fixed or permanent allergies), though not on such a constant basis as before.

3. Eat all the remaining nonallergic foods on a rotating basis. Most people eat a limited number of foods over and over again—which is one of many factors that may lead to allergies. On the Optimum Health Program you learn to eat many new foods and to eat each one no more frequently than once every four days. This highly varied diet, which you'll find very enjoyable once you get into the swing of it, will help prevent you from developing new food allergies. A rotation diet also has the effect of prodding you to eat more fresh, unprocessed, untreated food, to cut down on the consumption of saturated fats and processed vegetable oils, and to go light on sugar and dishes with numerous ingredients in them. You're also encouraged to eliminate alcohol and coffee, at least for these first three months.

If, as many people do, you've been having digestive problems (they're a common cause and side effect of allergies), there are easy steps you can learn that will restore proper digestion. And if you have withdrawal symptoms from giving up your usual food (many people do for a few days, for allergies can become addictions no different from those to alcohol or tobacco), we'll show you ways to minimize them. And we'll show you how to continue your diet after the first ninety days are up, adhering to the basic principles of rotation but on a more flexible basis.

4. Take a full spectrum of essential nutrients. It is impossible to get from our food—even if we think we're eating well—the full range of vitamins, minerals, essential fatty acids, and amino acids necessary for optimum health. There are too many chemicals in our food and in our environment, and too many stresses in our busy lives, for even a healthy diet to support. Nutrient needs vary widely according to individual health and biochemical makeup, but everyone needs across-the-board supplementation, often at levels well beyond the inadequate recommended daily allowances (RDAs) we hear so much about. Part III discusses the value of supplementation at length, detailing the many nutrients and itemizing the dosage range, therapeutic values, and symptomatic indications for each. All of Chapter 11 is devoted to the vital essential fatty acids that are lacking in most diets.

5. Exercise. Exercise goes hand in hand with good nutrition in the quest for optimum health and permanent weight control. Among its many benefits, it raises the metabolism rate, and that means that calories are *burned* rather than *stored.* It enhances the uptake of our most important nutrient, oxygen, stimulates the immune system, and is a natural mood elevator. Chapter 18 outlines exercise guidelines that will help anyone, regardless of age or present health, in planning a personal exercise program. See individual entries in Part V for special attention to exercise for those with asthma, arthritis, heart disease, diabetes, and other symptomology.

6. Learn about good health, especially about your own health needs. Education about the principles of good health and about your own body—its strengths and weaknesses, its ups and downs, its unique nutritional and exercise needs, its genetic inheritance—is your most powerful tool in the pursuit of optimum health.

FOOD MAY BE A HAZARD TO YOUR HEALTH

America is a nation obsessed with food, as the most cursory survey—of your neighborhood food shops, magazines, television advertising, and perhaps even your own refrigerator—will show.

Turn on the television. Hostess Cupcakes and Wonder Bread are official Olympic sponsors ("Official Junk Food of the 1984 Olympics," a *New Yorker* cartoon caption reads). The Dairy Council says that milk is the perfect food, and the Coffee Council says its product will calm you down when you're having a frazzled day at the office. Happy families are shown eating Sara Lee dinners or driving to Burger King. Friends hoist a beer after a sweaty softball game. Lovers celebrate with wine and candelight. Kids vie with one another for their share of the potato chips. Grandpa fixes his little darling her favorite sugared cereal. Athletes plug beer. Actors plug soda pop. Dancers relax with a cup of coffee.

This obsession, this inundation, with food is coupled dangerously with a head-in-the-sand attitude about the consequences of our diets, which are as plain to see as the golden arches of McDonald's. Overweight has reached epidemic proportions in this country. Weight loss is an $18-billion-a-year business. Hidden among the pizza parlors and gourmet takeout shops are thousands of diet clinics, exercise studios, health clubs, "fat farms," diet doctors, anorexia counselors, nutritionists, and psychologists whose mission it is to try to undo some of the damage done by too much of the wrong kinds of food. The supermarket itself yields up whole aisles full of low-calorie foods and a dozen brands of diet pills. Thousands of diet books have been published, and thousands more tout the benefits of health and fitness. The obsession with food coupled with the obsession with being thin constitutes a national schizophrenia.

Yet overweight is but one facet of the larger problem: the deterioration of our overall health, individually and as a nation. Even with all our marvelous medical technology, many degenerative diseases—most cancers, diabetes, obesity, arthritis, asthma, migraines, and other allergies—are on the rise. One in ten children is labeled hyperactive; many health professionals now recognize that food allergies, along with sugars and additives in food, are largely to blame. Juvenile delinquency can now, in part, be traced to junk-food diets high in milk and sugars. One study estimates that by the year 2000, one in three adult Americans will have diabetes. Even the majority of so-called healthy people complain of minor recurring health problems—colds, depression, headaches, runny noses, fatigue, aches and pains, indigestion. Just about everyone's got the "blahs."

How did we arrive at such a sorry state of affairs? The answer can be found not only in the way we eat, but also in our sedentary life-styles and in our increasingly toxic environment. The human species is not equipped to live the life we're living. Our diet, our environment, and our way of life have changed so radically in the last hundred years or so that our systems have not been able to evolve fast enough to tolerate the stresses we put on them.

Just since 1910, the fat content of our diets has doubled. Margarine, shortening, and other deadly partially hydrogenated oils were introduced to the American consumer in the 1920s. Protein consumption remains about the same, except that the protein that used to come mainly from grains now comes from meat (about 100 pounds per person annually) and dairy products (about 375 pounds per person annually) high in saturated fats. Complex carbohydrates should make up the bulk of our diet, but consumption has dropped, and where in 1910, 70 percent of our carbohydrate intake was complex carbohydrates, over 50 percent of our carbohydrates today are consumed as refined sugars. Today, Americans consume in excess of 125 pounds of sugar per person each year. Add to this the *thousands* of chemicals, additives, and preservatives we're served up in the name of better living, plus the coffee, alcohol, cigarettes, and drugs (both recreational and medicinal) we seem so fond of, and it doesn't seem hyperbolic to say that we are polluting our bodies.

THINGS ARE LOOKING UP

Fortunately, there are signs of change. People are finally starting to take seriously the dangers of a highly processed diet loaded with refined sugars, saturated fats, and hydrogenated oils. They've heard of binge eating and food allergy/food addiction. Many have become aware of set-point theory, which maintains that your metabolism will "set" in accordance with the amount of food and exercise you habitually take. The dangers of cholesterol and coffee and cigarettes are increasingly well-documented in the press. Fewer people are smoking. At last the American Cancer Society is recognizing the importance of diet in preventing cancer (they are now admitting that at least 30 percent of all cancers are diet-related). The Health and Human Services Agency now recommends that we eat less fat and more high-fiber food, such as fruits, vegetables, and whole grains. The government now says that a change of diet and life-style is the best medicine for high blood pressure and heart disease. There is, finally, a growing recognition of the direct cause-and-effect relationship between nutrition and health.

Though the dream of quick and painless weight loss doesn't die easily, people are finally coming to terms with the fact that the latest crash diet or miracle cream isn't going to work any better than the last one or the one before that. They no longer believe they can get by indefinitely without exercise. These days just about every town has a health food store (even if it's next door to McDonald's) and a health club where increasing numbers of people are getting into shape.

Finally, people are looking at the long-term effects of their diets, their not-so-pure environment, their high-stress lives—and the health risks that go along with them. They are facing up to the fact that some personal adjustment in their diets and life-styles is inevitable, and they are willing to tackle a serious program that will restore and maintain their health and solve their up-and-down weight problems.

WHY THE OPTIMUM HEALTH PROGRAM?

The Optimum Health Program is what they're looking for. It has proved so effective because it is based on sound principles of nutrition and exercise, because it addresses the root causes of the body's distress naturally, *and undoes the damage done.* It is not the latest fad diet.

The goal of the Optimum Health Program is simply to restore the body to the best possible health and keep it there. What is meant by optimum health? *Optimum health is the capacity of your system to cope with all the stresses of your life and environment—with plenty of room to spare.* (See Figure 1, page 11.)

Unfortunately most of us are in *average* health, which means that any unforeseen upset, any stress overload has the potential to tilt the tables in favor of disease. It could be any number of things—a prolonged period of anxiety or tension, surgery, pregnancy, the loss of a job, the breakup of a love affair, a lawsuit, a deadline, a long bout of virulent flu, a junk-food binge, recurring sleep disorders, or just the inevitable cumulative effects of age and inactivity.

Too many of us "average folks" fall into the huge yawning chasm *between illness and health.* Because we're not seriously ill, we make the mistake of thinking that we're healthy—even though we feel tired, stressed, and headachy, or bloated after meals, and our nose is stuffed up in the morning, and we feel grouchy in the middle of the afternoon. Our doctors can't be bothered with these "inconsequential" things; we take care of them ourselves with aspirin and decongestants and laxatives and over-the-counter sleeping pills.

But we're like walking time bombs. Sooner or later all those little things—or maybe one big thing—will push us over the edge, and we'll

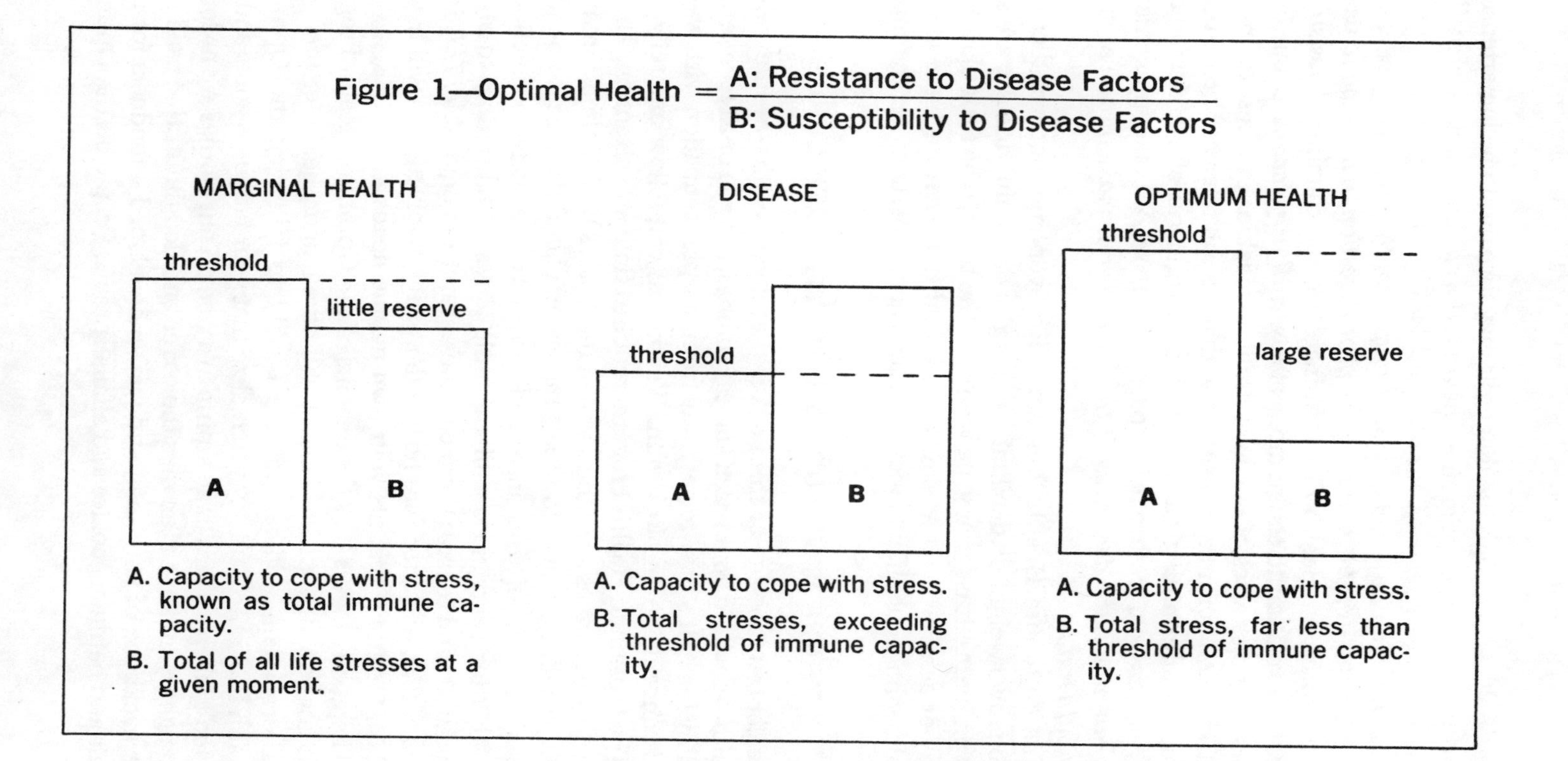
Figure 1—Optimal Health = A: Resistance to Disease Factors / B: Susceptibility to Disease Factors
MARGINAL HEALTH
threshold
little reserve
A
B
A. Capacity to cope with stress, known as total immune capacity.
B. Total of all life stresses at a given moment.
DISEASE
threshold
A
B
A. Capacity to cope with stress.
B. Total stresses, exceeding threshold of immune capacity.
OPTIMUM HEALTH
threshold
large reserve
A
B
A. Capacity to cope with stress.
B. Total stress, far less than threshold of immune capacity.

become ill. And though the diagnosis may turn out to be hypertension, arthritis, diabetes, or migraine, *the underlying cause may very well be the cumulative effects of our diet and lack of exercise—which undermined the immune system, which brought on the food allergies, which provoked the weight gain and the poor digestion, which made us ill.*

The Optimum Health Program increases the number of *resistance factors* in relation to the number of *susceptibility factors* in our lives. Many of the stresses of our lives are unavoidable. Our best defense is to strengthen our immune system so that we can tolerate these stresses without undermining our health. We *can* get rid of our debilitating allergies, *can* eat fresh, whole food, *can* exercise, *can* take supplements. *We can do a good deal to shift the balance and make ourselves much less vulnerable.*

The Optimum Health Program is for everyone, not just those for whom overweight or debilitating allergies or painful diseases are serious problems. It is for anyone who's got the blahs, who feels bloated or puffy or achy or tired or slow-witted. And it is even for those in good health who would like to increase their margin of safety for the future.

THERE IS NO SUCH THING AS A FREE LUNCH

The central message of this book is that good health—even excellent health—is within your reach and capabilities, but you must take responsibility for it. It's time to get away from our preoccupation with weight and concentrate on our health. Weight loss will follow naturally.

The Optimum Health Program requires time and attention. Though relief from serious symptoms will in most cases be felt almost immediately, it will take time to repair the accumulated damage, to build up a large margin of resistance, and to restore the body to functioning health after years of slow, often subtle abuse. It takes time to master new habits and to have them become natural and enjoyable. *This is not a crash diet,* and there are no wonder drugs involved. You will have to tailor a program that fits your own unique needs.

The good news is that the benefits of the Optimum Health Program will last you all your life—and it will be a longer, healthier life.

There is an insidious positive quality to following the Optimum Health Program. One day you realize that your fatigue is gone, and you haven't taken a Tums or an aspirin in a week. Your clothes are no longer too tight, you don't even miss the coffee and doughnuts that used to be the backbone of your diet, and you've developed a fondness for fresh fruit and oatmeal cookies and alfalfa sprouts. People on the Optimum

Health Program almost invariably report feeling more alive. They feel their stomachs calming down; they notice long-standing symptoms disappearing; they're no longer tired all the time. Just to get off the seesaw of weight loss and gain, of feeling good one day and lousy the next, is already a big improvement. As they feel and look better, they feel more confident and aware of their ability to make choices about their lives.

At OHL, I see people every day who can't quite believe how good they feel just because they're doing something as simple as eating better and exercising. I believe that on the Optimum Health Program anyone can take charge of his health, can learn the ropes, can make the changes and establish the habits necessary for a longer, healthier life. And all without counting calories!

2

Me, Modern Medicine, and the Optimum Health Program

I was a hyperactive child. However, they didn't have that name for it when I was growing up, so they labeled me a "problem" child. I certainly had many problems: migraine headaches, indigestion, fatigue, bed-wetting, nightmares, skin allergies, a constantly congested nose. I was often moody and irritable, and I walked around with a chip on my shoulder. Somehow I was spared the learning disorders and clumsiness many other hyperactive kids are burdened with, but I seemed to have just about every other thing going against me.

By the time I was thirty, some of these problems had run their course, but some remained, and I was not an easy person to be around. Irritability and chronic, recurring headaches and depression continued to be a problem, along with profound sleepiness after meals, mental fatigue, acne, and wide fluctuations in my weight. Predictably so, since hyperactive children, when the condition remains untreated, go on to become hyperactive adults.

So, I lived with my ailments as best I could. I knew, for example, that strenuous activity made me feel better, so I focused more on sports and exercise—which I enjoyed in any case. I ate what I thought was a fairly healthy, balanced diet (aside from drinking too much coffee). But inevitably the time came when, during a period of intense stress, my defenses and my system simply began to break down.

At the time, I was a practicing physician, terribly disillusioned with medicine. I couldn't escape the feeling that a certain amount of hoax—and not a high level of cure—was involved in its practice and that the whole profession had become seriously sidetracked. There seemed to me something unclean and dishonest about what I was doing, and I was seeking something else—without having a clear idea of what it might be.

Like most general practitioners, I prescribed drugs for my patients for relief of symptoms, though I knew that none of them addressed the underlying cause of their distress. The underlying causes, I assumed (and had been taught), were most likely of a psychological nature; I'd been trained to label even most physical ailments psychosomatic.

The irony, of course, was that now my own system was failing me, and I had lost faith in the power of my profession to cure my ills. I was a classic case. My assorted maladies and the cumulative stresses of my life —repeated nutritional mistakes, inattention to fitness, even what might be called spiritual mistakes—combined with my recent crisis of confidence about my career, were pushing me over the edge, into illness. My immune system, my defense against illness, was no longer adequate for handling the amount of distress I'd managed so cleverly to squeeze into my life.

Fortunately, I am an insatiable reader of scientific literature, and during this period I had the luck to come across writings by some of the pioneers in nutrition and allergy—Dr. Theron Randolph, Linus Pauling, Dr. H. J. Rinkel, Dr. William Rowe. I started experimenting with some of their very sensible concepts and soon found that by eliminating certain foods from my diet, *symptoms that had been bothering me all my life disappeared:* The mental and physical fatigue evaporated, the bloating and weight fluctuation ceased, along with the chronic stuffy nose and headaches and irritability. It was astounding. So after a couple of weeks of unexpected and not quite trusted well-being, doubter and doctor that I am, I switched back to my old diet. The symptoms returned, with a vengeance. That was pretty convincing, but just to be sure, I again repeated the experiment—with the same results. What a joke to learn that I was allergic to—among other foods—the half-gallon of milk I drank each day "for my health."

Thus began a very exciting time for me. I was feeling better—rather, I was feeling *healthy* for the first time in my life. Finally I had some answers to my own problems and to those of many of my patients. For the first time, I began really listening to my patients and understanding what was happening to them. For the first time, I felt I was actually *helping* them. Suddenly I didn't have a practice composed of 80 percent neurotics who needed tranquilizers and antidepressants or psychological counseling for their psychosomatic complaints. They were malnourished and allergic. Their digestive tracts and immune systems were out of whack. What my patients were telling me now made sense.

Now, if you've devoted your life and a great deal of mental energy, as I had, to a different point of view, and you've been searching for better answers, this kind of sudden reawakening is very exciting.

It transformed my approach to medicine. I wish it could transform that of other physicians. Often I find myself at odds with the medical community in which I was educated and its head-in-the-sand attitude toward nutrition and food allergy. I am deeply concerned about the ability and willingness of the medical establishment to respond to new knowledge about health and disease, and it would be gratifying to see it turn in the direction of nutritional and preventive medicine before the health of the nation is further endangered.

OLD MEDICINE AND NEW

Increasingly the medical community seems to be divided into two warring camps: the "charmed circle" of traditional medicine, and the "outsiders" of what has come to be called alternative medicine. Alternative medicine is a catchall term for everything that falls outside the ever higher and more protected walls of the establishment—chiropractic, nutrition, acupuncture, clinical ecology, sports medicine, preventive medicine, orthomolecular medicine, any discipline that relies predominantly on nutrition, exercise, and self-care rather than on physician-managed drugs and surgery. Increasingly, I find myself outside those establishment walls, and increasingly I feel I'm in the right place.

Traditional medicine has given us truly miraculous wonder drugs and ingenious surgical procedures that save and prolong life. But the exaggerated emphasis on advanced technology and on the pharmaceutical/drug-oriented approach to the treatment of disease has ruled out attention to other approaches as well—most particularly, to preventing the development of disease in the first place and to nondrug, nonsurgical therapies for its reversal.

The Information Bias

The premises on which modern medicine is based tend to screen out anything that doesn't conform to ever more strongly established biases. These biases are evident in the literature read by most health professionals. Each month there are some 8,000 scientific publications in the medical field: cases, abstracts, journal articles, research reports. Even the best-read physician misses 90 to 95 percent of what is published. However, an impressive body of scientific information is made available to physicians nationwide through much-consulted computer banks of medical information, such as MedLine and Medlars. This seems like an extraordinary source of information until you realize that only about 10 percent of what is published is included in the computer's stores, and that 10 percent is chosen by review boards of very prominent—but very traditional—physicians. So most of the information available through such services follows the established line of prejudice. Because those doctors don't consider the latest nutritional findings important, they don't include them in the material selected for the information bank. Instead their prejudices cause them to opt for publications on the latest drugs and up-to-date surgical procedures. Even though the last decade or so has produced an abundance of scientific study in the fields of nutrition, fitness, and allergy, little of it makes its way into mainstream channels.

There is also a double standard when it comes to research. Though only a small percentage of commonly accepted medical procedures and techniques have been subjected to the rigorous scientific testing and double-blind studies traditional medicine is so fond of, established medicine expects an extraordinarily high level of study and research for even the most innocuous procedures and treatments of alternative medicine. In 1978, the Office of Technology Assessment, under the authority of the Library of Congress, published a year-long study entitled, "Assessing the Efficacy and Safety of Medical Technology." What did they find when evaluating the effectiveness of modern medical procedures? The document stated:

> Only 10–20% of all procedures used in present day medical practice have been shown to be of benefit by scientifically controlled clinical trials. It was concluded that the vast majority of medical procedures now being utilized routinely by physicians are "unproven" when subjected to the same rigid standards these same orthodox physicians are demanding of alternative, nutritional practitioners.

For example, there have been no double-blind, placebo-controlled studies with coronary bypass surgery (177,000 operations in 1983, costing the public well over $4 billion), no double-blind placebo-controlled study for immunosuppressive therapy (radiation and/or chemotherapy) of cancer, etc. While alternative practitioners also strongly believe in meticulous research and testing, their feeling is that double-blind studies often measure only narrow and individual reactions that do not take into consideration the complex mix of factors involved in disease and thus cannot often be applied on a broad scale to large numbers of patients.

Two Views of Disease and Medication

Traditionalists believe that many diseases are biological in nature: Germs *cause* disease. This in spite of the fact that although everyone is exposed to germs, only a minority succumb to them. This premise leads to the next one: If the germs are the problem, then germ warfare in the form of drugs—chemical concoctions—is the remedy. The traditional physician, faced with a set of symptoms, will prescribe medication. Thus traditional medicine is *allopathic*—it is drug-oriented medicine. The average physician today writes over 3,800 prescriptions a year. With over 200,000 prescribing physicians, that's over 800 million prescriptions written annually—creating a monstrous $40 billion pharmaceutical industry.

Alternative medicine, certainly the kind practiced at OHL, begins with the assumption that to be successful in treating the underlying cause of disease, medication is necessary in only a *few* cases. Most prescription drugs, because they are compounded of chemicals foreign to the body, do not treat the causes of disease and are, by definition, potentially toxic. In fact, one alternative health professional defined medication with prescription drugs as "The use of sublethal doses of toxic chemicals in the attempt to suppress the expression of symptoms." If that sounds exaggerated, just take a look through the *Physician's Desk Reference* (or PDR) at your doctor's office or a local bookstore. This pharmaceutical "bible" lists over 2,700 prescribable drugs, and most of its 3,000-plus pages are devoted to outlining their potential, sometimes lethal, side effects. Ten to 15 percent of hospitalizations in this country are—primarily or in part—a result of toxic or allergic reactions to *prescribed medications.* Introducing foreign chemicals into the body may inhibit or divert certain undesirable biochemical pathways—may even provide much-needed temporary relief of symptoms—but the root problem is *not* a deficiency of these chemicals or drugs. Valium does not treat Valium deficiencies; aspirin does not treat aspirin deficiency; Tagamet does not treat Tagamet deficiency.

Where modern allopathic medicine is symptom-oriented, alternative medicine attempts to address the *causes* of illness. Alternative medicine operates on the belief that the answer is going to come through what we call "optimizing the internal environment" through the use of substances and activities *natural to the body.* This includes a variety of substances, among them unprocessed nonallergic food, digestive enzymes, vitamins, minerals, amino acids, essential fatty acids, accessory food factors, oxygen, water, stress-management techniques, and exercise. This sounds simple enough, and it is. But most people today are sorely lacking in the right balance of these natural activities and substances. Determining individual needs and restoring what's missing require expertise and time.

Most alternative medical practitioners also believe that the state of disease, like the state of health, is a consequence of *multiple factors or stresses* working together. Not all stresses are equal, of course; there may well be one that is predominant. In order to reverse disease, or to restore or substantially improve health, you usually have to deal with *all* the stress factors that led to that disease. And the reverse is true. To stay healthy, you must treat it as a multifactorial challenge, one with both physiological and psychological components. This is a very basic principle. Killing germs is not the answer. Since everyone is exposed to germs but only some people get sick, doesn't it make sense to make everyone as nearly healthy as those who are naturally able to withstand the exposure to germs?

The Passive or Active Patient

The traditional doctor/patient relationship is that of the ignorant, trusting, passive patient seeking cure from the all-knowing healer. Too many patients go into their doctors' offices desperate for help, prepared to describe their symptoms carefully, braced to ask questions. But they leave too embarrassed or intimidated by their doctors' busy schedules and abrupt, dismissive attitudes to have gotten the attention and answers they deserve.

Too many doctors are willing to play the role of demi-god healer and know-it-all authority, and too many patients are willing to sit still for it. It is a dishonest and dangerous situation. The patient puts too much faith in the doctor and too little in his own ability to understand his condition and its possible treatment.

Doctors and medicine are often held in such reverence that patients come to believe there is a medication or surgical procedure for just about everything. This encourages a false sense of security and discourages the patient from taking responsibility for his health. This illusory "comfort zone" encourages patient to believe that no matter how much they smoke or drink, no matter how badly they abuse their diets, no matter how stressful their life-styles, if they get really sick, the doctor can perform some miracle with drugs or sutures that will enable them to go back to living their health-destroying lives.

It's no wonder that doctors are often pretty pessimistic about their patients' ability to take care of themselves, even if they are partly responsible for perpetuating these attitudes. Statistics are high on patients who don't take their medication, who don't refill prescriptions, who all but ignore their doctors' advice on diet, smoking, and drinking.

However, such grim statistics don't tell the whole story. In my experience at least 10 to 20 percent of people *are* aware of the health and medical dangers in their lives and—given the knowledge, direction, and opportunity—have the inner strength and commitment to make basic and necessary changes. Then there's another 20 to 40 percent who want to become healthier but for whom that change is a real struggle. But with persistence, plus advice and guidance from a caring group of health professionals, these patients have a better than fighting chance to overcome illness.

There is an essential requirement for making changes, one central to alternative medicine. The "patient" has to be the primary, active, self-motivated, and committed participant. *The patient, not the doctor, is the healer.* The responsibility for healing is in his hands. The doctor—nutritionist, allergist, physician, osteopath, chiropractor, psychologist, physical therapist—is primarily an educator and director. His job is to provide accurate information clearly, and the patient's job is to apply the information consistently to his or her own life.

Nutrition, Allergy, and Exercise

Orthodox medicine begins with the premise that nutrition is of little importance in the prevention and treatment of disease. Nutritional therapy is considered unscientific and faddish—even though thousands of articles about nutrition can be found in the scientific literature if you choose to look. But if you start with the premise that nutrition is unimportant, you're not going to be reading in the right journals to begin with. Even doctors who consider nutrition to be of value tend to think in simplistic (and outdated) terms of "balanced" diets or cutting down on alcohol or high-cholesterol foods.

Exercise too gets little more than lip service from most doctors. They'll tell you it's good for you, but they probably won't have any specific recommendations and may be unaware of its crucial importance to people with specific diseases such as asthma, arthritis, diabetes, and heart disease.

The attitude is about the same when it comes to vitamins and other supplements. Many doctors tell their patients that if they eat right, they don't need vitamins; perhaps they throw in a scare about vitamin overdoses. Or maybe they recommend a multiple vitamin, with some extra C or E thrown in. Unfortunately the motivation here is not only ignorance about supplementation, but seemingly a desire to discredit nonestablishment practitioners and thus to maintain complete control over the medical field. The established medical community and the pharmaceutical industry are presently putting tremendous pressure on the government to regulate the sale of nutritional supplements and make them available only by prescription. This despite the fact that the number of toxic reactions to supplements *ever reported* doesn't equal the number of toxic reactions to aspirin in *one year.*

Finally there's the related and all-important issue of food allergy. To the traditional doctor, food allergy is another of those often psychosomatic complaints that affect only a small percentage of the adult population, which reveals itself in immediately obvious symptoms such as hives or breathing difficulties. To a nutritionist or allergist, food allergies are as common as colds. Most people have them, and they are often the unseen, misunderstood cause, or a contributing factor, of many diseases and symptoms.

To the alternative medical practitioner—especially to the nutritionist and allergist—nutrition and exercise are at the very center of good medical care; drugs and surgery are the treatment of last resort. Where the American Medical Association recognizes perhaps thirty nutrition-related diseases (scurvy, for example, is acknowledged to be the result of Vitamin C deficiency), it is probably closer to the truth to say that hundreds of diseases can be traced to suboptimal nutrition and nutritional deficiencies and that nutritional therapy is therefore the key to good health.

WHAT'S IN STORE FOR MEDICINE?

Is modern medicine failing us? The answer is probably yes and no. If you have a heart attack or stroke, chances are better and better that the miracles of modern medicine will keep you alive. On the other hand, the head-in-the-sand attitude of traditional medicine rules out the approach that might keep you from having a heart attack or stroke in the first place.

The function of medicine should also be to improve and optimize health; relief of suffering and disease should not cause further suffering and disease. One of the premises of medicine is "First, do no harm." Yet the available evidence is that modern medicine may be harming as many people as it's helping with drugs and medication. Remember that 10 to 15 percent of patients who are hospitalized as a side effect of drugs? That's about the same percentage as are helped. And research shows that as high as 40 percent of all patients who are hospitalized more than five days end up malnourished. Dr. Maurice Shils, director of clinical nutrition of the prestigious Sloan-Kettering cancer hospital in New York, states that by the time a nutrition consultant is called in, hospitalized patients have already become seriously malnourished. Barney Clark, the man who struggled so long to live as the first recipient of an artificial heart, had surgery performed while seriously malnourished—according to the consulting nutritionist. His doctors had been unaware of the problem. Sophisticated drugs and innovative surgical procedures are alleviating symptoms and eradicating some diseases, but other diseases are punishing and killing more people than ever. It seems to be a draw.

Modern medicine is failing because its foundation—albeit an impressive foundation in light of its technologic breakthroughs, its extensive hospital and research facilities—is based on many false premises. And I believe that alternative medicine, because it concentrates on wellness rather than on illness, because it is patient-centered rather than doctor-centered, because it emphasizes nutrition, exercise, stress management, and substances and functions natural to the body, because it emphasizes self-care, because it attempts to address root causes rather than symptoms, is based on a truer and more solid foundation.

And last but not least: If the drugs and surgery don't do you in, the costs of modern medicine will. At this writing, more than $1,080 is spent annually *per person* to fight disease in this country. Only 4 percent of that goes to preventive medicine, mostly in the form of vaccination and immunization. Almost nothing is spent on public education, yet studies show that patients who learn about basic health care make fewer visits to the doctor. The national medical bill in 1984 was over $360 billion, up from $27 billion in 1960. The increasingly sophisticated health-care consumer is already up in arms about the cost and quality of medical care and is demanding results.

Then there's the medical-insurance bias. Most insurance companies will reimburse you only for the "customary and usual" treatment the AMA endorses—and you know what that is and isn't.

Your insurance covers all manner of drugs and shots and lab tests and surgery, regardless of their effectiveness. But if you get well just through nutrition and exercise and education, you may have to foot much of the bill yourself. Why? Because alternative medical therapies are not "customary."

THERE'S HOPE

However, there are indications that the status-quo mentality of the medical establishment is loosening up. Young doctors today indicate that they are highly interested in nutritional and preventive medicine, and are eager to work with acupuncturists, chiropractors, exercise therapists, and nutritionists to round out their patients' treatment.

As of 1984, 100 of the 142 medical schools in Canada and the United States offered some sort of nutrition course (though it was required at only fifteen schools). This was up from only 25 percent of medical schools in 1979.

This is an exciting time of transition for medicine, but it is becoming apparent to all concerned that prevention and self-care are the only viable alternatives to an inflationary, cost-inefficient, disease-oriented health system. It is hoped that the not-too-distant future will hold a two-pronged health-care-delivery system: (a) a low-technology, low-cost, nutritionally oriented alternative to the medical approach, which views each patient as an individual and employs such therapies as nutrition, exercise, stress reduction, and life-style management; and (b) a highly specialized, high-technology (and high-cost) *disease care* system —i.e., traditional medicine as it now exists with its astounding pharmacological and surgical arsenal. This crossover and balanced sharing of responsibility will benefit everyone.

MEDICINE AT OPTIMUM HEALTH LABS

Much has happened in the years since I stumbled upon my own cures, since I started rejecting some of the sacred premises of traditional medicine. I am a healthier and happier man—as long as I practice what I preach. I exercise and supplement regularly. I have reintroduced into my diet all the foods that I was once allergic to, and I can tolerate them as long as I don't overdo them. I can truthfully state that I have not had a single headache and have not been depressed more than a day or two in the last eight years—and this used to be the on-and-off theme of my life.

These days I am medical director of Optimum Health Labs in California, a full-service nutrition/allergy facility, where we do scientific research and operate a licensed laboratory, in addition to offering clinical treatment and in-depth education. Since OHL was founded in 1980, more than 10,000 people have come to us for relief of everything from hay fever, asthma, hives, and obesity, to migraine headaches, high blood pressure, hyperactivity (in children), premenstrual syndrome, insomnia, rheumatoid arthritis, eczema, chronic pain, irritable bowel syndrome, psychological depression, and much more. The great majority of our patients get well or show significant improvement. It is incredibly satisfying and rewarding to see people who have been ill or in chronic pain leave treatment with smiles on their faces. I feel that I am finally doing the job for which my medical training was intended. The Optimum Health Program represents the continuing evolution of the simple program that so radically changed my own health, my beliefs, and my professional life.

3

Thirteen Commonsense Truths About Good Health

The Optimum Health Program requires change in the way one is used to doing things and thinking about diets and health. The thirteen basic points discussed here are meant to rout out the ignorance, myth, misinformation, and blatant propaganda about diet and good health that have for too long eroded the health and well-being of so many. I hope that when you read this, you will realize that the pieces of the puzzle of health fit together in a simple, logical, persuasive manner. There is no mystery to good health, just as there is no mystery to why so many people are unhealthy and overweight.

Good health is within everyone's reach, given the information and guidance needed to pursue it. Here are a few facts of healthy life:

1. You are responsible for your own health. Even if you are very young or are one of those rare specimens genetically blessed with a cast-iron constitution, you must pay attention to your health.

It is hard to focus on good health when we feel healthy without having made any special effort to achieve it, hard to focus on the eventual consequences of bad habits when there's so much to be enjoyed in the present. It's hard to deny ourselves when instant gratification is the American way. Too many of the things that are bad for us are made to seem glamorous, desirable, and safe. We've become suckers for instant remedies like crash weight-loss programs and instant-fitness regimes. And it's hard to rely on ourselves for health when we are told that doctors and pharmacies will fix us up if we get into serious trouble.

But we must stop kidding ourselves. A doctor can prescribe antibiotics to cure an infection, but he cannot make us do the things—exercising, eating properly, getting enough sleep—that would help prevent our catching the infection in the first place. It is the individual who must educate himself about good health.

2. Nutrition is extremely important. This sounds simple-minded, until we contemplate how careless most people are about what they put into their systems. What we put into our mouths is the fuel for our bodies; it is the most crucial determinant of our level of performance, of how well and how long we will live. Yet many people are more concerned with what type of fuel and oil they put into their cars than with fuel for their own bodies.

How can we be so blasé about the consequences of our diet, when evidence for the direct cause-and-effect relationship between diet and health is so overwhelming? When we eat a candy bar, we get a sugar "boost," and then, an hour later, a low hits us. When breakfast has consisted of two cups of coffee and a Danish, we feel an acute energy drain in midmorning. Sluggishness follows a steak-and-two-martinis lunch. Doesn't this demonstrate that *everything* we put into our system has a direct effect—whether it's an apple or a Coke, a cupcake or a slice of whole grain bread—even if we're not always aware of a reaction?

The effects of diet have been borne out by a number of studies. The Japanese, for example, have a very low incidence of heart disease and cancer—on a diet very low in red meat and dairy products, high in fish, vegetables, and fiber. The Greenland Eskimos might seem to be likely candidates for heart disease, with their extremely fatty, high-cholesterol diets, but in fact heart disease is all but unknown to this population. For the fat they consume is what is called an essential fatty acid, derived mostly from the fatty cold-water fish and other marine animals that are staples of their diet—and this kind of fat actually *reduces* the potential for heart disease. Studies of primitive cultures still living in Australia show that they remain free of the Western world's degenerative diseases on their highly varied regime—until they're introduced to "civilized," refined foods. Then it's all downhill—and fast. Another convincing study involves the Seventh Day Adventists, whose religious tenets dictate a diet of natural foods high in vegetables and fiber and grains, low in meat and dairy products—and, of course, they neither smoke nor drink. Heart disease is almost unknown, the cancer rate is less than one third that of the general population, and life expectancy exceeds that of the rest of the population by several years.

Diet affects mood and temperament and personality. There is growing consensus that hyperactive children are the victims of diets high in allergic foods, chemical preservatives, and colorings, which wreak havoc on the brain and nervous system. Studies show that juvenile delinquents eat diets considerably higher in milk and sugars and refined packaged foods than other members of their age group, and that when their diet is changed, repeat offenses drop dramatically.

Too, nutrition can solve health problems in ways that medicine and surgery cannot, and it can deal with problems that most doctors don't want to be bothered with. Doctors like problems with specific names and known remedies. Have you ever tried telling your doctor that you felt kind of "down" or tired? Chances are he told you he was tired too and to take it easy. Perhaps he suggested you see a therapist or prescribed a mild tranquilizer. But most of us are walking around with nonspecific symptoms—that is, conditions that indicate no known "diagnosable" disease. We feel fatigued or stuffed up, or our stomachs are upset, or we feel depressed and anxious, or our bones and muscles ache. Medicines may relieve and mask the symptoms, but they will not solve the underlying problem. In many cases, only proper nutrition will do the trick—permanently.

3. Food allergies are common (though often undetected), and they underlie much poor health and disease. The general public (and much of the medical profession) has very outdated ideas about allergy, which they usually associate with hay fever or a tendency to break out in hives from eating strawberries. In fact, sensitivities or allergies, especially to food, are common to about 60 percent or more of the population. There are a number of reasons for this (detailed in Chapter 4), most having to do with the way we live and eat and with our environment. Until recently, food allergies were difficult to diagnose and to test for, so they often went undetected for years. Ironically, the foods we crave and eat repeatedly are most likely to be the ones we are allergic to, in many cases, physiologically *addicted* to.

The consequences of allergies are serious. Food allergy may be a primary underlying cause—or contributing factor—of degenerative disease, which has become epidemic in America. Determining our food allergies and removing these allergies from our diets is a major step to restoring our health.

4. The fact that we eat a particular food does not mean that we digest it. There is often a big gap between what you ingest and what you digest. Your digestive tract may not properly digest (that is, absorb into the proper tissue) a food that it is allergic to. You may be consuming a well-balanced diet consisting of all the "right" foods and nutrients, but if your system is allergic to those foods—or generally weakened from fighting off allergens—the nutrients will never make it past the lining of the digestive tract and into the bloodstream in a form easily utilizable by your body. Even vitamin supplements, if they contain fillers and binders you're allergic to, won't do you much good.

Every dose of antacid, of Alka-Seltzer or Pepto-Bismol or Tums, is a sign that many people are not digesting their food properly. And poor digestion means that nutrients are not well absorbed, and poor absorption leads to malnutrition. Malnutrition is usually thought to be a problem only in poor, underdeveloped nations, but it's becoming apparent that subclinical malnutrition is a common problem in affluent America. We have all the food we need, but we're not getting the benefit of it.

Healthy people, who are digesting their food properly, are not bothered by gas, belching, nausea, indigestion, diarrhea, bloating, abdominal cramping, heartburn, smelly stools, or constipation. Many people accept these symptoms as natural or as predictable signs of aging. They are not. Once proper diet and exercise habits are established, once allergies are cleared up and the immune system is shored up, digestion returns to normal—that is, becomes symptom-free.

5. Good food may not be what you think it is. There are a lot of half-truths and outdated ideas about what constitutes a good diet. For one thing, a food that you are allergic to is not "good" for you, no matter how healthy or nutritious it is purported to be. Someone who is allergic to whole wheat may be better off eating refined white bread. Not all fats are bad—certain kinds of fats (lacking in most diets) are sorely needed to offset the effects of other fats. "Starchy food," in the form of complex carbohydrates, may be quite good for you. Sugar and coffee are worse than you think. Milk, long considered the healthiest of foods, is a common allergen and is not properly digested by *the majority* of people, causing all sorts of digestive upsets and allergic symptoms. And even the "healthiest" food may be bad for you if eaten too frequently—an apple a day, for example, or eggs for breakfast every morning or cottage cheese invariably for lunch. Learning more about proper nutrition is one of the first tasks in achieving optimum health.

6. There is no such thing as an "average" person. Many misunderstandings about good health start with a false premise: that there is an *average* healthy person. There's no such thing anatomically, physiologically, nutritionally, biochemically, or psychologically. Individual differences are the rule rather than the exception, and they are often striking. Young medical students are often shocked to realize that an individual heart may bear very little resemblance to pictures and photographs of "the human heart" and that each heart they see may differ remarkably from the ones that preceded it.

Each person is born with different physiological and psychological strengths and weaknesses, and each person is exposed to a different type and number of environmental stresses. One person has chronic sinus problems but never gets a headache or a cavity. Another never gets colds, but bleeds excessively when cut. Each has different allergies, and their reactions—their target organs—for those allergies are different.

We are always hearing reports about Recommended Daily Allowances for vitamins, but a simple blood test would demonstrate that your vitamin needs may differ greatly from those of most other people. It's been estimated that the official RDA—aside from being almost uselessly skimpy in the first place—would apply to only about 10 to 20 percent of the population.

Health statistics based on the "average" American are likewise illogical. These statistics fail to take into consideration one simple fact: Not only is the average American a phantom, but should he (or she) exist, he would not be in very good health. He is in borderline health—a pushover for disease. For "average" in this country is suboptimally healthy. We derive our standards of what's healthy from the normal (or average), which in turn is deduced from a malnourished, unfit, suboptimally well population.

It's a mistake to settle for *average* health. And it's a mistake to rely on information that assumes you are like everyone else. One important task in your quest for optimum health is to find out more about *you*—what *you* are allergic to, what vitamins and other nutrients *you* need, what makes *you* feel good (and bad), what kind and amount of exercise does the job for *you,* what stresses and relaxes *you.* (See Chapter 13 for help with finding out more about your own health and diet habits.)

7. Weight problems can often be solved permanently without counting calories—by getting rid of food allergies and eating properly. There are many reasons for the "fattening" of America and for the seesaw of weight loss and gain that plagues so many people. In this land of ease and plenty, in the context of a sedentary life-style, most of us just plain eat too much of the wrong kinds of foods—and far more than our systems are programmed to process if we're not exercising. And much of what we eat is the product of our sophisticated technology: processed, refined, high in saturated fats, oils, and sugars, and laden with chemicals that supposedly make the food safer and more attractive. Again, it is a far cry from the food our systems are designed to consume.

For most people, the "solution" to the inevitable weight gain on such a diet is to go on a strict, low-calorie crash diet from time to time and get their weight down to a point where they can return to their usual fare. This is a self-defeating cycle, for each time we go on such a crash diet, our body's sensitive adaptive censors slow down our rate of metabolism to match the new restrictive regime. When we return to the old diet, it takes the body time to readjust, and it seems never to return to the old metabolic rate needed to burn the higher calorie load. Also, with each crash diet, we lose muscle mass—valuable tissue with a higher metabolic rate than fat tissue—and each time we return to our old diet, we gain that lost weight back in metabolically sluggish *fat tissue.* So with each crash diet, we lower the rate at which we burn calories and decrease our percentage of muscle to body fat, making us more apt to store calories, rather than burn them. It should also be mentioned that the 500–1,200 calories allotted in most diets are not enough for proper nutrition. Malnutrition associated with chronic crash dieting may eventually lead to other degenerative problems.

Weight problems are seriously compounded by lack of exercise. Not only is exercise a prime means of increasing the metabolic rate—that is, the rate at which calories are burned—but it helps us to maintain and increase valuable muscle tissue. Research reveals that the metabolic rate of people who exercise remains elevated by 25 percent or more for as along as fifteen hours after exercising. That means that someone who exercises regularly is burning more calories than a sedentary person even while he is sitting at his desk or eating.

But perhaps the most crucial problem that traditional diets fail to address is food allergy/food addiction. Undiagnosed food allergy is probably the most common cause behind abnormal food cravings and bingeing, which keep so many people glued to their refrigerators. The reason that following a calorie-restricting diet is such torture is that, in the course of dieting, we often have to withdraw from foods we crave —foods that we are in fact addicted to.

Everyone who wants to lose weight permanently must find out what he is allergic to and eliminate those foods from his diet. Once that is done, cravings abate, appetite and metabolism return to normal, and the digestive system regains its ability to digest fully and properly absorb needed nutrients.

8. You cannot get by indefinitely without exercise and hope to remain in good health. Exercise—vigorous physical activity—is not a natural part of many people's lives. It is something we have to plan for and often to pay for. Despite the attention paid to physical fitness in recent years, far too many people still do not get enough exercise, or they get it—like their diets—in intermittent crash programs. Physical fitness cannot be attained in a month of daily aerobics classes. If the exercise is abandoned, the achievement of that month will quickly erode. The only sane and effective approach to attaining physical fitness is to accept the fact that it is a long, gradual process—a few months to see the first real gains, probably more than a year to reach a high degree of fitness.

The good news is that almost everyone, regardless of age or present physical condition, can achieve a high level of fitness—by starting slowly *and keeping at it.* Exercise raises the metabolic rate, stimulates the immune system, and increases the delivery and capacity rate of the body's most essential nutrient—oxygen. It is a great depression fighter and self-esteem builder. Regular exercise makes it possible to withstand a higher level of stress, to improve one's digestion and elimination, and to overcome allergies and improper nutrition.

9. Your food cannot supply all your nutritional needs. Most practitioners of traditional medicine are still paying little more than lip service to the tremendous importance of nutrient supplements. Those doctors who don't entirely dismiss the need for supplementation most often prescribe a daily commercial multivitamin capsule and perhaps some extra Vitamin C when a cold is imminent.

But there are many reasons that more aggressive supplementation is needed, for children as well as adults. Most people do not eat an adequate diet. They do not find time for three varied and balanced meals a day, and what they do eat is often highly refined, lacking in the nutrients necessary for good health. They consume too many things that compromise the nutritional value of their food—sugar, coffee, nicotine, and alcohol. They are allergic to many of the highly nutritious foods they eat, so their systems are not forwarding those nutrients through the bloodstream. Their lives are full of stress and illness. They don't get enough sleep. They are bombarded daily with toxic chemicals: in the air, at the office, in their homes, and of course in their food and drinking water.

The average American diet doesn't come close to providing the nutrition we need for optimum health, and in many cases it sabotages good health. Recent nutritional research shows that there are many vital nutrients—specific minerals, vitamins, amino acids, and essential fats—that are sorely lacking or suboptimal in most people's diets.

Supplementation is not a substitute for good food, but it takes up the slack between what we eat and what we need for optimum health. A daily regimen of balanced, allergy-free, chemical-free supplements is the best assurance that our nutritional needs are being met.

10. There's such a thing as too much of a good thing. In our enthusiasm to make changes or to get quick results, it's tempting to think that if a certain amount of something is good, more must be better. Conversely, if something is bad, less must be better. It isn't so. The optimum level of most things falls somewhere in the middle.

This principle is most vividly illustrated by the bell-shaped curve (see Figure 2, page 32), in this example showing desirable levels of serum

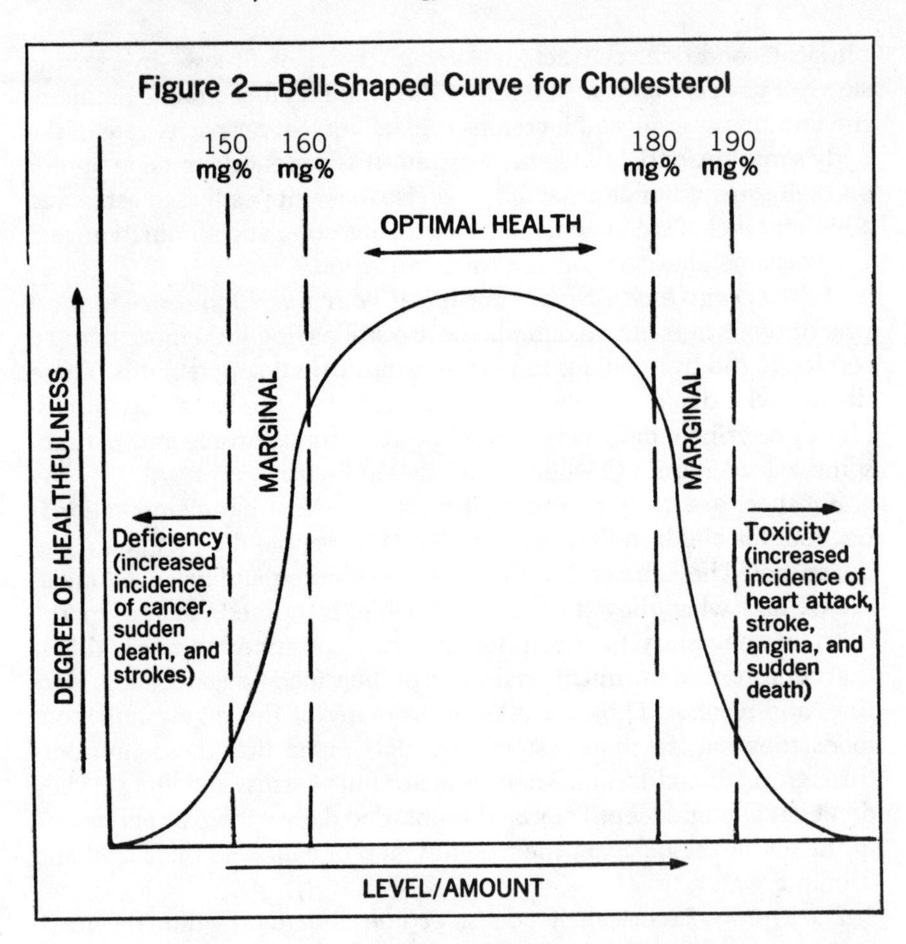

cholesterol. Popular mythology has it that cholesterol is bad for you; this is *partially* true. As the chart shows, any amount between 160 and 180 mg is a desirable level, and anything over 180 is associated with an increased risk of such diseases as hypertension and heart disease. What most people don't realize is that anything below 150 may indicate a cholesterol *deficiency*. At this level, the body may be lacking in the cholesterol vital to building up cellular membranes, Vitamin D, the nervous system, and steroid/sex hormones.

There are many other examples of the bell-shaped-curve phenomenon. The acceptable levels of fluoride may follow a very narrow curve —1 to 4 mg a day seems to be the acceptable range. Fluoridation of the water supply is said to provide major health benefits, but now that fluoride is being added to toothpaste, mouthwashes, and other hygiene products, there is a real danger of widespread fluoride toxicity—exceeding the optimal amount and registering in the downslope of the bell-shaped curve. Even exercise has its limits: Athletes who overtrain or exercise instructors who teach too many classes over a long period of time without proper rest and nutritional compensation become susceptible to the very stress fractures, overuse injuries, and infections that their superior training should protect them from.

11. Contrary to popular belief, your feelings of depression, achiness, or fatigue are probably not psychosomatic. It's become practically a convention of modern medicine to label inexplicable symptoms or unresponsive disease "psychosomatic." This is both a disservice to the majority of people, whose complaints are very real, and a cop-out for modern medicine. Whether doctors like it or not, many physical and emotional complaints that don't lend themselves to a specific medical diagnosis nevertheless have a treatable physiological and biochemical cause, and are entitled to receive treatment as such.

There is undoubtedly a strong mind/body connection in disease. There is no doubting the power of the mind and of the unconscious both to aggravate and to reverse illness. But rest assured that your migraine headaches or rheumatoid arthritis or peptic ulcers, even your chronic depression or spastic colon, are often more likely to be a product of undetected allergies, prolonged malnutrition, and/or some other very sensible and concrete explanation than of your demented mind.

12. Nobody's perfect. You may be thinking, as you read all this, that it's asking too much from a mere mortal that he should reform his entire life: change his diet, exercise, give up foods he loves. Maybe you're better off resigning yourself to periodic crash diets and exercise binges.

But the Optimum Health Program is not meant to be an all-or-nothing thing. It's not that you will never eat chocolate cake again or skip a day of exercise or take an extra drink at a cocktail party. But you will be slowly minimizing these things in your life and at the same time shoring up your body's ability to withstand their effects. You will not give up the foods you are now allergic to forever—only long enough for your body to be desensitized and rebuild its defenses against them. And all the time you are on the diet, you will be making small, cumulative, permanent changes toward better health.

You probably acquired this book because you already know in your heart of hearts that the diets you've tried before don't work or the medication you've been taking for arthritis has undesired side effects. If your malaise has gone on for some time, you have probably tried a number of doctors or diets or cures. You already know you should be exercising or cutting down on coffee. You know that any lasting benefits are going to be the result of time and effort.

You don't have to be perfect to follow the Optimum Health Program. You just have to be prepared to live your life a little differently. Chances are excellent that you'll end up enjoying your new health habits.

13. Optimum Health is possible for YOU. No matter what your present weight or state of health, you can, with time and effort, achieve your best possible health. You do not have to live with your allergies, with chronic pain, with overweight, with nagging, debilitating symptoms, with depression or insomnia.

PART II

How the System Works: Allergy, Digestion, and the Immune System

4

The Allergy Epidemic

The thinking of the majority of health professionals, including allergists and dieticians, is some fifteen to twenty years out of date when it comes to food allergy. The traditionalist's view is limited to the immunological events associated with the so-called Type I responses of inhalant and airborne allergies—the kind that fit a known, long-accepted pattern and are reasonably easy to detect by established testing methodologies. These are food allergies in which allergic symptoms may appear less than an hour after eating, affecting only limited areas of the body—the skin, airways, and digestive tract, for example.

Because of this extremely narrow view of allergy, these same experts have dismissed food allergy as a serious threat, especially to adults. They have concluded that it is rare; even among children, they claim, only 10 percent are affected by food allergy, and it is quickly "outgrown." Adult food allergies are not taken seriously unless they conform to the same symptomatic patterns seen in the immediate Type I allergic responses: stuffy nose, wheezing, hives, or gastrointestinal upset occurring shortly after eating the allergic food. Thus, most sufferers get little help from their personal physicians.

To add insult to injury, food allergy is so badly misunderstood that many allergy sufferers have to contend with the condescending professional conclusion that their allergic symptoms are psychomatic: It's all in the mind, and therefore compassion, tranquilization, and "talk therapy" are the best treatments. The only people who benefit from this treatment—in many if not most cases—are the psychiatrists and the pharmaceutical industry, which together treat the symptoms without treating the cause of the problem.

Mountains of research, numerous international symposiums on food allergy, and certainly our own extensive clinical experience with thousands of allergy sufferers at Optimum Health Labs show that these widely held ideas about allergy are distorted. The truth about food allergy is both exciting and rather shocking and tells us a radically different story.

WHAT ARE THE FACTS?

1. Food allergy is not rare. Food allergies are common, frequent reactions, in both children and adults, to an increasingly nutritionally depleted diet, to an increasingly stressful existence (often improperly treated with drugs and alcohol), to increasingly chemically polluted environment and food, and to hereditary disposition. *Food allergy clearly affects the majority of the American people.*

2. The effects of food allergy are not limited to just the air passages, the skin, and the digestive tract. Although these are common sites, food allergens, once in the bloodstream, travel throughout the body, their effects showing up anywhere that the blood flows and producing a wide variety of physical and mental symptoms.

3. Most food allergies are delayed reactions, taking anywhere from an hour to three days to show themselves, and are therefore much harder to detect. Because the immune mechanism is different, the customary tests used to diagnose airborne allergens are of little use in identifying food allergens. (More on this topic in Chapter 5.)

4. Delayed food allergy appears to be simply the inability of your digestive tract to prevent large quantities of partially digested and undigested food from entering the bloodstream. Once in the bloodstream, allergens may be deposited in tissue, causing the symptoms and inflammatory diseases we call by other names.

5. When allergic sensitivities begin to develop—for whatever reasons—they have far-reaching, unsuspected effects. The expression of allergy indicates that the balance of the system is undermined. For example, most people having allergic reactions to food are unable to digest and absorb what they're eating. As a consequence they become progressively malnourished. (You are not what you eat—you are what you eat, digest, absorb, transport, and utilize!) As time passes and your allergies go undiagnosed and the causes untreated, your primary defense against all diseases, the immune system, perhaps the body system most sensitive to malnutrition, begins to wear down from fighting off the influx of allergic substances. As a consequence the functions of the immune system become slowly more and more impaired (e.g., the ability to fight off infections, to prevent accelerated aging, to heal wound and injuries quickly, etc.), and you become significantly more prone to other diseases. The weakened immune system further impairs digestion. The whole organism weakens from lack of proper nourishment and can no longer defend itself.

6. Most of the causes of allergy are under our control and can therefore be minimized, corrected, or eliminated.

FOOD ALLERGY: A WIDELY IGNORED AND MISUNDERSTOOD ILLNESS

Up until the 1920s allergy was defined by much of the medical community in very broad, general terms—as an individual's symptomatic reaction to something in the environment, in a concentration or quantity that most other people could easily tolerate. Interestingly, with this less precise approach to food allergy, it was generally recognized that many people did in fact suffer from adverse reactions to food.

A "Scientific" Blunder

Then, about 1925, research in Europe turned up a mysterious substance scientists called *reagin* (related to the word "react"), which appeared to be involved in allergic responses in the skin. In the excitement of the moment the medical community decided that henceforth the only proper identification of an allergy *must* include reference to a skin response involving reagin. By this specious argument, if a tested substance did not provoke a skin response (if there wasn't reagin present), there wasn't an allergy; there must be some other explanation. Yet most food allergies do not provoke a skin response or an immediate reaction of any sort.

Consequently, in the absence of a scientifically verifiable method of identifying and naming any *nonreagin* reaction, delayed food allergy (which accounts for about 95 percent of food allergies) was ignored by most physicians for the next fifty years or so.

Reagin turned out to be, in present-day terminology, a specific antibody called immunoglobulin E (IgE). IgE is the antibody known to be the culprit in airborne allergies (such as those to pollen, dust, and animal dander) but only in a very limited number of food allergies. IgE response is what the allergist is looking for with skin testing (e.g., the prick test, the patch test) and the IgE RAST (radioallergosorbent test) blood test.

However, most food allergies are delayed responses, showing up one hour to three days after eating the allergic food, and involving a different antibody or antibodies, including immunoglobulin G (IgG). They may affect any system, tissue, or organ of the body. Unfortunately, the broad range and widely varying degrees of emotional and physical responses to non-IgE-mediated allergens are not so easy and convenient to pin down.

As a consequence of this uncertainty and prodded along by the new mystical influences of Freudian analytical concepts, the medical com munity found it fashionable in the 1940s, 1950s, and 1960s to label patients (especially women) with multiple, nonspecific physical and/or emotional complaints as neurotic housewives or just plain hypochondriacs. The *unprovable* psychological illness of the patient was a more palatable explanation for such medical mysteries than the ignorance or incompetence of the physician. Neurosis, hypochondriasis, and psychosomatic illness have been the diagnoses of choice for 50 to 80 percent of patients over the last forty years or so. Yet in many cases their chronically recurring symptoms were aggravated, if not caused, by food and/or chemical hypersensitivities. The guilt, the embarrassment, the medications, and the self-doubt were all unnecessary.

The premature, prejudiced dismissal by the medical community of all allergy responses that were not IgE-mediated (that did not have immediate reaction to skin tests) created a huge gap in the treatment available to a suffering public—a gap that is only recently being closed by nutritionally oriented medicine. This treatment is based on research and clinical studies conducted and published outside the mainstream of modern medicine. To this day, many if not most traditional allergists continue to work within the narrow confines of the reagin/IgE-mediated/immediate-response mentality, which confines them to recognizing fewer than 10 percent of food-allergy problems.

The Beginnings of Modern Food Allergy

Drs. Theron Randolph and Herbert Rinkel are considered the fathers of modern allergy, which has unfortunately acquired the ponderous and esoteric name of "clinical ecology." Clinical ecologists, or alternative allergists, are concerned with the body's immunological and nonimmunological responses to *all* substances in the environment: in the air, in the water, in medications, and most of all in our food. Drs. Rinkel, Randolph, and Zeller's classic 1951 book, *Food Allergy,* is an important starting point for much of what is properly understood today about allergy. Dr. Herbert Rinkel, father of the four-day rotation diet, began to lead other pioneers out of the Dark Ages of food allergy. He coined the phrase "hidden food allergy" and first talked about the allergy/addiction syndrome and the "masking" of symptoms, which are so basic to our present understanding of how food allergy works (more about this in Chapter 5, page 55).

About the same time Dr. Arthur F. Coca, another prominent allergist and former president of the American College of Allergists, created considerable controversy when he began to focus on the importance and frequency of food allergy. In his book, *The Pulse Test,* he stated that many people with allergies to food don't always demonstrate the usual overt, outwardly recognizable symptoms. In fact, one way in which they may initially show a reaction to food is simply by an increase in heart rate or pulse. He advocated a simple—but at that time highly controversial—self-test by which you could determine food allergy by checking your pulse just before eating a suspected food and then rechecking it every thirty minutes or so to see if the pulse has accelerated. If there was an approximate fifteen-beat increase during the next hour or so, not explained by exertion or emotional change, that was a clear indication of a hidden food allergy. Most of Dr. Coca's colleagues dismissed this as sheer heresy.

Pediatrician Dr. Arthur Black, Drs. William and Miriam Bryan of St. Louis, Dr. Charles Dickey, Dr. William Philpott, and more recently Dr. Marshall Mandell—through their focus on delayed rather than immediate allergic reactions, their focus on both food and chemical sensitivities, and their utilization of the theoretical constructs of Drs. Herbert Rinkel and Theron Randolph—are the other major contributors to the later developments in this field. Today the findings of these pioneers are being borne out by an ever-expanding wealth of new research and clinical evidence and a fuller understanding of the mechanism of food allergy—and of all delayed, IgG, immune-complex-mediated reactions (more about this in Chapter 6). With their help, and the more recent applications of nutritional biochemistry, this work is leading not only to the development of updated diagnostic tests and improved therapies, but perhaps to the *cure* for many allergies. *The elimination of food allergies is an important key to optimum health.*

THE SYMPTOMS OF FOOD ALLERGY

Food allergy is by definition an irritation of tissues or inflammation, caused by a food allergen. *Where* an allergen decides to deposit itself and do its damage is probably genetically predetermined. Everyone has his physiological and biochemical strong and weak points—diseases that he is resistant to and others to which he is especially susceptible. Ten people allergic to milk may react to it in ten highly individual ways. It may cause migraine headaches in one person, diarrhea in another, eczema or hyperactivity in another, anginalike symptoms in a fourth, or perhaps a flare-up of rheumatoid arthritis.

Keep in mind that the symptoms that appear are usually not sudden reactions but have probably built up over a period of time. In fact, one of the insidious aspects of most food allergy reactions is that the majority of symptoms, at least in the early developmental stages, are mild and seem to have no direct connection (timewise) to the food that brought them on. The full flare-up of symptoms may be the result of months or years of cumulative food-allergy damage.

As you can see from Table 1 on pages 44–45, many possible indicators of food allergy are the kind of discomforts we often tolerate without giving a thought to getting medical attention. It's highly unlikely that we will connect them to food allergy and therefore highly *likely* that we will continue to ignore them until they become intolerable.

Some of the symptoms listed in Table 1 are especially frequent indicators of food allergy. One is fatigue, mental or physical. Though many disease states may be associated with chronic fatigue, perhaps the most common cause is food and chemical hypersensitivity, particularly if the tired feeling shows up after meals, upon awakening in the morning, or in association with other symptoms of allergy, such as chronic depression and gastrointestinal disorders.

Another common sign of allergy is water retention or edema. People who have a tendency to gain or lose more than a couple of pounds a day, or whose weight bounces around unpredictably, unassociated with the quantity of food eaten, should at least suspect food allergy. One of the ways in which the body can reduce the irritation of allergy is to hold on to a lot of water, in order to dilute the tissue-bound allergens—hence, edema (water retention). Because your body will not release these fluids as long as it is defending against allergic attacks, it is very hard to keep one's weight down until allergies are eliminated from your diet. Bloating after meals is a common manifestation of water retention. Inappropriate thirst is yet another symptom related to water retention. (But excessive thirst could also indicate diabetes or a deficiency of essential fatty acids, so this symptom should be taken seriously.) Many women taking water pills or diuretics for chronic edema are targets for serious potassium and/or magnesium deficiencies and related cardiovascular risks. A safer, more effective therapy for chronic edema would be to identify and eliminate allergic foods from their diets.

"Allergic shiners" (dark circles under the eyes), swelling or puffiness under the eyes, wrinkles under the eyes ("Dennie's sign") are all usually traceable to allergy. So is the nose wrinkle (or "allergic salute"), a horizontal crease across the bridge of the nose that comes from habitually wiping the nose.

Yet another very common symptom of allergy is excess mucus formation—characterized by a chronically congested nose, postnasal drip, excessive phlegm (often coughed up after exercise or strong emotions), mucus in the stools, frequent nose blowing or nose picking, etc.

Digestive disturbances almost always accompany food allergies. These can include bloating after meals, belching, gas (flatulence), coated tongue, nausea, vomiting, diarrhea, constipation alternating with diarrhea, abdominal cramping, bad breath, symptoms of gallbladder disease, pronounced anal itching, mucus or blood in the stools. The digestive tract appears to be the first line of defense against food allergy; inversely, impaired digestion is often the first cause of food allergy as well. (Chapter 6 explains the role of the digestive and immune systems in more detail.)

Various chronic pain syndromes are caused or aggravated by allergy. Food allergy often contributes to rheumatoid arthritis, muscle aches and pains, and sore, achy joints. Migraine and related headaches such as cluster headaches (severe pain in the eye or temple, usually recurring) often indicate that delayed food allergy or chemical hypersensitivity is at work. The headache and cramping found in premenstrual syndrome (PMS) are yet another pain syndrome that responds to the elimination of food allergies.

How does food allergy bring on pain? When the food allergens deposited in tissues cause inflammation, the immune cells summoned to the inflamed area release large quantities of chemical mediators. Among these chemical mediators are several that seem to cause or exacerbate the pain response—bradykinin (probably the most painful one produced by the body) and PGE2 and PGF2 alpha, both thought to increase sensitivity to pain.

Then there are the many emotional, mental, and behavioral symptoms and signs: inability to concentrate, or to focus one's attention for any length of time, recurring mental fatigue, irritability for no apparent reason, inexplicable depression, free-floating anxiety, crying jags, mood swings, hyperactivity, confusion, perhaps indirectly even an alcohol hangover, acute schizophrenia, bulimia, and some phobias.

Frequent, recurring infections, especially in children, are common signs of associated food allergy. Chronic upper respiratory infections, such as sore throats, colds, and middle-ear infections, may be the result of reduced immunity as a consequence of food allergy. Modern physicians, myself included, believe that you don't catch colds, you eat them.

Table 1 (on the following pages) covers only a partial listing of the symptoms that may be associated with or caused by food allergy. Food

Table 1 — Common Symptoms Associated with Food Allergies	
Physical Symptoms	
Head	Dark circles under eyes, swelling and wrinkles under eyes (Dennie's sign), cluster headaches and other "vascular" headaches migraine headaches, faintness, dizziness, feelings of fullness in the head, excessive drowsiness or sleepiness soon after eating, insomnia, frequent awakenings during the night, early A.M. awakening (usually between 2 and 4 A.M.) with inability to return to sleep.
Eyes, ears, nose, and throat	Runny nose, stuffy nose, excessive mucus formation, postnasal drip, watery eyes, blurring of vision, tinnitus (buzzing, roaring, popping, ringing of the ears), earache, fullness in the ears, fluid in the middle ear, hearing loss, recurrent ear infections, itching ear, ear drainage, sore throats, hoarseness, chronic cough, gagging, canker sores, itching of the roof of the mouth, recurrent sinusitis, persistent nose picking.
Heart and lungs	Palpitations, arrhythmias, increased heart rate, rapid heart rate (tachycardia), asthma, congestion in the chest, exercise-induced anaphylaxis and asthma.
Gastrointestinal	Mucus in stools, undigested food in stools, nausea, vomiting, diarrhea, constipation, bloating after meals, belching, colitis, flatulence (passing gas), feeling of fullness in the stomach long after finishing a meal, abdominal pains or cramps, irritable bowel syndrome, colic in infants, failure to thrive in infants, extreme thirst, inflammatory bowel disease (Crohn's disease and ulcerative colitis, e.g.), anal itching, coated tongue, apparent symptoms of gallbladder disease (which may turn out to be of allergenic nature instead).
Skin	Hives, rashes, eczema, dermatitis herpetiformis, pallor, dry skin, dandruff, brittle nails and hair.

Table 1 *(Continued)*	
Physical Symptoms	
Other symptoms	"Growing pains" in children, symptoms of PMS, chronic fatigue, weakness, muscle aches and pains, joint aches and pains, arthritis, swelling of the hands, feet or ankles, urinary tract symptoms (frequency, urgency), vaginal itching, vaginal discharge, abnormal craving and its close ally binge eating, epilepsy in children with migraines, obesity, rapid weight fluctuation from day to day (2–10 pounds or more).
Psychological Symptoms	
	Anxiety, "panic attacks," depression, crying jags, aggressive behavior, irritability, mental dullness, mental lethargy, confusion, excessive daydreaming, hyperactivity in children and adults, restlessness, learning disabilities, poor work habits, slurred speech, stuttering, inability to concentrate, indifference, perhaps certain types of autism and schizophrenia, perhaps bulimia/anorexia nervosa.

allergy is a great masquerader. We are only beginning to recognize it in its many guises.

WHY WE HAVE ALLERGIES

Allergies develop for a number of reasons. For many, *heredity* plays a role. The tendency to develop allergies is often passed down from parent to child, either as a genetic tendency or as a nutritionally induced tendency transmitted to the fetus during pregnancy. Asthma is commonly passed from generation to generation; so are hay fever, eczema, and migraine headaches. The immune system and digestive tract, weakened through inheritance or congenital malnourishment, will not take as much abuse before they start to shut down and malfunction, unable to deal with the environment and a poor diet.

But most reasons for our allergic tendencies have to do more with the way we live and eat. It is not farfetched to say that allergies are a side effect of modern life: of what we eat and don't eat, of the manner in which we eat, of our polluted environment, of our stressful life-styles, and of our lack of exercise. Let's look first at the way we eat.

Dietary Indiscretions

The Wrong Food. At the turn of the century, only 10 percent of our diet was refined, chemically "enhanced" food. By 1950, 25 percent of our foods were processed, devitalized, and chemicalized. Today that figure is very close to *90 percent.* Most Americans are eating too many highly processed foods, too much of the wrong kinds of fats, too much salt and refined sugar, too many chemical additives and contaminants, and too little fiber, essential nutrients, complex carbohydrates, and fresh, unprocessed foods.

What are the dangers of an overrefined, chemical-laden diet? Processing removes much of the valuable fiber in foods, fiber that assists in the digestion and absorption process, in the elimination of undigested foods and toxins, and in the reabsorption and elimination of cholesterol. Refining, preserving, and processing leach many of the nutrients out of our food, and the "enrichment" processes fail to put them back in proper amounts, if at all. Nutrients that are not removed are often changed in processing to chemical forms not recognized or utilized as nutrients once they enter the body.

Refined foods often pass too quickly and indiscriminately into the bloodstream. This may be the reason that so many people react allergically to highly refined foods—alcohol, sugars, coffee. Excessive consumption of refined sugars (such as in pastries) has been demonstrated to inhibit the protective effect of white blood cells directly and to exert undue stress on both the pancreas and adrenal glands. Excessive salt intake (sodium chloride) in conjunction with an imbalance or deficiency in other minerals such as potassium, magnesium, and calcium can become a major factor in high blood pressure. And the high saturated-fat content of meats, dairy products, and egg yolks—staples of the American diet—aside from being a common allergy provoker, is a powerful metabolic inhibitor and contributor to the epidemic of coronary heart disease, strokes, kidney failure, diabetes, obesity, and cancer. Ironically, at a time when we are finally learning the dangers of a high-fat diet, we are learning that there are *beneficial* fats that must be in our diets to balance the impact of the undesirable ones. These are the essential fats found naturally in vegetables, seeds, nuts, cold-seawater fish, and certain cold-weather plants. (More on essential fatty acids in Chapter 11.)

There is a growing suspicion among informed nutritionists and nutritional biochemists that an important root cause of food allergy may well be a deficiency in certain essential fatty acids or an imbalance of hormonelike chemicals called prostaglandins and prostanoids derived from these fatty acids. The symptoms of food allergy in these cases could really be the expression of this imbalance of prostaglandin, induced by a nutritional deficiency.

The "Leaky Gut" Contributors. Over 3,000 chemicals (that is, substances produced by a chemical process) are added to the American diet today, plus over 10,000 chemical contaminants, not intentionally added but there nonetheless, thanks to our polluted environment. All told, it weighs out to about 8 to 15 pounds of potentially harmful chemicals consumed per person annually. It is now well established that some of these chemicals actually have the ability to change the digestive process and distort the permeability of the intestinal lining, the last barrier between the outside world and your bloodstream.

Foods that you consume at the same time you have an alcoholic drink or a cup of coffee appear to be much more likely than usual to pass into the bloodstream in an only partially digested state. Such macromolecules, too large to be recognized as nutrients, are treated by the bloodstream's immune system as foreign invaders, or allergens, and provoke an antibody response as the immune system desperately tries to fight and clear these "undesirables" from circulation. People who drink, who smoke cigarettes or marijuana, or who consume several cups of coffee daily (these things are often found keeping company, aren't they?) are more likely to have food allergies.

As we'll see in Chapter 6, susceptibility to allergy has to do primarily with the ***permeability,*** the "leakiness," of the digestive tract—the tendency of the gastrointestinal tract to allow unwanted substances through the mucosal barrier of the intestines. The recently documented phenomenon called the leaky-gut syndrome, associated with even moderate alcohol consumption, is helping explain the nature of allergy (and addiction), both to food and to alcohol in general.

Too Much Food. Another factor in the development of allergy is that we just plain eat too much. We are overtaxing our digestive and immune systems with the sheer quantities of food that we consume—an average of 500 to 1,000 calories more each day than we need to maintain good health. That excess food leads to immune-system suppression is well-established in animal studies: Simply by being fed reduced calories—without malnutrition or starvation—animals often live at least twice as long as nonrestricted animals, with a lower incidence of cancer and other degenerative diseases of aging. As Chapter 5 points out, it's not just the availability of food that leads us to gluttony. Often we eat too much because we are literally addicted to some foods, and as a result, we binge on them. ***This may be the single most common reason for overeating in the Western world: food allergy/food addiction.***

Too Few Foods, Too Often. The next most damaging aspect of our modern diets is that ***we eat a very limited number of foods, and we eat them far too often.*** A national survey found that, with well over 100 to 200 distinctly different foods to choose from year-round, most people in the United States get about 80 percent of their calories from only eleven foods. Table 46 on page 230 lists the most commonly diagnosed allergic foods: wheat, rye, eggs, milk and other dairy products, nuts, soy, some fruits and vegetables. They are the staples of many a diet.

Eating the same food over and over again, especially if you are allergy-prone—if your gut is "leaky"—is a sure way to develop allergies to those foods and provoke symptoms. When you continually bombard the body with the same foods, containing the same nutrients, it eventually cries "uncle."

In other words, we become immunized against and sensitized to certain foods in our diet. Unaware that immunization and food allergy are involved, we become philosophical or stoical about the chronic recurring mental, emotional, and physical fatigue: the weight gain, the aches and pains, the insomnia, the swelling under the eyes, the congested nose, the bouts of irritability and depression for no apparent reason. We may go on for years, or a lifetime, not feeling up to par, never suspecting that food allergy and the malnutrition associated with it are at the root of the problem. And the longer the problem goes untreated, the more the digestive and immune systems weaken from having to cope with allergy and associated overconsumption and malnutrition. When serious illness strikes, the immune system, busy fighting the allergy battle, has little energy left to combat it.

One of the many reasons we can go so long without being aware of our food allergies is that our body, lacking intelligent alternatives, soon finds maladaptive ways to cope with the repeated assaults from the same foods and chemicals. It releases a rush of stress hormones, narcoticlike chemicals, and a wild assortment of chemical mediators in an attempt to minimize the suffering and stress caused by the allergic foods. These chemicals and hormones may give us a temporary rush or "high," often accompanied by a temporary amelioration of symptoms, relief from pain or discomfort, elevation of mood, and a feeling of relaxation. This maladaptation leads to physiological addictions, and we begin to crave the allergic food for the temporary relief it brings.

However, the time soon comes when we crave the allergic food to get us "up" from the low feeling of depletion that follows, rather than for the high that got us addicted in the first place. We become literally addicted to the food, not so much, ironically, for how good it makes us feel, but rather *so that we don't feel miserable.* This phenomenon, known as the allergy/addiction syndrome, is at the heart of many food allergies. In such cases, it is through breaking these addictions that we get rid of the allergies. Chapter 5 explains more fully how the allergy/addiction syndrome works.

Malnutrition in the Land of Plenty

With maldigestion and malabsorption accompanying all food allergies, what all this boils down to is that many of us are actually malnourished, even on a theoretically well-balanced diet. Malnutrition can come from a variety of directions, only one of which is inadequate intake of nutrients. The digestive tract's natural tendency is to try to fend off any substance the immune system perceives as harmful or toxic. When a food becomes allergenic, the digestive tract will do what it can to short-circuit it and prevent its absorption. By attaching antibodies to the allergen while it's still in the intestinal lumen, the body will try (often successfully) to eliminate the food through the small and large intestines before it can pass into the bloodstream. However, this unabsorbed food provides no nourishment to the body. The body also tries to prevent allergic, overeaten foods from being absorbed as nutrients by suppressing the production of digestive enzymes and acids necessary for complete digestion. If a food is incompletely digested, its nutrients cannot be used by the system, and again the body is deprived of its nutritional value. If the food does pass through the weakened intestinal lining only partially digested, the body will treat it as an allergen and not a nutrient. Again malnutrition.

Exercise and Allergy

Then there's exercise or rather the lack of it. Adequate exercise is more important than ever in our mechanized and polluted world. The oxygenation and immune stimulation provided by prudent, regular exercise are needed for proper metabolization and neutralization of the many toxins we take in and for working off all the excess calories we consume. It is well known that athletes can get away with worse nutritional habits than the general sedentary population, without the symptoms and diseases to which the latter are prone. A sedentary life is allergy-promoting.

Chemical Bombardment— in the Air, in the Water, in Our Medications, and in Our Food

Our polluted environment is yet another contributor to the high incidence of allergy. Let's examine more closely the issue of chemicals and toxins in the environment—the actual number of which, not so incidentally, has passed the 12,000 mark. No matter where we live and no matter what we eat, we are all to one degree or another eating, breathing, drinking, or coming into physical contact with many potentially harmful substances. To stay healthy, our bodies must develop and sustain defenses to neutralize and purge these metabolic and enzymatic poisons. This means that our systems are constantly being taxed. If we are well-nourished, fit, and healthy, or genetically fortunate, the impact of our environment will only slowly and subtly take its toll. With knowledge of how to prevent chemical overexposure and detoxify the body, we can buy time in which to strengthen our systems further and to minimize the damage.

Others aren't so prudent or lucky and suffer greatly from metabolic poisons in the air, food, medications, and drinking water. They become so hypersensitized to their immediate environment that they end up having to avoid tap water or all clothing except specially laundered cotton. Perhaps they have to stay indoors in the spring and get rid of the rug and the dog, the gas stoves, the air conditioner, the smoking spouse, and the houseplants. Every season and every new petrochemical brings a new threat. Without relief, increasingly restricted in the way they live, they spiral downward, seemingly ever more susceptible to more and more environmental agents. Their lives and their diets are often limited and joyless.

Seriously allergic and chemically sensitive people are essentially no different from everyone else—it's a difference in degree, not kind. They just have a lowered defense and tolerance to the same environment that the rest of us are slightly more successful in dealing with. Their suffering is a clear warning to the rest of us about the incredible invisible dangers of our surroundings.

There's not much we can do to avoid contact with most environmental pollutants, though it does help to be aware of what they are and how to avoid excessive exposure, and to be forewarned about possible sensitivities. Some environmental hazards can be avoided to a significant degree: other people's cigarette smoke, on-the-job chemical pollutants, certain allergy-related medications, chlorinated tap water, certain household cleaning products, and others.

With vigilance, it is possible to avoid many of the most troublesome chemical additives and contaminants in food. There is a considerable level of pesticides and herbicides in all produce and some traceable level of antibiotics and hormones in many commercial animal proteins. Nevertheless, the danger of food chemicals can be greatly minimized by consuming our foods before they have been canned, packaged, dried, smoked, heated, or otherwise abused. With care we can also sidestep the processed and refined foods that are chock full of artificial flavorings, colorings, antifungal drugs, antioxidants, anticaking and antifoaming agents, extenders, blenders, bleachers, antibacterial agents, flavor enhancers, and preservatives. Such common additives as MSG (monosodium glutamate), tartrazine (FD&C Yellow No. 5), sodium benzoate, BHT, and metabisulfites (sulfites) are among the most widely used. All are known to cause a wide variety of allergic reactions for hundreds of thousands of Americans, and all can be generally avoided if you are cautious. Reading labels and voting with your consumer dollars may be the very best ways of forcing the manufacturers and restaurateurs to take seriously our need for more chemically free foods.

At Optimum Health Labs we do not attempt to treat airborne allergies and chemical sensitivities *directly,* for a number of reasons. First, we do not test for chemicals as we do for foods, because we are not convinced that a reliable test exists, and there are thousands of chemicals that would have to be identified. Second, if those multiple chemical sensitivities could be accurately diagnosed, most of them are not avoidable without major—sometimes unacceptable or impossible—life-style changes. Instead, the Optimum Health Program treats airborne allergies and chemical hypersensitivities *indirectly* and quite effectively. Because the diet gets rid of food allergies and because the total program results in improved nutrition, a stimulated immune system, and an optimally functioning digestive system, general health improves, and the body becomes much less sensitive to the environment. Airborne allergies and chemical sensitivities abate considerably in most cases.

The Stress Factor

The last major factor in our susceptibility to allergies appears to be excessive stress—not only dietary stress, but what Hans Selye called the stress of life itself. "The stress of life." It's such a simple phrase, but it says so much. It often seems that the day-to-day struggles of contemporary life are piling up—accumulating—as fast as the chemicals in our environment and the fat on our bodies.

The level and quality of stress in our lives can make a big difference in our health. Our body needs to be well-nourished, fit, and strong—mentally as well as physically—to be able to handle the demands we put on it. Stress in excess, stress gone wrong, is *distress,* and it is destructive. Unfortunately, distress appears to be increasingly the consequence when all the accumulated responsibilities, indulgences, traumas, and chemical toxins in our lives pile up. Even those people who seem to thrive on stress and pressure are chipping away at a finite amount of resistance, unless they are actively working to counteract those pressures through diet, exercise, supplementation, rest, relaxation, supportive and loving companionship, etc.

Each year 230 million prescriptions for tranquilizers are written. There are 20 million problem drinkers in this country, with a total of 82 percent of adults admitting to frequent alcohol consumption. Polls show that almost half the population expresses a need to learn how to relax. This is the consequence of too much stress—stress pushed beyond the point where a Valium, an aspirin, or an Alka-Seltzer will take care of the problem.

Most people are doing their best to cope with the stress of life, and many are aware that there is a threshold beyond which lies illness and serious mental disturbance. Often the very awareness of the possible consequences of their stressful lives is itself an added worry, and rightly so. Distress, disease—it is a continuum. These days it is often that extra unexpected or unavoidable trauma that pushes us over the edge, into illness. A patient comes into OHL and says: "I ran a marathon a year ago, and I wasn't in condition for it. I've been symptomatic with allergies ever since." Or "I was perfectly healthy until I had my baby" or "I didn't have all these symptoms until my divorce." Then suddenly each crossed over his or her own *individual* stress threshold, and their symptoms, which until then had been evidenced only on a mild, tolerable not-to-worry level, suddenly bloomed into disabling illness.

There is not an organ in the human body you cannot overstress, whether it's your heart, your brain, your muscles and joints, your liver, or your immune system. If you go beyond that limit, there will be a malfunction, inhibition, or breakdown. Many of the stresses of our lives are unavoidable. But how we are able to cope with those stresses can be improved immeasurably by beneficial changes in our life-styles and diets. And chief among these is to address the roots of certain major stresses—the allergies, bad diet, and general poor health habits that undermine the digestive and immune systems that are our health centers.

5

The Allergy/Addiction Syndrome and the Dilemma of Diagnosis

Diagnosing allergy can be devilishly tricky, not only because the symptoms show up in so many shapes and forms or because so many foods and chemicals may be the provocateurs. There are two other factors, both basic to the understanding of how food allergy works, that compound and confuse the problem of diagnosis. One is the fact that food allergies are often *delayed* reactions and thus hard to connect to the food that originally provoked the symptoms. The second, and more insidious, factor is that food allergies often become addictions, the signs of which are "masked" to make them bearable. Let's look at these two problems.

THE DELAYED RESPONSE: EAT NOW, SUFFER LATER

One of the common misconceptions about allergy, and one which has left the diagnosis of allergy in the Dark Ages for far too long, is the orthodoxy that it is easy to identify the allergic substance, since it provokes an obvious reaction. However, this applies only to the Type I, or IgE-mediated, immediate allergic reactions: angioedema (pronounced swellings of the skin, face, or mucous membranes), hives, asthma, hay fever. You can't do much about them, so the traditional allergists tell us, except try to alleviate the patient's suffering with hyposensitization shots and/or medication. But at least you know what you're dealing with.

The majority of the allergens that bring about allergic response, however—and that includes almost all food allergens—do not reveal themselves with obvious or immediately distressing symptoms. The immunology is quite different: different antibodies, produced by different tissues of the body, working in different ways. (The antibodies involved in food allergy, which have names like IgG, IgM, and secretory IgA, will be explained in Chapter 6, in a full discussion of the mechanics of allergy and the part played by the digestive and immune systems.)

The crucial point is that our reaction to the majority of allergens doesn't usually show up right away. Because cause and effect are often separated by a few meals, the food that provoked the reaction often proves difficult to identify. The splitting headache, the achy joints, the crying jag, or the irritability may occur hours, or even a couple of days, after eating the allergic food.

There are still other tricky differences between IgE- and non-IgE-mediated reactions. Most Type I allergies flare up from just a small exposure to the offending food. But the amount of food involved in delayed non-IgE-mediated reactions varies considerably and is often influenced by the amount eaten, by what is consumed *with* the food, or by the amount of stress you're under at the moment. And it doesn't help matters that people with food allergies—and that's most of us—are usually allergic to an average of five to fifteen foods, compared to only one or two for those with IgE-mediated allergies. If all this is sounding just too complicated, Table 2, on pages 56–57, will help you distinguish between what *is* and what is *not* likely to be symptomatic of food allergy.

THE PROGRESSION FROM ALLERGY TO ADDICTION

Now we come to the heart of the problem. One of the most insidious and confounding things about food allergy is that, until the damage to our health becomes obvious, the symptoms are usually hidden or "masked." In other words, we are often unaware that we have food allergies because we cover up symptoms.

How does this happen? We cover up the symptoms by frequently eating the food that we are allergic to. If we stopped eating it, we would feel withdrawal symptoms—pain, nervousness, discomfort. Similarly, many alcoholics continue drinking to keep hangover at bay.

This doesn't take place on a conscious level, of course. We are not usually keenly aware of "craving" the allergic food; we think that we choose to eat it so often because we like its taste. But consciously or not, we tend to crave foods we're allergic to because we need them to keep withdrawal symptoms at bay. When we reach this point and need a particular food in order to feel good—or, rather, in order not to feel bad—we are addicted to it.

This topsy-turvy phenomenon is called the allergy/addiction syndrome. Simply put, allergic reactions may lead to an addiction to food that is bad for us, because eating the food temporarily relieves the discomfort it caused in the first place. It follows that the foods that we are allergic to are often likely to be our favorites—the ones we eat

Table 2—An Allergy-or-Not Checklist	
Yes, this probably *is* an allergic symptom	**No, this probably is *not* an allergic symptom**
Head	
Migraine headache. Cluster headache. Sinus headache. Muscle-tension headache especially after eating the wrong food.	A headache that's worse when you awaken in the morning but rapidly improves when you sit upright. A headache associated with stiff neck and fever. A headache associated with loss of muscle control, especially in anal sphincter or bladder.
Eyes	
Blurred vision associated with eating certain foods or smelling certain odors. Visual changes associated with specific geographic locations. Visual changes preceding migraines.	Double vision when looking hard to the right or left. Protrusion of both eyes. Loss of vision in one or both eyes. Unequal size of pupils. Yellowness in the eyeballs. Pain or swelling in one eye only. Rapid deterioration of vision.
Ears	
Ringing or buzzing. Recurrent infection. Blockage. Itching. Sounds too loud or very soft. Intermittent hearing losses.	Pain in one ear only. Infection accompanied by fever, pain, and swelling below or behind the ear. Deafness, vertigo, nausea, and a tendency to fall in one direction.
Nose	
A thin, clear discharge. Excess mucus buildup. Sneezing fits. Itchy nose and palate. Nose picking.	A thick yellowish-green discharge (infection). Severe nosebleed with high blood pressure.
Mouth and Throat	
Difficulty swallowing. Chronic sore throat with no known causes. Chronic dry feeling. Cold sores. Chemical taste in the mouth. Sudden change of voice.	A painless lump in the throat. Sore throat associated with fever. Persistent cough without fever in smokers. Chronic sore on the tongue or lips. Gradual change in voice.

Table 2 *(Continued)*	
Yes, this probably *is* an allergic symptom	**No, this probably is *not* an allergic symptom**
Neck	
Stiff neck not associated with injury, fever, or trauma.	Stiff neck associated with infection or fever. Painful lymph glands down front or back of neck. Bulging neck veins, which become worse when you are lying down.
Chest	
Wheezing (both lungs). Coughing associated with exercise.	Wheezing from one lung only. Chest pain associated with fever. Chest pain or pressure associated with sweating, clammy skin, and fainting. Chest pain or pressure associated with exercise. Shortness of breath associated with nausea and/or palpitations. Labored breath that is worse when you are lying flat and is associated with swollen ankles or belly.
Abdomen	
Diarrhea alternating with constipation. Chronic or temporary diarrhea not associated with infection. Bloating after meals. Excess gas. Indigestion.	Blood in stool. Pain that starts below the breastbone and radiates to the back. Severe pain with or without fever. Pain that starts below the breastbone and radiates to the right of the rib cage. Pain that starts at or above the navel and descends to the right lower quadrant of the belly.
Muscles and Joints	
Pain, stiffness, and swelling of joints. Muscle aches and/or pain; "growing pain."	Sharp muscle pain. Arthritic symptoms of gouty arthritis, psoriasis, lupus erythematosus, infections, etc.

frequently because they make us feel good. Addiction to food is biochemically and physiologically identical to the relationship between an alcoholic and liquor or a junkie and drugs. It causes the same cravings and drives, and has the same potential for withdrawal symptoms.

This requires a bit of explanation. Comparing food cravings to drug addiction may sound like nonsense to you. But let's look at different examples. Do you ever wake up at night and raid the refrigerator? Do you just *have* to have ice cream every day? Or a steak? Do you always eat the same thing for lunch? Do you just *love* pasta? Or find yourself standing in front of the open refrigerator without realizing how you got there? Do you have trouble falling asleep without a bedtime snack? Do you ever feel better after eating a particular food? If you can answer any of these questions in the affirmative, you may very well be addicted (in addition to being allergic) to certain foods.

How It Works

As illogical or farfetched (and unfair) as this may seem, there is a logical sequence of events leading from food allergy to addiction. The body is an adaptive mechanism, always coping in physiological, biochemical ways with whatever demands you or your environment place on it. The natural inclination is to keep things in balance at all costs. The body cannot function well or, in the long run, survive when things are out of whack.

It's already been noted that the body's natural reaction is to reject or throw off any substance it perceives as harmful or toxic—which is how it perceives any food or chemical that it is presented with too often and in excessive quantities. The addiction response is only one of several actions your body takes to cope with allergic foods.

As we'll see in Chapter 6, the first line of defense against an unwanted food is in the digestive tract, where the system employs several tactics in the hope of passing the food through the body before it is broken down sufficiently to allow it to enter the bloodstream. But because the digestive and immune systems of a person with food allergy are likely to be impaired, what actually may happen is that the allergic food will make its way into the bloodstream in a highly irritant form—as macromolecules of incompletely digested food.

This alerts the immune system, which dispatches antibodies to the rescue, antibodies developed specifically to fight off the unwanted foods. These antibodies attach themselves to the macromolecules of incompletely digested food; together they form immune complexes, which, if not cleared from circulation, travel throughout the body, depositing themselves in tissues, where they cause irritation and inflammation.

Here's where the addiction comes in. To cope with the resulting discomfort, the body sends out a rush of chemical mediators, including a group of narcotic-like substances called opioids, to tranquilize the body so that it can withstand the onslaught of the circulating immune complexes. For a short time after this reaction takes place, there is a real high, a physical and emotional boost. Thus the very substance that is punishing your system seems to be giving you pleasure. Later, when the danger has passed, the system returns to normal (though with some cell damage done and eventually vague symptoms that we don't necessarily connect to eating the allergic food). But perhaps we're left feeling a bit depleted or down.

Consuming the toxic food is now provoking a high that makes you feel good. You crave the lift it seems to give you, so you have some more of it or perhaps another allergic food that produces the same results.

But the good feelings are only temporary. Although the allergic food causes the brain to release the opioids that stimulate you and raise your spirits, it doesn't increase the brain's ability to produce a greater supply of these chemicals. In fact, as the assault of the allergic food is repeated over and over, it depletes this ability. In addition, the stress hormones from the nervous system and adrenals, which at first produced a surge of energy to make you feel better during an allergic attack, at higher levels can cause weakness, fatigue, shakiness, nervousness, and anxiety.

As this process repeats itself over time, the depleted feeling that follows the pleasurable feeling gets stronger, and without noticing the change, you're unconsciously eating the allergic food *in order to avoid the symptoms that would show up if you didn't eat it.* As depletion increases, you eat those favorite foods ever more frequently and perhaps in larger amounts. You're *bingeing* on these foods; *you are addicted to them.* The body has become so accustomed to functioning *with* the addictive food that it suffers *without* it. The need to eat frequently, the craving for a particular food, and the very fact that it provides a lift or amelioration of withdrawal symptoms are signs of addiction to that food.

A Dangerous Maladaptation

Cigarette smoking provides a vivid illustration of how allergy/addiction works. No one ever enjoys that first cigarette—most people remember feeling nauseated and dizzy. But cigarette smoke (like coffee and alcohol and certain foods) is a particularly powerful allergen and poison, and the body must go into high gear to fight it. After the first few cigarettes, the smoker becomes aware of the pleasant high of smoking—which is most likely the effect of the increased stress hormones and opiates the body needs in order to tolerate the powerful irritant tobacco. But after a brief "honeymoon" stage, the body has learned to cope; it is ready for the nicotine/sulfur oxide/carbon monoxide assault, and its reaction is barely perceptible. Now the smoker is aware only of the relief and relaxation of smoking—and the low he feels if he has to wait too long for a cigarette. Now he craves a cigarette more and more frequently and feels depleted until he satisfies that craving.

On the surface, this technique the body uses to cover up its suffering seems quite a clever adaptation. But it is dangerous and almost always disastrous. Because of this *masking* phenomenon, we're kept in the dark about what's really going on. The body may perpetuate an addiction for months or years while the damage accumulates silently and slowly, until the constant sinus headache turns into migraine, until the mild aches and pains become full-blown arthritis, or the psychological malaise accelerates into a serious mental disorder.

You can see how easy it is to be fooled by allergies. It's not until we stop eating the allergic foods and go through withdrawal and then relief of symptoms that we see how addicted we've become and how much harm we've been doing to our health.

The majority of people who give up foods they are allergic to go through a mild to moderate withdrawal phase, lasting one to five days, while the body detoxifies itself. Their usual allergic symptoms—runny nose, migraine, arthritic aches and pains, fatigue—may get worse. And they may suffer the usual symptoms of narcotic withdrawal—cravings, irritability, jitteriness, depression, and general malaise. Since the usual remedy for this discomfort—eating more of the offending food or drink—is not desirable, there are powerful nutritional tactics to soften these physiological withdrawal symptoms. (They are outlined in Chapter 16, page 261.) Of course, once the withdrawal phase has passed, the cravings also abate, and the allergy sufferer is free of dependence on that food, free of the both physiological and psychological desire to consume it so frequently and in such great quantities.

ADDICTION AND THE DIETER'S DILEMMA

It should now be clear why restrictive calorie-counting diets don't work and why they can be dangerous for some people. *Hidden or delayed food allergies (and their associated malnutrition) may be the single most common factor in binge eating, overeating, depressed metabolic rate, and obesity.* It is the addiction itself that *causes* the overeating—the abnormal cravings and binges are the result of trying to keep symptoms from getting out of control and causing discomfort. Once the allergen is removed from the diet, when the craving (and thus the overeating) disappears, the digestion and immune systems have a chance to recuperate from prolonged abuse; uncontrollable hunger abates, the metabolic rate increases, and weight loss usually follows.

Overweight people are often accused of lacking willpower and discipline. But look at what is actually happening on the usual calorie-restrictive diet. The dieter is often asked to perform the Herculean feat of having every day just a little bit of the foods to which he is physiologically and psychologically addicted—the equivalent of insisting that the alcoholic take one small drink every day. *No wonder only one out of 200 dieters loses unwanted weight and keeps it off.*

Another danger of most diets (aside from the poor nourishment inherent in consuming only 500 to 1,200 calories a day) is that in eating the same foods over and over, many people are either perpetuating existing allergies or are developing new ones. Most diets ignore the crucial factor of food allergy and the need for an *individualized* nutritional program. Even a basically sound diet like that of the late Nathan Pritikin, which does take up important questions of good nutrition and exercise, fails to address the problem of food sensitivity. Eventually this causes significant health problems for some people on this otherwise effective program.

The only lasting answer to weight problems—and not so incidentally to general health problems—is to break those food addictions and thus restore the efficient functioning of the digestive tract and immune systems, normalize the body's metabolism, and bring calorie intake back into line with the body's needs. Weight loss is an almost inevitable bonus of the Optimum Health Program.

THE DIFFICULTIES OF TESTING FOR ALLERGIES

Figuring out what you're allergic to takes some serious snooping around. Procedures for food-allergy testing have long been an issue of controversy and confusion in the medical community. The tests traditionally used to diagnose IgE-mediated allergies (usually costly, painful skin tests) are reliable for diagnosing airborne allergies but don't work at all for most food allergies—though some doctors insist on using them for that purpose.

It is only in the last decade or so that attention has been focused on accurate ways of determining non-IgE-mediated sensitivities. Until recently, the best non-IgE test was the cytotoxic food-allergy test. The cytotoxic test employs blood samples from the patient in a kind of litmus test. It measures the degree of damage done to white blood cells when they are put in contact with extracts of each potentially allergic food. Since a highly allergic food can damage and even destroy blood cells, the test thus shows which foods the patient should avoid in the future.

The cytotoxic test, if done properly, appears to be more reliable for diagnosing food allergies than the skin test or the IgE RAST test, but it suffers from many potential shortcomings, especially the problems of false positive readings and poor reproducibility. Too, it is very delicate and time-consuming, since strictly controlled lab procedures are an absolute must; few labs are up to the task, thus nearly all cytotoxic labs are unlicensed and poorly supervised. Yet another problem with the cytotoxic test is that it must be performed within three hours of taking the blood sample. This means that only those people with access to a lab could take advantage of the test.

But now OHL's licensed clinical laboratory has introduced the Food Immune Complex Assay, or FICA,* which measures the actual presence in your blood of food-specific antibodies and food-allergen-containing circulating immune complexes for each of the foods tested. So far, this fully automated test is available only at Immuno Nutritional Clinical Laboratory in Van Nuys, California. It was developed by professors of immunology and a pediatric allergist at the University of Kansas Medical School. It is much more reproducible, more sensitive, and more accurate than the cytotoxic test, and safer and quicker than elimination/challenge tests. Another major advantage is that it is capable of measuring both immediate (Type I) and delayed (Types II and III) allergic reactions to over a hundred different foods. Finally, it can be performed with blood samples sent through the mail from a physician or blood lab anywhere in the world.

*Registered trademark.

6

Digestion and the Immune System

The immune system is the body's primary defense against disease, and an immune system that is malnourished and/or exhausted from continual efforts to ward off repeated assaults from allergic foods is a weakened defense. Since the front line of the immune system's defenses against unwanted dietary allergens or toxins is in the digestive tract, the digestive system and the immune system are intertwined and interdependent in their tasks as the body's defenders.

An understanding of how this process works makes the logic of the Optimum Health Program crystal clear. The purpose of this chapter is to examine the workings of the digestive tract and immune systems and to illustrate the double-whammy way in which allergy sabotages our health. For allergies are associated with maldigestion and malabsorption and can further undermine the immune system, while impaired digestion and an overwhelmed immune system in turn lead to allergies.

TRACKING THE GASTROINTESTINAL TRACT

The gastrointestinal tract (see Figure 3, page 64) is a tube 25 to 32 feet long (everyone is different) that begins with the mouth, followed by the oral pharynx at the back of the mouth, and the esophagus, which is the food tube leading from the back of the throat down into the stomach, a pouch located in the upper abdominal cavity.

Digestion continues from the stomach into the small intestine, the longest section of the gastrointestinal tract, 10 to 15 feet in length. The small intestine is composed of three segments—the duodenum, the jejunum, and the ileum.

From the ileum, food and other materials proceed through the ileocecal valve into the first part of the large intestine called the cecum (where the appendix is attached).

The final segment of the gastrointestinal tract is represented by the large intestine: the ascending colon, the transverse colon, the descending colon, into the rectum and out the anus.

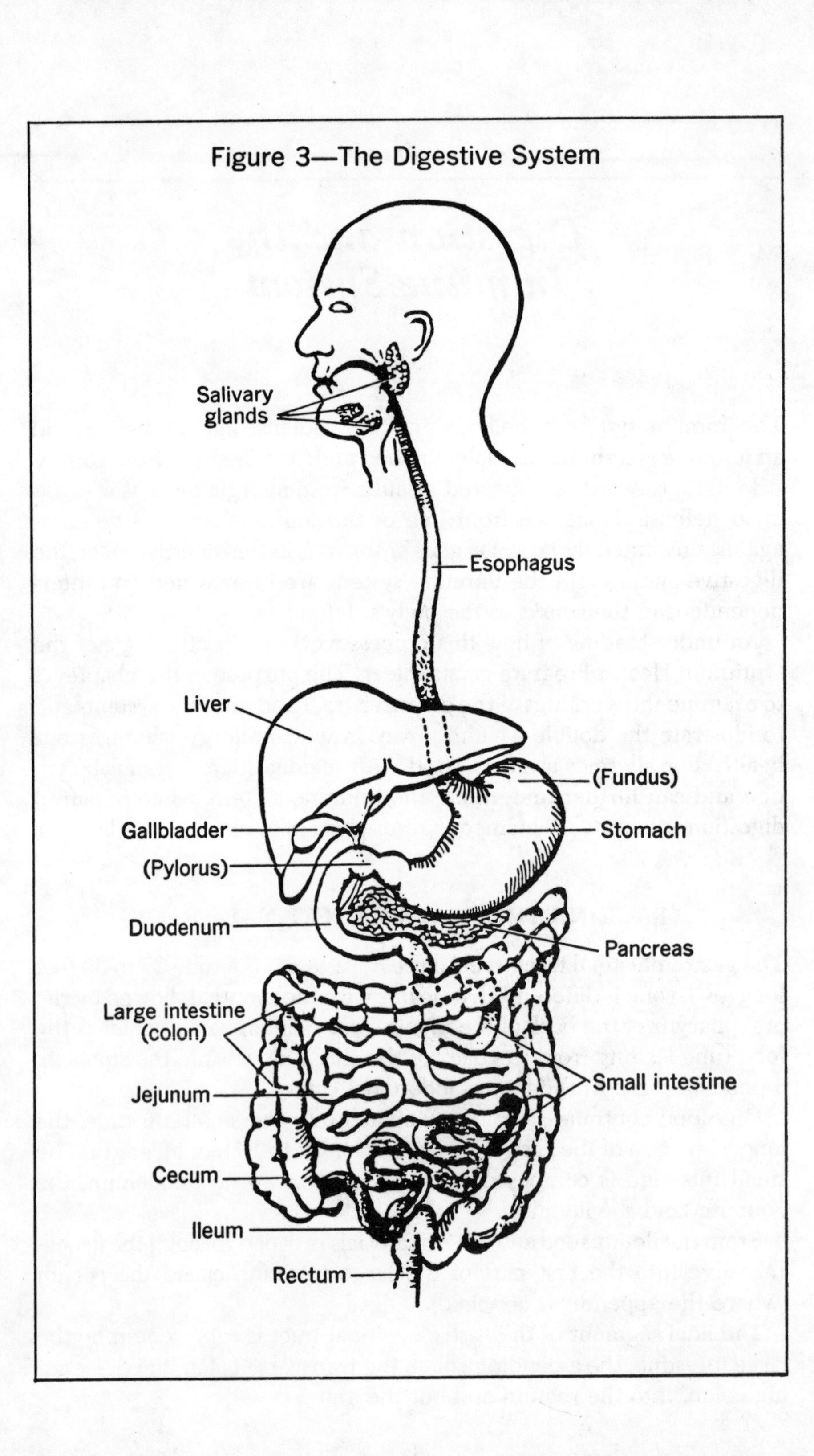

Figure 3—The Digestive System

What Happens En Route?

The primary part of the digestive process involves the mouth, the stomach, and the small intestine.

The process of digestion is prepared for even before you put food into your mouth. The brain, registering hunger or anticipating food, does two things: It provokes the first secretions of pepsin (a protein-digesting enzyme) and hydrochloric acid into the stomach, and it makes your mouth water (salivate). But when you eat in a rush or when you're not hungry or when stressed, this anticipatory phase is neglected, and this neglect can be a first step in poor digestion.

The immune response and digestive process proper begin when you put food into your mouth. Chewing the food increases its surface area, so that it mixes better with saliva, which contains the enzymes that start the digestion of *carbohydrates.* (Saliva also contains antibodies that attach to bacteria, toxins, and presumably allergens.) You swallow, and the food-saliva mix passes through the esophagus into the stomach.

The next event is the digestion of *protein* by means of secreted hydrochloric acid and pepsin. A diet deficient in protein will not provoke sufficient gastric (stomach) secretions for proper digestion, and this in turn will cause insufficient release of pancreatic enzymes.

Anywhere from fifteen to forty-five minutes later, this mixture of digestive enzymes, acid, and food—called chyme—leaves the stomach through the pyloric valve and enters the first section of the small intestine, called the duodenum. At that point, two additional organs are stimulated:

The gallbladder releases bile juices that help break down, or hold in suspension, the *fat* content of the food. This fat suspension can then be digested down to fatty acids by pancreatic fat enzymes.

The pancreas—perhaps the most crucial target organ in the expression of food allergy—functions in a number of ways:

1. Stimulated by digestive hormones and the acid pH of the chyme arriving from the stomach, it releases digestive juices into the first part of the duodenum. The pancreas produces up to 2½ quarts of digestive juice daily, which contains three specific types of enzymes for digesting protein, fats, and carbohydrates.
2. At the same time, the pancreas sends out bicarbonates. Pancreatic enzymes cannot function in an acid medium; since the food coming from the stomach is saturated with

> hydrochloric acid, bicarbonates are needed to neutralize it. Without this acid neutralization, no further digestion can take place in the small intestine.

In this now alkaline environment, the food is broken down more completely, until it reaches a state in which it can be absorbed by the tissues. These digested (rendered absorbable) food molecules then pass through the lining of the small intestine and into the circulation, which transports them to various sites in the body.

Each nutrient is absorbed along a *specific* stretch of the intestinal wall. This may be one reason that an individual may absorb some nutrients but not others. If certain areas of the intestinal wall are inflamed or irritated, the nutrients normally absorbed there will pass into the large intestine and be eliminated.

Hazards Along the Route

This is a simplified explanation of how the digestive process is supposed to function. But many things can go wrong with this intricate and continuous process. And if at any point along the route some function falters, we will not be able to absorb all the nutrients that we eat.

Then we are in serious trouble, for the inevitable consequence of chronic digestive problems is malnutrition and undermining of the immune system, both from lack of proper nourishment and the continual bombardment of the bloodstream with macromolecules of incompletely digested foods.

In addition, much of the food eaten will pass—undigested—into the large intestine or colon, where it can upset the delicate balance of bacteria and other microorganisms. This can result in endotoxin production and absorption, inflammation, and common bowel disorders such as constipation, diarrhea, diverticulitis, or colitis. *The negative impact of food allergy begins with its effect on the digestive process.*

THE IMMUNE SYSTEM: THE GREAT DEFENDER

How does the body determine whether or not a particular food should be digested? The immune system appears to make these decisions.

The immune system is the body's internal defense against all disease processes—unwelcome invaders that may cause infection, cancer, communicable disease, heart disease, accelerated aging, delayed healing of wounds and injury, allergies, autoimmune disease, and abnormal blood clotting. It is through the immune system that substances foreign to the body or potentially harmful are recognized. It responds in similar protective ways whether this foreign substance is a bacteria, a virus, a parasite, a toxin, drugs, pollen, dust, mold, dander—or an incompletely digested macromolecule of food.

The immune system is our sentinel or barrier against the world. Its importance was poignantly and eloquently illustrated by "David," the boy forced to live out his twelve years isolated in a plastic bubble, deprived of human touch, because he was born without a functioning immune system. It was hoped that bone-marrow transplant surgery would establish a competent immune system, and this necessitated his removal from the bubble. Once outside—even under the most carefully sterilized conditions and the aggressive use of antibiotics—he quickly fell prey to the germs and ordinary environmental hazards that most human bodies repel easily. David was unable to fight off the army of invaders entering his system, and he died.

The rest of us are blessed with a barrier between us and a world of hostile substances outside our bodies. Our skin and the mucosal linings of our air passages, genitourinary tract, and digestive tract—in short, all the parts of us that come in contact with the outside world—are guarded by the immune system. It is designed not only to fight off disease but also to handle stress. As long as it remains capable of screening out dangerous invaders, our inner self stands a good chance of remaining healthy and whole.

How It Works

The immune system includes a master gland—the thymus—plus the spleen, tonsils, adenoids, appendix, specialized lymphoid tissues, bone marrow, lymph nodes, white blood cells, mast cells, and an arsenal of antibodies, complement proteins, and dozens of chemical mediators.

It is through the bloodstream and lymphatic system that this arsenal works to incapacitate whatever the system decides is toxic. One type of white blood cell, the T-lymphocyte, produces interferon, which renders certain viruses unable to reproduce. Certain of these T-cells also stimulate and regulate other immune cells (called B-lymphocytes) to produce antibodies against other unwanted substances. Yet other white blood cells called phagocytes (macrophages and neutrophils) have the ability to locate and destroy bacteria. Every potential invader is guarded against by some part of the immune system.

The Vulnerable Thymus

The immune system is dependent on its overseer, the thymus, to do its job. But although the thymus maintains its size and activity until adolescence, thereafter it decreases. Until recently, the atrophied, relatively inactive thymus found in most "average" American adults was thought to be normal. However, it is now acknowledged that the thymus remains crucial in the maintenance of a healthy immune system and that its shrinking may be the result of improper diet—a diet missing certain vitamins and minerals (Vitamins A, B6, and C, and the minerals zinc, iron, and selenium), essential amino acids, and especially *essential fatty acids.* When these essential nutrients are restored to the diet, the thymus quickly regains its youthful size and function, and as a consequence the rest of the immune system is reactivated.

Recent evidence suggests that the thymus may play a major role in AIDS (Acquired Immune Deficiency Syndrome), a condition associated with rare infections and a rare cancer with a 90 percent mortality rate called Kaposi's sarcoma. Upon autopsy, the thymus glands of AIDS victims have been found to be severely altered in appearance and structure.

The Adrenals and the Stress Factor

Before we go on to a discussion of the mechanics of food-allergy response, another organ system—the adrenals—should be mentioned, because it is also tied in to the proper orchestration and functioning of the immune system. The adrenal glands are very small—perched atop the kidneys, they weigh just ⅛ ounce apiece—but are essential to life. The adrenals produce, among other hormones, adrenaline, noradrenaline, and cortisol, important stress hormones that seem to stabilize and regulate the immune system. A striking experiment was done in which the adrenal glands of dogs were surgically removed. Predictably, all the animals died, but before that, every one of them developed a wide variety of "human" allergies: asthma, hay fever, eczema, arthritislike pain and stiffness in the joints. (It is worth noting that veterinarians are reporting higher incidence of allergies in pets as people feed them more and more of their "human" diet.)

Dr. Hans Selye has mentioned how the physiological response of the body to demands placed on it often results in the overstimulation, swelling, and eventual exhaustion of the adrenal glands. (One study showed that in solving a simple list of mathematical problems, Type A personalities—impatient, tense, ambitious people—have forty times as much cortisol and three times as much adrenaline circulating in the blood as more relaxed, laid-back Type B people solving the same problems.) Allergy sufferers—that is to say, most people—seem to have a significantly lowered threshold to stress, in part *because of* the physiological and psychological overstimulation of their adrenals.

HOW FOOD-ALLERGY REACTION WORKS

To understand the dynamics of food-allergy reactions, we can start by looking at how airborne allergies work.

It is known that when an unwanted substance enters the body's tissues for the first time—be it a virus, bacteria, toxin, drug, pollen, or an incompletely digested food the body has decided doesn't belong there—the body will begin the process of manufacturing antibodies specific to that substance, to use against it *the next time it shows up.* Meanwhile the body begins to repair itself, using the immune system's numerous other defenses.

The active antibody in airborne allergies (and a small number of food allergies) is IgE. Once these specific IgE antibodies have been produced, they attach themselves to a very basic cell of the immune system known as the mast cell. Tens of millions of these mast cells line the air passages, skin, digestive tract, and small blood vessels throughout the body. Each mast cell is coated by hundreds of thousands of IgE antibodies, specifically formed to counter the effects of certain allergens, such as pollen, animal dander, toxins, dust, or an allergic food. When that allergen enters the system and encounters the antibody-coated mast cells, the contact causes the cells to release substances to ward off the unwanted allergen. These substances, called chemical mediators (histamines are the best-known mediators, but there are many other more potent ones), trigger a multitude of allergic symptoms: watering eyes, rash, running nose, itching, etc.

Food Allergy Is Much Different

What hasn't been recognized until recently is the existence of a different type of mast cell in the connective tissue lining *the intestinal tract.* Whereas IgE-mediated allergy more often initiates reaction in air passages, on the skin, and in the bloodstream beyond the intestinal barrier, food allergy starts to work *in the digestive tract itself.*

So you don't get deathly ill each time you consume the offending food, a type of free-floating antibody called secretory IgA is released into the digestive tract, apparently by way of the gallbladder. From there it trickles down through the bile ducts into the upper duodenum, where it coats all of the offending food particles entering the small intestine from the stomach. When the IgA antibody and allergic food combine within the intestinal lumen, it stimulates the secretion of a thick protective coating of mucus from the mucosal lining. The function of secretory IgA antibodies therefore appears to be protective—keeping these allergic or too frequently eaten foods from coming in contact with this lining of the small intestine and presumably with the troublesome intestinal mast cells. But although secretory IgA does block release of chemical mediators, it also prevents the food from being digested.

So far, so good. No real harm has been done, although those nutrients are not getting into our bloodstream. However, if we continue to eat these allergic foods, that overtaxes the immune system. Its ability to produce all those IgA antibodies (and perhaps other antibodies like IgG and IgM) breaks down, and once that secretory IgA protection is lost, foods that the immune system has recognized as toxic will come in contact with those hostile mast cells.

The Heart of the Problem

When the allergic food binds chemically with the mast-cell antibodies specific to it, you get the sudden release of powerful (and often painful) chemical mediators from the mast cells: histamine, bradykinin, inflammatory prostaglandins, leukotrienes, heparin, serotonin, and many more.

What happens? One very damaging long-range consequence is that these inflammatory prostaglandins cause the stomach to secrete less hydrochloric acid. Thus proteins aren't completely digested, and food entering the system is not properly sterilized. Moreover, insufficient hydrochloric acid sets up a chain reaction. When the food from the stomach passes into the small intestine, it is in an *underacid* state. This, paradoxically, causes the pancreas to underproduce the bicarbonates necessary to alkalinize the food for complete digestion. It also fools the pancreas into cutting down on the production and release of digestive enzymes, its other important function. Thus, the small intestine remains relatively *overacidic* and unable to complete proper digestion.

The most damaging long-term effect of releasing these chemical mediators is that, in addition to inhibiting the complete digestion of food, the mediators can weaken the impermeability of the vital ⅛-inch-thick mucosal membrane barrier that lines the intestinal wall. And this membrane is all that stands between the intestinal tract and the bloodstream. In other words, the release of chemical mediators greatly compromises the barrier that normally prevents the incompletely digested food from passing through and into the bloodstream.

Poisons in the Bloodstream

If such incompletely digested particles do reach the bloodstream, the bloodstream's response is to "clear" them from the system.

An antibody called IgG, also produced by the immune cells, quickly attaches itself to *all* oversized macromolecular food particles entering the bloodstream. This is not in the traditional sense an allergic reaction; it seems to be a way of "tagging" the unwanted macromolecules, so that other formed elements of the bloodstream, liver, and spleen (certain specialized white blood cells and perhaps even red blood cells and platelets) can easily identify them as potentially harmful invaders. The white blood cells (whose function is to combat such enemy invaders) can then devour and digest these "marked" macromolecules intracellularly and "clear" them from circulation.

However, the immune system, especially when undernourished, can take only so much. When large quantities of macromolecules, bound to IgG, regularly enter blood circulation, their abrasive bulk and sheer quantity may overwhelm the clearing mechanism. It becomes impossible to purge them from the system. Traveling around through the body, these circulating immune complexes (CICs) eventually penetrate the walls of capillaries and are deposited in tissue. All body tissues are susceptible. Wherever they are deposited, CICs cause inflammation and interfere with optimal function.

They do this by attracting an immune protein substance called complement, which in turn promotes the release of chemical mediators and free radicals (oxidized reactive atoms, highly destructive to tissue), leading to irritation and inflammation of tissue, the aggregation of platelets, pain, swelling, and damage and destruction of cells. Thus habitually poor diet can lead to such apparently unconnected disorders as arthritis, hyperactivity, insomnia, hypoglycemia, migraine, gallbladder problems, and innumerable others.

With concomitant nutritional imbalance—especially essential-fatty-acid disturbances, digestive suppression, and the resulting metabolic acidosis/protease deficiency—the allergic inflammatory response to CICs becomes ever more intense and chronic.

On the Optimum Health Program, this destructive pattern is reversed. The patient no longer eats the foods that activate hostile mast cells, allergic foods do not penetrate the intestinal wall, and there is no CIC formation. Thus no new deposits are made in tissue. Meanwhile, the immune system, strengthened by better eating habits, is no longer overwhelmed and is able to clear the remaining toxins from the patient's system.

Immune-Complex-Generated Diseases: A Provocative New Theory

It is worth noting here that a great deal of recent research seems to be converging on the idea that the immune-complex mechanism may explain much not only about allergy, but about allergy's connection to the basic nature of disease.

Once these immune complexes (macromolecules) are deposited in the surrounding tissues, they cause irritation, activating the sensitized tissue mast cells, which trigger a dramatic outflow of potent chemical mediators. It is these chemical mediators that are then responsible for delayed inflammatory or allergic symptoms and ultimate damage to surrounding organs and tissue. And this immune-complex-mediated damage can take any of a number of forms: pain, swelling, tenderness, increased sensitivity to pain; itching, redness, and cell proliferation (eczema); destruction of collagen connective tissue and bone demineralization (rheumatoid arthritis); vessel wall constriction (elevated blood pressure); excess mucus (allergic rhinitis), bronchospasm (asthma), fever, scarring; decreased hydrochloric acid production and decreased pancreatic secretions (digestive disorders); pancreatic dysfunction in regulating blood sugar (diabetes); smooth muscle replication (atherosclerosis); and more. All these, thus, may be conditions generated by activated immune complexes—allergens.

IT ALL STARTS WITH MALNUTRITION

There is a vicious cycle at work here, in which improper diet (including the eating of undetected allergic foods, overconsumption of alcohol, excess consumption of saturated and overly processed oils, and the improper metabolism or underconsumption of essential fats in the diet) causes profound digestive problems—the underproduction of secretory IgA, the easily destabilized gastrointestinal mast cell, the underproduction of hydrochloric acid, the malfunctioning pancreas, and the weakening of the mucosal barrier. And this in turn leads to poor absorption of nutrients, to massive penetration of undigested macromolecules into the bloodstream, and to an assault on the entire body of released chemical mediators. Eventually the immune and digestive systems wear down from trying to clear the toxic invaders and become still less able to process our food fully and extract its nutrients.

As long as allergic foods remain in the diet, the damage is progressive. The system starts reacting to more and more foods, including previously nonallergic foods that enter the system in conjunction with already allergic foods, foods eaten with coffee or alcohol, refined and processed foods that require little digestion to pass through the gut and into the bloodstream. Soon, very little of nutrient value—and a great deal that is toxic and allergenic—is absorbed. Eventually, weakened by such chronic stress and malnutrition, the immune system is overpowered by disease.

GETTING WELL AGAIN

In order to get well and maintain good health, it is necessary to digest properly and completely. Yet many ostensibly healthy people evidence digestive disturbances of one kind or another: hypochlorhydria, diarrhea, gastric pain, indigestion, heartburn, gas, nausea, constipation, undigested food in the stools, sudden weight fluctuations, symptoms of hypoglycemia, coated tongue, flatulence, halitosis, belching, fatigue or bloating after meals. Many people accept these conditions as normal, probably because everyone they know seems to suffer similar symptomology. But truly healthy digestion takes place *with an absence of symptoms.* Persistent symptoms indicate that something is wrong, and that something is often related to food allergy.

It was Dr. Aubrey Katz, a gastroenterologist at Harvard, who said that a good set of bowels is more important than a good set of brains. From what we've learned about the steamroller effects of poor digestion, this is certainly true. If we digest properly—assuming we are eating foods high in nutritional value—our bodies receive the proper nutrients, the system is fortified against disease, and everything—*including* the brain—functions at optimal levels.

But as long as we are eating allergic foods, we cannot absorb nutrients properly. Eighty percent or more of food-allergy sufferers have differing degrees of *hypochlorhydria,* the underproduction of acid in the stomach, which, as we have seen, leads to the pancreas' inability to secrete enough digestive enzymes and alkalinizing bicarbonates. And because, in response to the underacid stomach, the pancreas is not producing enough alkalines, we have a paradoxically hyperacid system.

Hypochlorhydria leads to poor digestion of protein, poor sterilization of food, poor activation of the pancreas and consequently poor performance of its functions—secretion of digestive enzymes and bicarbonates necessary to alkalinize the food for digestion—and poor activation of Vitamin D and absorption of B12 and most minerals. Hypochlorhydria also deactivates Vitamin C, an important natural antiallergy, antihistamine vitamin, which also stimulates the immune system.

Once we've reached this intestinal hyperacid stage—technically known as metabolic acidosis—there is trouble. The consequential buildup of acid in the small intestine has far-reaching repercussions. There will almost certainly be a breakdown in other metabolic systems throughout the body, for all the enzymes that make chemical reactions possible—for chemical A to become chemical B—are pH dependent. The body tries to maintain a pH balance that is a little on the alkaline side—a pH factor just above 7. (Everything below that is on the acid side.) Anything that throws this balance off—such as an overacid small intestine—can inhibit many of the 20,000 different enzymes in the body that are necessary for proper biochemical reactions.

The pancreas, undermined by hypochlorhydria and also under attack from inflammatory prostaglandins and other chemical mediators, perhaps weakened by essential-fatty-acid deficiencies, is also inhibited in its function as the regulator of blood sugar (glucose) in the body. Blood sugar is in large part handled by two pancreatic hormones, glucagon and insulin. It is the most important fuel of the body; a healthy pancreas will work to keep the blood sugar stable regardless of diet fluctuations and energy needs. The culprit in diabetes and hypoglycemia may very well be a pancreas that is malfunctioning as the result of food allergy and malnutrition, especially essential-fatty-acid deficiency.

Digestive treatment consists mainly of eliminating food allergens from the diet, correcting the effects of hypochlorhydria with hydrochloric acid capsules and pancreatic digestive enzyme supplements, stabilizing the gastrointestinal mast cells with Vitamin C in crystal or powder form before meals, assisting the buildup of the gastrointestinal mucosal barrier with essential fatty acids, Vitamins A, B, C, and zinc, and buffering the small intestine after meals with bicarbonates like Alka-Seltzer Gold. Digestive treatment is discussed in more detail in Chapter 16.

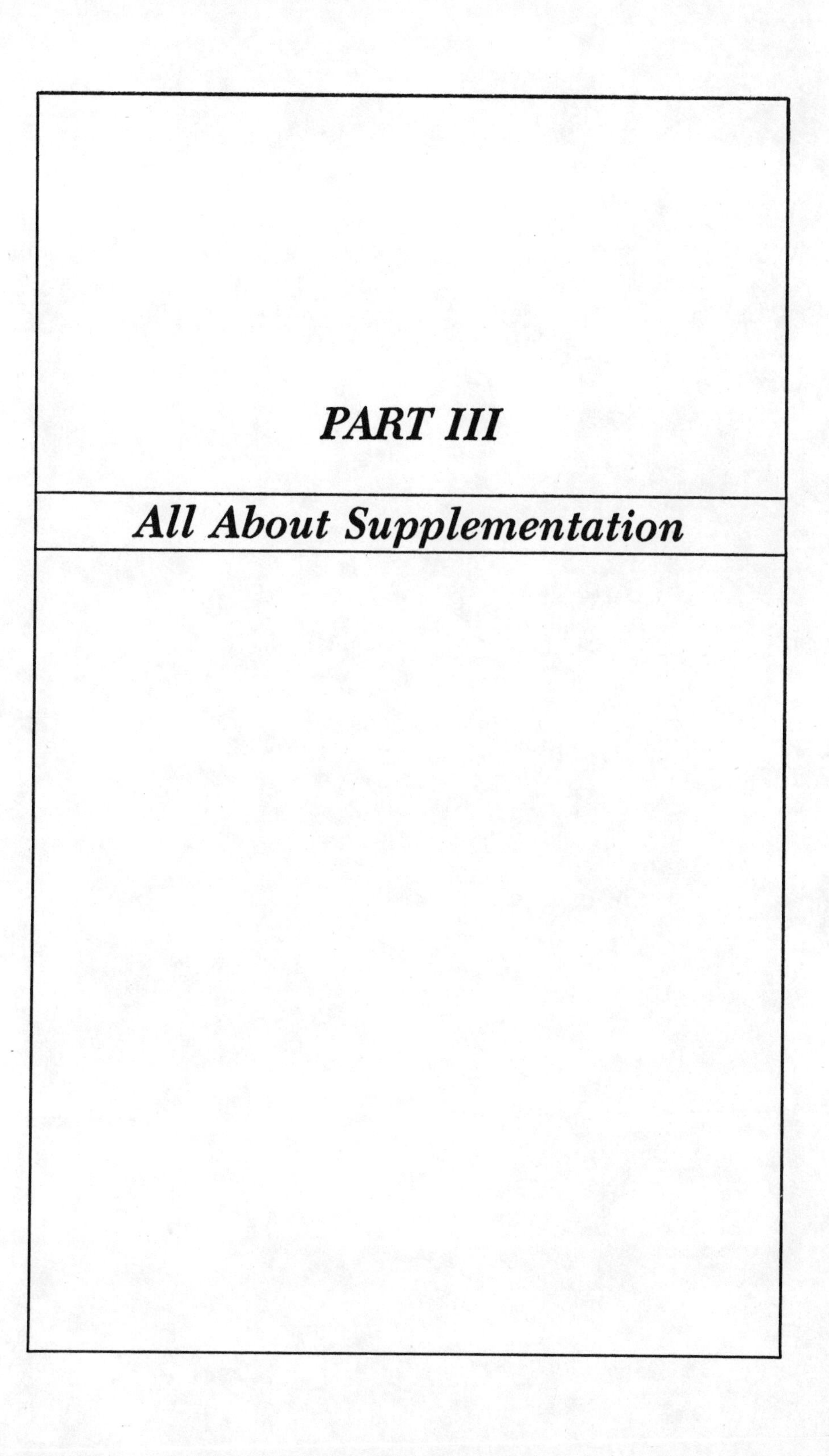

PART III

All About Supplementation

7

Supplementation: Your Nutritional Safety Net

Did you know that the recommended daily allowance of Vitamin C as currently calculated by the Food and Nutrition Board of the National Research Council is 60 mg, although *the law requires* that laboratory monkeys (our anthropoid relatives) be given 2,000 mg a day? That most "healthy" Americans with no diagnosed illnesses have at least one vitamin or mineral deficiency, and perhaps the majority are deficient in essential fatty acids? That our diets and the quality of the food we buy have declined so badly that while in 1955, 80 percent of Americans got their daily RDA of Vitamin A, in 1972, that figure had dropped to only 28 percent? That in a classic study done in 1965 by Leevy et al., involving randomly selected hospital patients, 80 percent had one or more low blood levels of vitamins, 60 percent had two, and 10 percent had five vitamin deficiencies? That individual differences are so great that one person's need for a specific nutrient may be twenty or more times that of another?

Sometimes it seems that the myth and mumbo jumbo and ignorance about good health are piled on the thickest in the area of supplementation. As recently as 1980, Dr. Victor Herbert, outspoken critic of nutritional medicine, was saying that "a normal, well-balanced American diet provides all the vitamins and minerals necessary for the average person to maintain his or her health." Chances are that this is your physician's position, unless he or she happens to be nutritionally enlightened. This attitude, in light of the overwhelming scientific evidence to the contrary, is simply outrageous, the more so because its loudest proclaimants are those people we entrust with our health.

What do traditional doctors have against vitamins and other nutrients? The kindest answer I have is that they're too caught up in their drugs and surgery to pay attention to the rapidly growing body of scientific evidence that deficiencies are rampant and that supplementation could actually *cure* some of their patients' ailments. There is also a less kind answer: Establishment medicine doesn't like nutrient supplements because you are not obligated by law to go to a doctor to get them; no prescription is required. Now that more and more people are seeking advice from those in alternative medicine and taking nutritional supplements, the medical profession and the pharmaceutical industry are lobbying hard to get the government to make these supplements available only by prescription.

Why do they do this if they don't believe in them? And why do most doctors ridicule supplementation for patients who are merely unwell but use megavitamin therapy for those same patients once they're hospitalized? Are vitamins good when you're overtly sick but not when you're healthy? Are they safe and/or effective in massive doses but not on a daily basis?

And—the $64,000 question—are vitamins really dangerous? Can you really overdose on vitamins if you're not very, very careful? Is it unsafe to take vitamins without a doctor's advice, much less a prescription? Here is the answer: *In 1983 alone more people succumbed to aspirin toxicity than have* ever *been reported to suffer vitamin toxicity.* In fact, aspirin in 1983 exceeded the all-time vitamin rate *by more than 1,000 to 1.* Perhaps it is aspirin, the most widely used over-the-counter drug in the world, that should be made available only under a doctor's prescription.

You will see in the supplement tables in the ensuing chapters that those nutrients that have been shown to have toxic effects are harmful only at *extremely* high levels. And even so, most toxic effects are not serious, and they are reversed as soon as the intake level is reduced. Nutrient *deficiencies* on the other hand are epidemic and are certainly doing far more harm than "overdoses." Supplements are not at all like heroin (or prescription drugs, for that matter), no matter what your doctor says. And they are a necessary ingredient in the recipe for optimum health.

WHY DO YOU NEED SUPPLEMENTS?

Very simply, you need nutrient supplementation because it is very unlikely that you can get the nutrition you need from your diet. When you're symptomatic or ill, I'm confident your diet alone can't handle the job. Over and over we hear that if a well-balanced diet is consumed, vitamins and other supplements are unnecessary. This is just not true, for a number of reasons.

1. It is nearly impossible to eat a diet that provides for all your nutritional needs. For one thing, most people are just too busy to be careful about what they eat and to prepare fresh, wholesome meals at all times. And it is all too human to eat the same limited number of foods over and over, which (in addition to the risk of developing food allergies and the maldigestion/malabsorption problems that go along with them) means that some nutrients are likely to be substantially missing from our diets.

Processing and refining robs our food of much of its vital fiber and nutrient content. Take the vitamin assay on a package label: That RDA percentage is often based on an analysis of that food when it is *fresh* and on the assumption that it has been carefully handled. It does not take into consideration the toll exacted by the canning or refining process or any shortcomings in growing and shipping. The actual RDAs of two different specimens of exactly the same food item can vary considerably. Two oranges, for example, can vary as much as 100 percent in their Vitamin C content, depending on

(a) time of year they were picked
(b) total sun exposure during growing season
(c) age of the orange when bought and consumed
(d) distance between orange trees in the orchard
(e) amount of rainfall and wind during growing season.

Other factors that can negatively affect the quality of that orange are the quality of the trees, the site on which they're planted, how well the trees are maintained (irrigation, fertilizers, cultivation, pesticides used, when and how the tree is harvested). Then, there are additional handling factors—transportation, storage, processing, packaging, and eventual preparation—that determine how much Vitamin C you end up getting from that orange. In the end, you may not only have lost the value of many of the vitamins, enzymes, trace minerals, and flavor factors, and much of the fiber from that orange; you may have gained chemicals and additives you hadn't bargained for, which may in turn interfere with the utilization of other nutrients in the body.

2. A poor diet is not the only reason that a person may be malnourished. Even if we manage to eat only highly nutritious foods, we may not digest or absorb those foods properly. There are literally millions who do not digest food well and who do not absorb all that they digest and who as a consequence become poorly nourished—even on a so-called well-balanced diet. The result is low blood and tissue levels of nutrients. *We are not what we eat, but what we digest, absorb, and utilize.*

3. Our high-stress lives often demand higher levels of nutrition than our diets provide. Excess stress increases the need for certain nutrients—particularly Vitamins C, A, E, the B vitamins, the minerals calcium and magnesium, and the amino acid tryptophan. Lacking optimum levels of these nutrients at times of stress, we're often thrown into a vicious cycle in which our ability to handle stress is weakened, so the impact on the tissues and organs of the body is progressively greater. This in turn causes decreased nutrient utilization, malabsorption, and/or deactivation, which further weaken an already impaired ability to handle stress effectively.

4. Illness and disease increase the nutritional demands on the body. Illness has at least three effects on the body's vitamin levels:

(a) Certain nutrients, most notably the "stress" nutrients listed above, are used in greater quantity during an illness, so the body needs an additional boost at such times.

(b) Unfortunately, many illnesses (e.g., cancer) also decrease the body's absorption of nutrients from the digestive tract and increase loss of nutrients in the urine, making it more difficult to get vitamins into the system. Conditions that irritate or inflame the digestive tract or that cause diarrhea are the most obvious examples of the former. Decreased absorption can also be brought on by thyroid dysfunction, food allergies, protein deficiencies, and more. Conditions leading to systemic hyperacidity (food allergy is one) are thought to inactivate Vitamins C and D. In other words, there is a wide range of illnesses during which, despite the fact that you may be eating a nutritious "well-balanced" diet, you are unlikely to be getting a high enough dose of the nutrients you need, to be absorbing what you do get, or to be making use of what you absorb. What complicates matters even more is that a relative deficiency of any one nutrient in the body will often impair the absorption and utilization of other nutrients.

(c) Medication prescribed by doctors to combat illnesses can often affect vitamin absorption. Drug-induced folic-acid deficiency is the most frequent form of vitamin deficiency due to pharmacological agents, but there are many others. Here are some examples of chemical- and drug-induced vitamin deficiencies:

- *Aspirin* can interfere with folic-acid utilization.
- *Anticonvulsants* prevent absorption of B12 and folic acid.
- *Birth control pills* can cause a deficiency of B6.
- *Methotrexate* can impair folic-acid use and increase loss through the urine.

- Certain *antibiotics* can interfere with the synthesis of Vitamin K and some of the B vitamins.
- *Mineral oil,* used as a laxative, can result in malabsorption of the fat-soluble vitamins A, D, E, K, and beta carotene.
- *Potassium chloride,* used to prevent potassium depletion in people taking water pills (diuretics), can cause loss of Vitamin B12.
- *Colchicine,* used to treat gouty arthritis, can result in malabsorption of Vitamin B12 and beta carotene.
- *Drugs used to lower blood cholesterol, such as cholestyramine,* can result in malabsorption and deficiencies of fat-soluble vitamins such as A, D, E, and K.
- *Hydrazide drugs, such as INH,* can cause excess loss of Vitamin B6 through the urine.
- *Alcohol, anticonvulsants, tetracycline, birth control pills, and aspirin* all can produce Vitamin C depletion in the body tissues.
- *Chlorine* in drinking water deactivates Vitamin C.

5. Environmental hazards place additional nutritional needs on our bodies. These include everything from inclement temperatures, sunshine, fluorescent lighting, noise, pollen, dust, and mold, to the chemicals of commercial and industrial pollution. Environmental pollution is a factor in every part of the country, not just certain urban areas. One of the side effects of these chemicals is that they act as oxidizing agents to the fats in the diet and in the body. This means that they alter the way that oxygen is used in the body, preventing oxygen-bound chemical substances from interacting as they should. Instead, they bring about the creation of free radicals, oxidized substances that move through the bloodstream into all parts of the body, creating chemical imbalances. This creation of free radicals is now seen as a major cause of immune-system impairment and cellular damage.

6. Even the healthy trend toward daily exercise and fitness places extra nutritional stress on the body. The nutrient needs of an active person differ greatly from those of someone who leads a sedentary life. The muscles, tendons, ligaments, heart, blood, immune system, and endocrine glands—particularly the adrenals—need extra nutritional support if exercise is to produce its full benefits and not end up instead exceeding one's threshold to stress, leading to injury, infection, or exhaustion. Because many people get involved in strenuous fitness programs without adjusting their intake of nutrients, they unwittingly expose themselves to added risk of overuse injuries, exhaustion, and harmful strain on the heart, lungs, and immune system.

The Danger of Deficiencies

Supplementary nutrients have traditionally been used to prevent well-documented deficiencies: scurvy as a result of severe Vitamin C deficiency, beriberi from lack of thiamine, pellagra from severe niacin depletion, rickets from lack of vitamin D, kwashiorkor as the result of protein/calorie deprivation, and night blindness from Vitamin A deficiency. But judging by studies of "healthy" people, vitamin deficiencies are rampant and not only in the ill and the elderly.

- One in three American households shows diets deficient in calcium and Vitamin B6.
- One in every four households shows diets deficient in magnesium, one in five deficient in iron and Vitamin A.
- Teenage girls are deficient in their intake of calcium, iron, magnesium, and B6.
- Half of all women have an inadequate calcium intake.
- In spite of enriched breads and cereals, iron deficiency in the blood is widespread in all age, sex, race, and income groups. Nine out of ten women have inadequate iron in their diets. Close to 100 percent of competitive women athletes and 25 percent of competitive male athletes are iron-deficient.
- More than 50 percent of men and women in a Michigan test were deficient in Vitamin A. In a California study, over 33 percent were deficient in riboflavin (B2). In Texas and Washington, over 25 percent were deficient in Vitamin A.

Chronic deficiencies from lack of adequate nutrition can lead to all kinds of ailments and general suboptimal health. Supplementation supports the health of six basic bodily systems: the immune system; the muscular/skeletal structure; the digestive system; the neurological network; the cardiovascular system; and the endocrine system. Lifelong substandard operation of these systems leads to many degenerative diseases. Allergies, chronic viral infections, even heart disease and cancer can arise from a suppressed immune system. Osteoporosis, muscular weakness, arthritis, bursitis, and overall lack of vigor result from lack of nutrient supply to muscles and bones; heart disease in all its manifestations appears to be a direct result of an imbalanced and inadequate dietary routine; the common cold, sore throat, headaches, carpal tunnel syndrome (pain or tingling in the fingers and hand, caused by pressure on the median nerve of the wrist), angina pectoris, and other complaints major and minor are all tied to nutritional inadequacies. Even emotional disorders such as depression, insomnia, hyperactivity, and PMS are created or worsened by faulty diet.

The Case for Optimal Supplemention

Optimal supplementation not only prevents the development of illness, it can cure it. Symptoms and ailments can be turned around by correcting deficiencies and boosting dosages of vitamins known to correct *specific* symptoms. (See the nutrient tables in the following chapters.) *Specific* nutrients can do truly miraculous things. Buffered Vitamin C can prevent or lessen an allergic reaction. Vitamins A, C, and zinc can literally increase the size of the thymus, the "master gland" that controls the immune system's functioning. Essential-fatty-acid supplements will profoundly lower the blood cholesterol and triglycerides, lower blood pressure, and prevent platelet aggregation.

Supplements can often be used in place of many over-the-counter drugs. Isn't it smarter to replace these chemical compounds with a *natural* laxative (in the form of Vitamin C or fiber tablets), a *natural* diuretic (such as B6), a *natural* painkiller (DL-phenylalanine)? Nutrient "medicines" can do many of the same jobs as prescription drugs, and in addition they have a broad range of safety and contribute to your overall health.

It is outrageous to me that nutrient supplementation continues to be a matter of controversy. To me, it is dangerous *not* to supplement the diet prudently, given the burden our systems have to tolerate. The veil of apparent health is very thin—nutrient supplements are a sure, safe, easy way to give ourselves a margin for health. A long-term study of 12,000 individuals of diverse backgrounds conducted by the Food and Drug Administration found that half the people studied were getting even less than the stingy federally recommended RDAs; the elderly, women, and children were the most severely deprived. And since the study began in 1969, the trend has worsened every year.

Nutritional deficiencies have genetic consequences. In tests on lab animals, it has been found that a zinc deficiency in parents causes the next two generations to suffer from a lowered immune-system function. Feeding children diets that contain normally adequate levels of zinc does *not* reverse this malfunction; it's too little and too late.

Food and supplements complement each other—neither can do the whole job alone. Food provides the calories that we need for fuel. Food is needed for the digestion, absorption, and metabolization of our nutrient supplements, which take up the slack between what we eat and what we actually need for *optimum* health.

HOW MUCH SUPPLEMENTATION DO WE NEED?

This is the crucial—and irrationally controversial—question. The answer is, very simply, that we often need far, far more than the RDAs indicate. They are way off the mark, for a number of reasons.

First, let's consider again that "average, healthy American eating a well-balanced diet" on whom those RDAs are based. We've already seen that the "average American diet" is hardly adequate—if such a diet even exists. What about that "average, healthy American?" He (or she) doesn't exist either—for two simple reasons:

1. There is no such thing as an average person. Nutritional research has shown that, contrary to what the RDAs would have us believe, individuals have *very different* nutritional requirements. Furthermore, the nutrient needs in the same person can vary widely under different circumstances—changes in health, stresses, activity, environment, age. Instead of paying lip service to the concept of an "average" human being, needing an "average" amount of nutrients to get through life, we have come to identify and respect the existence of something quite different in nutrition—*biochemical individuality.*

There are tremendous genetic differences that separate people. Over 2,000 well-known genetic defects can cause severe deficiency diseases. What is less known—but of greater importance—is the widespread variation in nutritional needs from one individual to another. This variation, genetically and environmentally determined, can mean that one man needs more than "normal" amounts of certain nutrients while another needs more of certain other nutrients. In the case of the zinc-deficient lab animals mentioned above, although "normal" amounts of zinc didn't correct their problem, *aggressive* amounts of zinc did, enhancing and stimulating the impaired immune system in subsequent generations.

People differ in age, size, body type, stress levels, physical activity levels, allergies, illnesses, medications taken, sleep patterns, resistance to stress of different kinds, the ability of their digestive tract to absorb and utilize certain nutrients. Those RDAs may apply only to about 3 percent of the population. Your needs for a particular nutrient may easily be twenty times or more that of the person who lives next door.

2. Not only is there no "average" American; there is no typical "healthy" American. The RDAs are designed to help that "average healthy" American eating a well-balanced diet. But how do you define health? Is it nothing more than the absence of well-defined deficiency states? Is it that mythic state of being "average" or "normal"? For as we've said, most "healthy," "average," "normal" people have aches and pains, headaches and fevers, excess body fat, blood pressure above 110/70, serum cholesterol above 160 mg, upset stomachs, and the blues. They're the walking wounded, targets for more serious disease.

And where are the RDAs for those recovering from the trauma of surgery, from burns or infections, for those under emotional stress or who suffer from obesity, digestive problems, arthritis, or cardiovascular disease, for those who are pregnant or who exercise strenuously?

The RDAs were developed as a rough guideline for food-service management, for hospitals and the armed forces. They need to be challenged and questioned very seriously. For one thing, some vital and frequently deficient nutrients are entirely missing from the list of RDAs—most glaringly, certain essential amino acids and fatty acids.

We have to start thinking about nutrient needs based on our individual requirements for *optimum health* rather than worry about staving off beriberi, or overdosing on too many health-promoting nutrients.

GUIDELINES FOR YOUR PERSONAL SUPPLEMENTATION PROGRAM

What Should You Take?

Since nutrients work together, anyone who supplements should take a comprehensive across-the-board regimen of daily vitamins, minerals, essential fatty acids, and amino acids. The routine supplementation program suggested for every adult on the Optimum Health Program is as follows:

- 1 multivitamin capsule two–three times a day with meals.
- 1 multimineral capsule two–three times a day with meals.
- An additional 1,000–3,000 mg of Vitamin C in crystal, powder, or encapsulated form, with each meal.
- 1 400 IU* capsule of Vitamin E daily with the morning meal.
- 3 capsules of evening primrose oil just before two meals daily.
- 2 capsules of MaxEPA just before two meals daily.

Table 3 on page 86 shows what your supplement schedule should look like through the day.

The following chart shows the daily adult dosage range and the

*International Unit: a quantity that produces a particular biological effect (activity equivalent) agreed upon as an international standard

Table 3—Adult Daily Routine Supplementation Schedule

	Before Meals	During or After Meals
BREAKFAST	3–4 capsules evening primrose oil 2–3 capsules MaxEPA	1 multivitamin capsule 1 multimineral capsule 1–3 grams Vitamin C 1 400 IU capsule of Vitamin E
LUNCH		1 multivitamin capsule 1 multimineral capsule 1–3 grams Vitamin C
DINNER	3–4 capsules evening primrose oil 2–3 capsules MaxEPA	1 multivitamin capsule 1 multimineral capsule 1–3 grams Vitamin C

recommended daily dosage of each of the vitamins and minerals. This will help you in finding multivitamin and multimineral supplements that give you the daily dosage you want.

The above is a basic suggested regimen for establishing optimum blood levels of all nutrients. To tailor this to meet your personal needs, you should be guided by your weight and body type, your age, you activity level, your health and particular symptoms, any hereditary disposition you may be aware of, and, most important, what objective laboratory tests show your *actual* nutritional needs to be.

If you are physically very large or very small, you may want to increase or decrease the routine amounts accordingly. As you get older, it is very likely that your digestive system won't absorb nutrients as well as it did when you were younger, and you will need higher doses (perhaps even periodic injections of certain nutrients) to ensure that enough of these nutrients make it into the system. Specific symptoms call for specific nutrients, as do changes in your life or habits—pregnancy, stringent work deadlines, competitive sports, hospitalization, illness.

Take the time to read the discussion of each nutrient in the following chapters for information on its therapeutic uses and its major food sources, and for any special advice regarding its supplementation. You should also look up each of your symptoms in Part V to determine exactly what additional supplementation is recommended for your problems.

Table 4—Recommended Daily Dosages of Vitamins and Minerals

Supplement	Daily Adult Dosage Range	Recommended Routine Dosage	% of USRDA
Vitamin A	10,000–25,000 IU	10,000 IU	200
Beta carotene	20,000–50,000 IU	25,000 IU	—
B1 (thiamine)	10–75 mg	50 mg	3,333
B2 (riboflavin)	10–75 mg	50 mg	2,941
B3 (niacin, niacinamide)	25–200 mg	50 mg as niacin and/or 200 mg as niacinamide	250 1,000
B5 (calcium pantothenate)	50–1,000 mg	200 mg	2,000
B6 (pyridoxine)	10–500 mg	200 mg	5,000
B12 (cobalamin)	100–1,000 mcg	400 mcg	6,664
Biotin	50–3000 mcg	80 mcg	26.6
Choline	50–2,000 mg	200 mg	—
Folic acid	500–5,000 mcg	400 mcg	100
Inositol	100–1,000 mg	250 mg	—
PABA (Para-amino-benzoic acid)	40–400 mg	100 mg	—
Vitamin C	250 mg—90% bowel tolerance (page 114)	3,000 mg routinely; 6,000–10,000 mg under stress	4,998
Vitamin D	100–400 IU	not routinely supplemented	—
Vitamin E	50–1,200 IU	400 IU	1,333
Calcium	1,000–1,500 mg	1,000 mg	100
Chromium	100–600 mcg	200 mcg	—
Copper	1–2 mg	1 mg	50
Iodine	50–200 mcg	not routinely supplemented	—
Iron	18–30 mg	not supplemented without proven deficiency	—
Magnesium	300–1,000 mg	750 mg	175
Manganese	5–50 mg	10 mg	—
Phosphorus	500–800 mg	not routinely supplemented	—
Potassium	50–300 mg	100 mg	—
Selenium	50–400 mcg	200 mcg	—
Sodium	—	not routinely supplemented	—
Zinc	10–50 mg	20 mg	133
Gamma linolenic acid	80–400 mg	6–8 capsules evening primrose oil	—
Eicosaphentaenoic acid	180–1,800 mg	4–6 capsules MaxEPA	—

Ideally, you should work closely with a nutritionally oriented physician for periodic evaluation and adjustment of your individual dietary and supplementation needs.

Note: Recommended children's dosages are on pages 294 and 297.

Blood Vitamin and Mineral Analysis

Since there is often a vast difference between what we ingest and what we absorb, it is very hard to tell exactly how much of our food and supplements is getting into the bloodstream. Because so many factors can affect the absorption of nutrients, taking supplements can be an expensive guessing game. The best way to ascertain that you are achieving optimum blood levels of nutrients is to have a blood vitamin analysis and blood mineral analysis to pinpoint those levels.

The blood vitamin analysis (BVA), developed at our licensed clinical laboratories, tests at present for blood serum levels of seven vitamins. Blood mineral analysis (BMA) determines levels of iron, magnesium, calcium, potassium, phosphorus, sodium, selenium, zinc, chromium, and manganese. Not only do the BVA and BMA detect blood levels of vitamins and minerals, they attempt to break these levels into five categories: severely deficient, suboptimal, adequate, optimal, and excessive. Notice that there are no nonsensical and archaic categories of "normal" or "abnormal."

When and How to Take Supplements

Here are a few simple guidelines to help you maximize the benefits of your supplementation plan.

- Most supplements should be taken in divided dosages for maximum absorption, and they should be taken with meals. Food aids the absorption of supplements and is in many cases necessary for the subsequent metabolism of certain nutrients—especially the water-soluble vitamins. Studies show that absorption and utilization are *far greater* when supplements are divided up through the day—*68 percent absorption for a divided multiple dosage, as compared to only 12 percent when taken in a single daily dose.* The few exceptions to this are as follows: The fat-soluble vitamins A, E, and beta carotene and the essential fatty acids can be taken once a day—preferably with breakfast—in a single dose. Iron and certain individual amino acids should be taken by themselves, between meals.
- Another area of much misunderstanding and ignorance has to do with combinations of supplements. If you believed every-

thing you heard and read, you'd think that many supplement combinations cancel one another out, unless you go through very elaborate precautions, so why bother to take them? There are only a few precautions. Here's an important one: Don't take a combined multivitamin/multimineral capsule. Though most vitamin and mineral combinations can be taken together, they should not all be *stored* together, for they drain one another's potency. For example, Vitamin E and certain forms of iron do not belong in the same pill, nor apparently do Vitamin B12 and copper. Iron should not be consumed with other minerals, especially calcium and magnesium.

- Vitamins and essential fatty acids keep best when tightly closed and refrigerated. But do store your supplements where they're accessible. Don't make it a chore to get to them at each meal. It is helpful to make up daily "packages" of your supplements, so that they are available when needed.
- There is an ongoing controversy about the difference, if any, between "natural" and "synthetic" supplements. Since natural and synthetic compounds have basically the same biochemical or molecular structure and the same biological activity in the body, I find the controversy specious. Until further scientific evidence proves the superiority of "natural" nutrients, I use either or both, depending on purity, dose, and hypoallergenicity.
- Make sure you are taking hypoallergenic supplements. Many supplements are made with highly allergenic food or chemical substances or contain highly allergic binders and fillers such as yeast, wheat, corn, soy, gums, food colorings, preservatives, and other additives. What's the use of rotating your diet if you're going to be ingesting an allergen several times a day? OHL supplements contain no allergy-causing binders and fillers. Our Vitamin C is derived from sego palm starch or tapioca starch rather than from the more common corn, which is potentially highly allergic, and our Vitamin B is from a purified, hypoallergenic synthetic source rather than from the highly allergic brewer's yeast. In general, it is a good idea to buy name-brand supplements and to read labels carefully. A case in point is evening primrose oil, which is marketed under many names and brands: Few brands contain the vital gamma linolenic acid in sufficient amount to warrant their high price.
- Take vitamins and minerals in loose capsule or powder form when possible. A huge hard horse tablet of a multivitamin is so tightly compressed that it cannot dissolve enough in the digestive tract in time to be completely absorbed; it is usually passed along into the large intestine incompletely absorbed and ends up in the toilet. Too, the heat involved in the compression process can destroy some of the B vitamins.
- MaxEPA, which is a fish oil, causes uncomfortable belching for

some people. If this problem persists, taking the MaxEPA with meals instead of before should do the trick.

- Because many people have problems absorbing the fat-soluble vitamins, Vitamin A and E in *micellized* form are preferred. "Micellized" indicates a liquid form in which the molecular structure is gently miniaturized to enhance absorption. If you are able to locate the micellized A and E—available from a few distributors—you will have to take only a fraction of the usual amount to get the same benefit. One ml (or 20 drops) of Vitamin E (150 IU) can be taken in place of the usual 400 IU capsule. For those wishing to take extra Vitamin A, 1 drop equals 3,000 IU; 1–2 drops daily is adequate routine supplementation.
- Timed-release supplements are a waste. Most supplements are maximally absorbed in short segments of the gastrointestinal tract and need food for absorption. Anything released in the wrong segment of the digestive tract, or released at a time when there's no food in the GI tract, will mostly go to waste.

Complete supplement tables and a full discussion of the properties and uses of the most important supplements appear in the following chapters. Supplement tables appear at the end of the supplementation section; they begin on page 158. Recommendations for specific symptoms and ailments can be found in Part V under the Optimum Health Program protocols. But the routine supplementation is a good place to start. Don't worry about overdosing; toxic levels are very rare at these adult supplementation levels—the important thing is to guard against deficiencies and give yourself that optimum health margin.

8

Vitamins

Before the official discovery of vitamins in 1910, it was known that certain "accessory factors" were needed in the diet—in addition to proteins, carbohydrates, and fats—in order to avoid nutritional deficiencies. These accessory factors, known to prevent such diseases as scurvy and beriberi, were finally identified as vitamins: organic compounds necessary for life, which cannot be produced in the body and thus must be obtained from the diet.

The discovery of vitamins (and minerals, too) was one of the most important medical achievements in history. But although most nutritional biochemists will tell you that all the vitamins have probably been discovered by now, they will also agree that knowledge concerning all the subtle workings of these substances in the human body is still in its infancy stage. We have much yet to learn about getting the most from our diet and supplements.

For one thing, because they were identified in connection with their *absence* in nutritionally caused diseases such as pellagra, scurvy, kwashiorkor, and rickets, their role was first seen as a preventive one. Unfortunately, this got vitamins off on the wrong foot, for it fixed the notion that vitamins were needed only in amounts that would forestall dramatic at-death's-door problems. The concept of minimum daily allowances was born of this thinking and got stuck there.

However, in spite of continuing resistance from the established medical community, attitudes about the role of vitamins have begun to change. Things haven't been the same since Linus Pauling in 1970 caused a sensation when his experiments showed that Vitamin C, in megadoses up to a thousand times that of the RDA, may play an important role in the prevention or cure of just about everything from the common cold to cancer. Today research is constantly turning up new *therapeutic* as well as preventive applications for vitamin supplementation.

Vitamins are organic compounds. In most cases these compounds are found in the food we eat, but some vitamin compounds are made by intestinal bacteria from food. Vitamin D can come from our diet, but we get most of our Vitamin D from a chemical transaction that takes place as a result of exposure to sunlight. Seventeen vitamins have been identified and numbered (including K), plus a few as yet unclassified nutrient substances that may turn out to be vitamins, too.

Vitamins are used to carry out the chemical reactions involving enzymes and thus are involved in tens of thousands of biochemical actions. Every bodily process, from cell metabolism to muscle power, from thought to the sensations of the five senses, requires the presence of vitamins.

THE NAMES AND NUMBERS GAME

Don't get confused by the names and numbers of vitamins. Though the original intention was to give them logical, orderly designations, this system fell apart fast, as nutrients were classified and declassified or were found to exist in several forms or under yet other names. Even the dosage units can be confusing; some are given by weight, others by units of biochemical activity (IU).

It is probably useful to know that most vitamin dosages are given in terms of milligrams (mg) or thousandths of a gram. There are 28.3 grams to an ounce. The dosages of vitamins needed only in trace amounts are given in micrograms (mcg) or millionths of a gram. Dosages for vitamins usually taken in larger amounts, such as C, are given in terms of grams. These large doses are often referred to as megadoses.

FAT-SOLUBLE/WATER-SOLUBLE

A distinction is also made between fat-soluble and water-soluble vitamins. Water-soluble vitamins—C and the B-complex vitamins—are dissolved by body fluids and excreted through the urine. Thus they must be constantly renewed. Because any excess of these vitamins is flushed out of the system (unless taken at *very* high doses), there is little chance of building up toxic levels in the body.

Any excess intake of the fat-soluble vitamins—A, E, beta carotene, D, and K—is stored by the body's fat cells and retained for use on demand. Therefore, they can be overdosed. However, it should be noted that toxic side effects are as a rule easily eliminated by cutting back on dosage, and if identified have no real long-term consequences as far as is known. The one exception to this rule of reversibility may be the toxicity of Vitamin D overdose. However, assuming weekly exposure to sunlight (twenty to thirty minutes twice weekly), supplementation of

Vitamin D is rarely needed. It is easily supplied by "enriched" foods in the American diet and is also manufactured in the body, in a process triggered by the exposure of cholesterol in the skin to sunlight.

Because fat-soluble vitamins are not absorbed as easily as water-soluble vitamins, people with food allergies and other inflammatory intestinal disorders are often unable to absorb them in the quantities needed. For example, even healthy individuals are able to absorb only about 25 percent of oil-based Vitamin E. Those who have trouble with fat digestion because of bile and pancreatic imbalances take in even less. Because of this problem, Vitamins A and E are now available in *micellized* liquid form. This process so greatly reduces the size of the fat molecule that it will even dissolve in water, making it more easily transportable into the lymphatic system and blood. Also, because of the greatly enhanced absorption, only a fraction of the usual amount need be taken —as a general rule, one third to one half of the usual dose.

Note: Vitamin Tables begin on page 158.

VITAMIN A—RETINOL

The term "Vitamin A" correctly refers to preformed Vitamin A, or retinol, and is found only in the animals or fish that form it. The precursor vegetable source of Vitamin A is beta carotene (also called Provitamin A), which must be converted to Vitamin A. Thus we can get Vitamin A in our diets by eating the fish or animals that make it naturally or by converting beta carotene from the vegetables we eat. Beta carotene is converted to A in the liver and small intestines on demand, when Vitamin A supplies fall short, so excess beta carotene does not appear to lead to Vitamin A toxicity, only to a harmless (and easily reversible) yellowing of the skin. Beta carotene may be transformed into any of three forms of Vitamin A: retinol, retinal, and retinoic acid. All act in essentially the same way within the body, and all can be considered part of the same biochemical processes.

Functions of Vitamin A

Vitamin A is an extremely important antioxidant and immune-system-enhancing vitamin. Its functions in the body are the following:

- Maintenance of mucous membrane and skin health, and thus the prevention and treatment of infection, eczema, psoriasis, and acne. Vitamin A also aids in healing wounds.

- Promotion of effective night vision. Vitamin A deficiency is the leading cause of blindness in the Third World (as diabetes is in the West).
- Control of highly destructive free radicals via its antioxidant effect.
- Maintenance of a healthy thymus gland, the master gland of the immune system.
- Development of normal reproduction and lactation cycles.
- Synthesis of the genetic material RNA.
- Metabolism of tissue.
- Prevention of excessive inflammatory prostaglandin release.
- Production of secretory IgA and protective mucus in the digestive tract.

Vitamin A's powers are still being discovered, but there is indication that it is also required for adrenal cortex and steroid hormone synthesis, bone development and the maintenance of myelin nerve sheaths, and protection against some types of cancer.

Therapeutic Applications of Vitamin A

- Hormone functions. Hormonal imbalances are implicated in the development of acne, in premenstrual syndrome, excessive menstrual bleeding, osteoporosis, and cystic mastitis.
- Acne. Acne is often treated by external application of retinol and high oral doses of A. It not only strengthens tissues and skin; it seems to moderate the hormones—especially the estrogen-to-progesterone ratio in women, closely linked with fatty-acid and prostaglandin metabolism—that can trigger eruptions.
- Excess menstrual bleeding. This problem can have many causes, but one study group of fifty-two women demonstrated significant improvement when given 30,000 IU of A twice daily for thirty-five days.
- Birth defects. Animal experiments have shown that Vitamin A deficiency during pregnancy can lead to birth defects.
- Cancer. Many studies have suggested the correlation between certain cancers and Vitamin A intake. Many precancerous conditions are similar, if not identical, to the effects of Vitamin A deficiencies. Further, when A is in short supply, tissue abnormalities and lack of mucous-membrane strength can cause lesions that are similar to cancer. Vitamin A may fight cancer-cell development in the same way that it boosts the immune system and fights infection: by making the immune system

and all its antibody functions more durable, and by reducing the production of inflammatory prostaglandins (e.g., PGE2, PGF2 alpha). One National Cancer Institute study showed that A administered in large doses stimulates the anticancer activities of white blood cells in people already suffering from cancer. Vitamin A may not only control cancer once it is present, but may actually *prevent* the growth of cancer from occurring.

- Asthma. In conjunction with Vitamins C and D, zinc, and essential fatty acids, A is effective in the control of asthma. It helps soothe and heal fragile, irritated lungs damaged by asthma attacks.
- Allergy. Allergies show themselves in many ways, but all seem to involve an immune system response, which produces chemical mediators released from irritated mast cells of the airways and digestive tract. Vitamin A appears to aid in such allergy-related disorders as migraine, rheumatoid arthritis, inflammatory bowel disease, cystitis, sinusitus, rhinitis, and eczema.

Vitamin A Supplementation

As with all fat-soluble vitamins, there is the possibility of toxicity from overdoses of Vitamin A. Individual tolerance levels depend on metabolic demand and general state of health. Too much Vitamin A is most commonly indicated by dry skin, but also by irritability, tenderness or aching in the long bones of the body, headaches, cracking at the edges of the lips, hair thinning or loss, and abnormal liver-function tests. Decreasing the dosage will relieve the symptoms.

Megadoses of A should be taken only under a physician's supervision, after tests for liver function, blood levels of A, and red-blood-cell sedimentation rate tests; and follow-up tests should be repeated at four- to six-week intervals.

However, understanding and recognizing the possible side effects of Vitamin A supplementation should not scare you away from including substantial amounts of this vital supplement in your program. I personally take 25,000–50,000 IUs a day, and have experienced no side effects other than occasional dry skin. A basic dose of 25,000 IU a day is very safe for most adults, and 10,000 is really minimal. Toxic levels are usually reached at rather rarefied levels: upward of 100,000–300,000 IU daily for several weeks or months. And remember, toxicity can be avoided if you learn to recognize the early signs of overdose and immediately reduce your intake when they first appear.

BETA CAROTENE—PROVITAMIN A

For years, beta carotene was seen as nothing more than the precursor to the formation of Vitamin A in the body, and as such it was considered an important nutrient, though not necessarily a vitamin in its own right. Now, however, independent functions of beta carotene are being uncovered. It is for this reason that I consider beta carotene a vitamin in its own right.

Functions of Beta Carotene

Beta carotene appears to be a participant in prevention and control of some degenerative diseases, particularly as an anticancer agent. A nineteen-year study involving more than 3,000 men has produced evidence suggesting that carotenoids (especially beta carotene) may be capable of significantly reducing the incidence of lung cancer in both smokers and nonsmokers.

A potent antioxidant, it blocks the formation of potentially destructive free radicals and also seems to act as an internal sunscreen against the damaging effects of ultraviolet light from the sun.

It aids in the prevention of inflammatory prostaglandin formation.

Therapeutic Applications of Beta Carotene

As noted above, the most exciting application for beta carotene therapy may prove to be in the prevention of cancer. One theory is that cigarette smoke destroys Vitamin A in lung tissue, making the membranes more vulnerable to disease. But beta carotene, which is converted slowly and continuously, can provide a continually replenished source of Vitamin A and protect the tissue from Vitamin A depletion.

Another study, conducted in 1974 at the Albert Einstein College of Medicine, showed that the antitumor effects of beta carotene combined with chemotherapy can be quite potent, effecting remission much more thoroughly than chemotherapy alone.

Beta Carotene Supplementation

It is also possible that the beneficial properties of beta carotene have a great deal to do with the fact that foods high in beta carotene are also high in fiber and additional nutrient antioxidants; thus food sources may be preferable to supplements. Papaya, carrots (particularly carrot juice, because the dense cellular structure of the carrot has been broken down), sweet potatoes, spinach, collard greens, and cantaloupe are high in beta carotene.

Too much beta carotene will cause a yellowing of the skin, most noticeably in the palms of the hands, soles of the feet, and earlobes. It is not dangerous (it is not related to jaundice) and reverses itself when intake is reduced. Recommended supplementary intake is 20,000–50,000 IU.

THE B COMPLEX

There are eleven B vitamins, but until the mid-1930s Vitamin B was thought to be just one big happy vitamin. A reasonable mistake, since they all come from the same dietary sources and are dependent on one another for proper functioning. In the course of recognizing the different B vitamins and sorting out the confusion, the Bs ended up with all sorts of baffling names and numbers, which tends to complicate rather than clarify things.

The important thing to remember is that the B vitamins—sometimes called the stress vitamins—should be taken together in a balanced supplement if they are to function at their best. A lack (or an extraordinarily high dose) of any one B vitamin can block the absorption and/or utilization of others and cause long-term deficiencies. Since food allergies and digestive problems can interfere with proper uptake of individual vitamins, this balanced supplement makes a difference.

When a B-complex supplement is taken orally, it is broken down in the body and joined with a phosphorus molecule before it can be assimilated into the bloodstream. Optimum Health Labs' B-complex supplements have already been joined to phosphorus through a process known as *phosphorylation,* which eliminates the extra step the system must perform, thus assuring an optimal absorption. It is also advisable to buy B vitamins that are not in the usual yeast base, since yeast is potentially highly allergic and may inhibit the absorption of the B vitamins in adequate amounts.

VITAMIN B1—THIAMINE

It turns out that thiamine was the specific B vitamin instrumental in curing beriberi, which gave the whole group of vitamins its "B" designation. But it has other valuable uses. B1 is essential for the metabolism of the three basic food groups—fats, carbohydrates, and proteins—and is instrumental in the utilization of energy from carbohydrates. It is required for energy production and tissue respiration and for the maintenance of heart function. Along with A, B5, B6, C, E, and cysteine, it is a primary antioxidant and thus combats destructive free radicals.

Therapeutic Applications of Thiamine

Thiamine works to combat infection and to strengthen the immune system. Because it is involved in producing healthy nerve sheaths, it may (along with other nutrients such as evening primrose oil, eicosapentaenoic acid, and octacosanol) aid in the management of multiple sclerosis. *The Journal of Speech and Hearing* has reported its possible effectiveness in helping children overcome stuttering problems.

Thiamine Supplementation

There are no toxic effects from thiamine intake known to us at this time. However, it is important to bear in mind that excess intake of any individual B vitamin may cause imbalance in the metabolism of the other B vitamins. Therefore, thiamine is best supplemented as part of a B complex vitamin, in a suggested range of 10–75 mg daily. It is rarely supplemented alone.

VITAMIN B2—RIBOFLAVIN

Riboflavin is essential to cell respiration. Working with other energy-releasing B vitamins, it assures the cells of ample oxygen to metabolize other nutrients. Cells cannot function without B2; the adrenal gland is weakened, arteries can become clogged with fat, and eyesight may become impaired. Few bodily systems are not dependent on an ample supply of riboflavin.

There are four major areas of riboflavin activity:

- Tissue and cell strength. Its ability to aid in cell respiration makes it vital for endurance, particularly for athletes.
- Enzyme and hormone production. The thyroid is regulated by

B2, as is the manufacture of the enzyme glutathione reductase, vital in preventing the creation of destructive free radicals.
- Skin, hair, and mucous-membrane activity. The delicate balance of fluid and proteins necessary for these functions is regulated by B2.
- Metabolism of blood sugar (glucose). It plays a major role in the production of bodily energy.

Therapeutic Applications of Riboflavin

Because of its essential contribution to cellular functioning and its role in hormone and enzyme production, B2 has powerful therapeutic effects, especially when combined with general supplementation and a healthy diet. Current research has highlighted several areas of special effectiveness:

- Athletic endurance. Supplementation with B2 increases the muscles' ability to resist fatigue. A 1976 study in *Nutritional Metabolism* demonstrated that just 10 mg of B2 increased resistance to fatigue by 11 percent. Experiments with lab animals showed that it increases resistance to cold weather.
- Control of cholesterol levels and prevention of atherosclerosis. Since B2 helps the liver in clearing cholesterol and is vital to the metabolism of fat, it plays an important part in any program to reduce serum cholesterol and reverse arterial clogging. Further, it helps detoxify pollutants as they pass through the liver.
- Overcoming digestive problems. B2, in conjunction with other supplements (such as Vitamins A and C, zinc, evening primrose oil, and MaxEPA), is effective in reducing inflammations of the intestine and irritable bowel disorders caused by food allergy, poor diet, and excess psychological or physiological stress.
- Acne control. Hormonal fluctuations are often associated with acne. Riboflavin (along with Vitamin A, zinc, and essential fatty acids) helps stabilize skin cells and regulates hormonal function.
- Control of alcoholism. New research indicates that alcoholism can be both triggered and caused by faulty metabolism of sugar and other carbohydrates, by essential-fatty-acid deficiencies, and by adrenal gland deficiencies. B2 (in conjunction with glutamine, Vitamin C, and the elimination of food allergens) helps stabilize these functions and may decrease the cravings that lead to alcohol abuse.

Riboflavin Supplementation

Individual riboflavin requirements are determined by caloric intake, body size, physical activity, and metabolic rate. You can test to see if you are absorbing riboflavin by taking a 50 mg tablet with your normal supplementation. An increased level in the body will normally produce bright yellow urine about twenty minutes later. (This also shows you how fast water-soluble nutrients pass through the body, which is why these supplements should be broken into three daily doses.) The usual range of supplementation is 10–75 mg daily.

VITAMIN B3—NIACIN

A devastating deficiency disease known as pellagra plagued many parts of the world up until the 1930s. Characterized by the four "D's"—dermatitis, diarrhea, dementia, and death—plus malaise, sensitivity to light, tremors, and sore, swollen tongue, it was finally traced to a lack of niacin.

Known variously as nicotinic acid and nicotinamide, B3 is converted (in conjunction with B1 and B2) into an important coenzyme called NAD. NAD is absolutely essential to allowing energy (calories) to be released from food. Without NAD, the body would cannibalistically consume its own energy stores, bringing on tissue breakdown and severe nutritional deficiencies.

Acting alone, niacin (but not niacinamide) plays a major role in reducing elevated serum cholesterol and in dilating the capillaries. It is this process of dilation that causes the "niacin flush"—the warming, tingling, sometimes itching sensation and reddening of the body soon after taking niacin. This seems to occur because niacin, or nicotinic acid, releases histamines from their storage depots in the mast cells, sending them into circulation. It is not a serious side effect and has no medical repercussions other than those mentioned. Continued use of niacin builds up a tolerance, which eliminates the flush. Some people are fond of their niacin flushes. Those who find it uncomfortable can get their B3 in the form of niacinamide; however, they will forfeit niacin's powerful dilation and anticholesterol effect.

B3 further functions to promote healthy skin and to stimulate the production of HCl (hydrochloric acid) in the stomach; as such it is used in therapy to aid digestion. Finally, B3 plays a significant role in the production of the anti-inflammatory health-promoting prostaglandins PGE1 and PGE3.

Therapeutic Applications of Niacin

Because niacin plays such an important part in the maintenance of the circulatory system and the prostaglandin balance, and in control of the psychosis (dementia) aspect of pellagra, it is recognized as having profound applications in the treatment of brain and mental disorders.

- Schizophrenia. Niacin was the first vitamin to be used by psychiatrists. Combined with Vitamins C, B6, and other orthomolecular substances, it has been shown to be as effective as some tranquilizers (Valium, for example) in reversing depression and anxiety, but without the notorious side effects of prescription tranquilizers. Studies done since 1953 confirm the effectiveness of niacin therapy in this disorder.
- Mental and learning impairment. Probably due to B3's impact on essential fatty-acid metabolism and prostaglandin balance, both hyperactivity and the mental infirmities of old age respond to niacin therapy. Over a dozen double-blind experiments have found that hyperactive kids with learning disorders have a subpellagra condition that improves with niacin. Likewise senility is diminished by a program that combines niacin with B6, B12, C, zinc, magnesium, and other essential-fatty-acid-to-prostaglandin cofactors.
- Vascular disease. Vascular disease and the resulting defective blood supply to the brain, heart, kidney, and other organs may be helped by niacin (nicotinic acid) because of its ability to dilate the blood vessels and prevent abnormal platelet stickiness, thus preventing sludging of the blood flow and abnormal clotting. This sludging may cause the buildup of atherosclerotic plaque, obstructing blood flow and leading to strokes and heart attacks. Such cardiovascular events may be prevented with niacin because niacin increases the negative charges on the surface of red blood cells, decreases the abnormal platelet aggregation, and disperses the red blood cells and platelets through the circulation. Niacin has also proved to lower cholesterol significantly and promote the production of HDL cholesterol (high density lipoprotein).
- Arthritis. Today cortisone and ACTH are two of the drugs most commonly prescribed for arthritis. But as early as 1945 it was known that niacin is more effective and less harmful than these. However, this inexpensive, unpatentable therapy has received little notice, presumably because, as it is a nutrient and not a drug, it cannot be turned to profit by the pharmaceutical companies. Because arthritis has many causes and is part of a complicated syndrome, niacin alone will not help every arthritis sufferer. But it is effective in many cases, especially in conjunction with other therapy to enhance digestion and the immune system. See page 326.

- The immune system. Although it is difficult to pinpoint all the causes of immune system diseases such as lupus, multiple sclerosis, myasthenia gravis, thyroid disease, and muscular dystrophy, there is evidence that niacin may play an important role in their treatment.
- Sleep disorders. Due to tryptophan's conversion both to niacin and the sleep-enhancing brain neurotransmitter serotonin, high supplemental doses of niacin lead to increased serotonin and thus better sleep.

Niacin Supplementation

To get the vasodilating benefit of the niacin "flush," be sure to supplement with niacin or nicotinic acid, *not* niacinamide. Niacinamide is preferable for those who want B3 supplementation but wish to avoid the flushing.

Niacin supplementation should start at a very low level and be increased slowly as the system builds up a tolerance for the flushing. A suggested beginning dose is 25 mg daily, building up in small increments to a maximum of 1–2 grams daily. Those at risk for cardiovascular problems, peptic ulcers, and diabetes, and pregnant women should take niacin only under a doctor's supervision.

Persistent intake of niacin over 2 grams daily may lead to complications ranging from mild nausea and vomiting to abnormal liver function, and a benign and temporary brown skin discoloration (niacin usually gives the skin a healthy glow).

VITAMIN B5—PANTOTHENIC ACID

Pantothenic acid, from the Greek word meaning "from all sides," is found in an enormous variety of foods, from organ meats and grains to fish and green vegetables. It wasn't until 1940 that it was isolated and identified by the pioneering nutritional biochemist Roger Williams, Ph.D. Since then its importance in a wide spectrum of vital processes has been slowly uncovered.

The functions of pantothenic acid can be broadly divided into five categories:

- Strengthening the immune system. Adrenal gland functions are contingent on an ample supply of B5, which affects the ability of the whole system to manage stress and, through the action of the adrenals on the immune system, to resist infection. B5 also interacts with B6 to produce healthy antibodies from certain white blood cells. This, combined with its ability to stimulate the production of cortisol and adrenaline, makes it an important part of an allergy-control program.

- Conversion of calories into energy for the cells. B5 is essential in the synthesis of Coenzyme A, a product of several vitamins and amino acids working together. It is a primary factor in the conversion of carbohydrates, fats, and proteins into energy. ATP, another substance essential for cellular metabolism and thus energy production, is also produced in part by the action of pantothenic acid.
- Support of neurotransmitter function in the brain. As a link in the conversion of the B vitamin choline into acetylcholine, B5 contributes to memory enhancement.
- Control of cholesterol and free radicals. In conjunction with Vitamin C and other antioxidants, B5 prevents the oxidation of fats and helps optimize cholesterol levels.
- Maintenance of normal uric-acid levels in the blood. By acting as a chemical component in the conversion of uric acid and ammonia into urea and ammonia before it is passed out of the body, B5 (along with Vitamin C) helps prevent gouty arthritis (arthritis associated with gout).

Therapeutic Applications of Pantothenic Acid

B5 is almost always used therapeutically in conjunction with the full spectrum of B vitamins. It appears to play an instrumental role in athletic endurance and the ability to handle stress of all kinds.

- Rheumatoid arthritis. Research at our laboratory confirms that rheumatoid arthritis may improve when treated with therapeutic doses of B5 in combination with other anti-inflammatory supplements and a strictly controlled nonallergic diet.
- Healing. As a vital part of the immune system's ability to fight infection and accelerate the healing process, B5 has been demonstrated to play an active role. Patients in a hospital study who were given 500 mg of B5 a day after abdominal surgery healed and recovered more quickly than those who were not.
- Fertility. Pantothenic acid is instrumental in the conversion of serum cholesterol into sex hormones. Without its active part in this process, hormonal levels may fluctuate, causing fertility problems.
- Allergy. As part of a general allergy-control program, therapeutic doses of B5, along with other B vitamins and C at 90

percent bowel tolerance (see page 114), provides powerful adrenal support and control of histamine reactions. It also lessens inflammation of the intestinal mucosa and digestive ability, both of which are affected by food allergies, and helps correct possible metabolic defects in the intestines that can lead to inflammatory bowel diseases such as Crohn's disease (regional enteritis) and ulcerative colitis.

Pantothenic Acid Supplementation

In a balanced ratio, it is possible to take up to 1,000 mg daily of B5 without harmful side effects. As with Vitamin C, the problem of loose bowels at high dosages can be alleviated by cutting back on the amount taken.

VITAMIN B6—PYRIDOXINE

B6 is the term used to identify a complex of three closely related vitamins: pyridoxine, pyridoxal, and pyridoxamine. Pyridoxine, in addition to being a major free-radical scavenging antioxidant, plays a big part in the metabolism of essential fatty acids to prostaglandins, and therefore has far-reaching effects on the cardiovascular, digestive, neurological, and immune systems. There is also a well-documented connection to learning, behavioral, emotional, and mental processes.

Pyridoxine's importance was made startlingly clear in an unfortunate incident in the 1950s, when infants all over the country were felled by mysterious convulsions. These otherwise healthy babies were all found to have consumed a brand of infant formula totally lacking in B6. Since that time, a wide variety of B6 functions have been identified in addition to the control of seizures, and immunological research is uncovering still more.

The two most important functions of B6 are its role in the metabolism of essential fatty acids and as a coenzyme for many biochemical reactions involving amino acids. Amino acids are metabolized and converted into proteins so they can be ingested by the body's cells; B6 helps this process along. For example, B6 is essential for the conversion of tryptophan into serotonin and niacin. Some additional functions:

- The production of hydrochloric acid (along with niacin and zinc) and thus healthy digestion.
- Formation of hemoglobin, the part of the red blood cell that transports oxygen. B6 deficiencies can result in anemia, similar in appearance to iron-deficiency anemia.

- The conversion of amino acids into neurotransmitters and neurohormones such as serotonin, dopamine, noradrenaline, adrenaline, and GABA (gamma amino butyric acid). B6 aids the development and function of the central nervous system (brain and spinal cord).
- Aid to glucose release and therefore energy production. Through its effect on glucose stores in the liver and muscles, B6, along with other B vitamins, aids in assimilation of carbohydrates.
- Maintenance of proper potassium/sodium balance in the cells.
- Aid to the absorption of B12.
- Stimulation of the thymus gland. B6 thus contributes to the formation of immune system antibodies and optimally functioning immune cells.
- Formation and function of the genetic materials RNA and DNA.
- Assurance of proper magnesium levels in red blood cells.

Therapeutic Applications of Pyridoxine

The cardiovascular system, psychological disturbances, and female hormonal distress all respond to B6 supplementation. Here are some additional functions of B6:

- PMS. Because of its role in the metabolism of essential fatty acids and thus the production of anti-inflammatory PGE1 and PGE3, pyridoxine alone has been effective in relieving both the physical and mental symptoms of premenstrual syndrome in perhaps 80 percent of sufferers.
- Rheumatoid and gouty arthritis. Because of its effect on the immune system and antibody production, plus its general anti-inflammatory benefits by way of PGE1 and PGE3 production, B6 is often used, along with other supplements, in the treatment of inflammatory arthritides. Preliminary research seems to indicate that people with rheumatoid arthritis have lower than normal levels of B6.
- Heart disease. There is a direct link between blood cholesterol levels, platelet aggregability, high blood pressure, atherosclerosis, and B6, again because of its connection to essential-fatty-acid and prostaglandin levels. Further, along with Vitamin C, it helps maintain collagen integrity in the connective tissue of artery and vein walls and thus contributes to overall vascular health. A diet high in saturated animal fats (arachidonic acid) is more likely to cause cholesterol-laden atherosclerotic plaque when levels of pyridoxine and essential fatty acids are low. This happens because such a diet stimulates

excess production of prostaglandins of the 2 series (PGE2, PGF2 alpha, leukotrienes, thromboxane A2, HETE, HPETE). B6 in sufficient quantities can help reduce these inflammatory, disease-enhancing chemical mediators. In the absence of enough B6, arterial-wall damage (secondary to abnormal platelet aggregation and vessel constriction) can occur.

- Calcium oxalate kidney stones. A deficiency of B6 and magnesium can lead to the production of excess oxalate crystals from Vitamin C (ascorbic acid) and consequently the formation of kidney stones.
- Psychological disorders. The brain's natural tranquilizer, serotonin, which is manufactured in the brain only in the presence of adequate B6 levels, is often found to be abnormally low in hyperactive children. B6 (along with essential-fatty-acid supplements) is very effective when combined with an overall nonallergic nutritional program.

  B6 can be very effective in treating certain depressions, in conjunction with an adequate intake of tryptophan or DL-phenylalanine.

  Orthomolecular psychiatrists use megadoses of B6 in treating schizophrenia. The theory is that it increases the production of PGE1, PGE3, serotonin, and niacin, which seem to be deficient in some schizophrenics. It also counteracts what is known as the mauve factor, involving increased levels of a toxic chemical with the name kryptopyrrole.
- Blood sugar disorders. Poor blood sugar regulation often stems from B6 deficiency, in conjunction with essential-fatty-acid/prostaglandin imbalance. Likewise, diabetics also have lower B6 levels than the general population. There is some research to confirm that both disorders are alleviated by aggressive B6 and essential-fatty-acid supplementation as part of a more comprehensive program.
- Tooth decay. Along with zinc, it prevents dental caries, apparently via stimulation of secretory IgA production.

Pyridoxine Supplementation

B6 deficiency is one of the most common nutrient deficiencies in this country. Yet the RDA for B6 is pitifully low—2 mg a day, with a recommended increase of ½ mg for lactating women. Some research biochemists believe that the proper intake should be eight to forty times that. Depending on symptoms, 10–500 mg are recommended on the Optimum Health Program. The only scientifically recorded cases of B6 toxicity occurred in seven individuals taking 2,000 mg or more a day for several months. Even then, the symptoms, which included numbness of the feet and hands, lack of balance, and coordination defect, faded when dosage was reduced. To prevent toxicity, B6 dosage should not exceed 500 mg daily, and this should always be taken with other B vitamins.

VITAMIN B12—COBALAMIN

Vitamin B12 is unique in two ways. It is the only vitamin that contains and functions in conjunction with a metal: cobalt. And unlike other vitamins, small amounts of B12 can be stored for months or years in many tissues of the body, especially the liver, kidneys, heart, and bone marrow. This storage facility can be enough to forestall severe deficiency for up to five years after the diet has ceased to provide adequate B12. For this reason, a severe B12 deficiency is always a sign of long-term malnutrition or malabsorption and is usually coupled with many other nutrient deficiencies. B12 is also commonly associated with iron and folic-acid deficiency; B12 shots are a popular therapy for people who are run down and fatigued, often because of long-running digestive disturbances.

B12's functions are legion. It is important in the metabolic actions of cells, in the maintenance of a healthy immune system, nervous system, and circulatory system, and in general well-being. Specifically, it is connected with

- Cell metabolism in the digestive tract, the bone marrow, and the nervous system.
- Growth in children.
- Synthesis of DNA and RNA.
- Formation of red blood cells.
- Formation of myelin, the protective insulating sheath of the nerves.
- Utilization of iron and the absorption and cellular uptake of folic acid.

Therapeutic Applications of Cobalamin

Besides the treatment of pernicious anemia and iron deficiency, there are several applications for B12 therapy, including asthma, bursitis, calcium bone spurs, chronic fatigue, alcoholism, and GI tract disturbances. The following also respond positively to B12 supplementation:

- Mental disorders. Because pernicious anemia involves severe mental disturbance, there has been interest in determining if other mental disorders, such as paranoia and depression, might be the result of low B12 blood levels. Research in Norway determined that fifteen percent of patients admitted to mental hospitals have abnormally low B12 levels; symptoms are alleviated with B12 injections. Other studies have reported that B12 injections assist even severely mentally disturbed patients, and one study documented the fact that B12 injections increased the test subjects' feeling of well-being and self-esteem while placebo injections did not.

- Immune system insufficiencies. People suffering from chronic immune deficiency respond to B12 supplementation.
- Chronic physical and mental fatigue. These syndromes often respond to periodic B12 injections.
- Allergy. A recent study from La Jolla's Scripps Institution (part of the University of California, San Diego) indicates that 1,000 mcg daily of oral B12 effectively prevented hypersensitivity reactions to the widely used restaurant preservative metasulfite. B12 worked as well as medication, but with no reported side effects.

Cobalamin Supplementation

Again, the 100–600 mcg of B12 recommended at OHL is a far cry from the 3 mcg RDA, but it is a safe and useful dosage in combination with routine supplementation.

Vegetarians should be particularly careful to get enough B12, since its sources are chiefly animal products. B12 deficiency is not common in vegetarians, however, because B12 is provided in fermented foods such as miso and tempeh, in brewer's yeast, and in sprouted beans and grains, whose natural bacterial activity produces B12.

FOLIC ACID

Now we come to the B vitamins without numbers—folic acid, biotin, para-aminobenzoic acid (PABA), inositol, and choline.

Folic acid was originally distilled from spinach and got its name from the Latin *folium*, "leaf." It is essential for many important physiological functions:

- The basic maintenance of the blood and immune system.
- The synthesis of the genetic materials DNA and RNA.
- The production and maturation of red and white blood cells and the production of antibodies.

- The metabolism of amino acids.
- Good digestion and the production of hydrochloric acid.
- The formation of collagen, in combination with other nutrients.
- The prevention and treatment of certain anemias in close relationship with B12 and iron.

Therapeutic Applications of Folic Acid

Because of its role as an essential building block in so many vital biochemical processes, folic acid is important as a component of general supplement therapy in a wide range of disorders, including folic-acid-deficiency anemia, circulatory problems, atherosclerosis, menstrual problems, ulcers, and alcoholism.

While folic acid in large doses can relieve the *symptoms* of fatigue and weaknesses that come with pernicious anemia, it does not cure the primary cause, which is reduced ability to absorb B12. Because of this false healing effect, it is illegal (and more to the point, dangerous) for a nonprescription tablet to contain more than 1,000 mcg of folic acid. Injectable B12 is needed for control.

When taken in sufficient quantity, folic acid appears to be effective in treating the subtle problems of learning disorders and anxiety.

Folic acid is especially needed during pregnancy. Deficiency can lead to toxemia, premature birth, and anemia in both mother and child. Folic-acid deficiency may also cause birth defects, especially neural tube defects such as spina bifida.

Folic-Acid Supplementation

The adult RDA for folic acid is 400 mcg, with a jump to 600 for lactating women and 800 for pregnant women. Depending on its therapeutic use, 500–5,000 mcg can be taken safely.

BIOTIN

The micronutrient biotin is needed in very minute traces. However, these small amounts are required for the metabolism of essential fatty acids and for the synthesis and conversion of many amino acids. Many of the other B vitamins cannot function optimally without the presence of biotin, and it is necessary for the metabolism of carbohydrates, fats, and proteins.

Taken with a balance of B vitamins, biotin contributes to overall maintenance of the cardiovascular system and to healthy skin, nails, and hair. Its most controversial therapeutic application, though, may be in the treatment of *Candida albicans* overgrowth (candidiasis) and all its far-reaching, potentially devastating effects.

A significant amount of biotin is manufactured by intestinal bacteria. The optimal amount has not been established.

PABA, OR PARA-AMINOBENZOIC ACID

PABA is actually a vitamin within a vitamin, in that it is found in nature only in combination with folic acid. In conjunction with folic acid, it is necessary for cell growth. On its own, it makes a contribution to viral resistance and has reportedly been successful in treating Rocky Mountain spotted fever.

PABA is needed to form red and white blood cells, and for stimulation of intestinal bacteria, which in turn produce folic acid, biotin, and other B vitamins. It functions in the metabolism of protein and is a prime antioxidant. Many people are familiar with PABA as the active ingredient in sunscreens, as it shields the skin from harmful ultraviolet solar radiation.

In addition to its purported therapeutic use with Rocky Mountain spotted fever, skin and tissue disturbances and general GI tract irritations call for PABA supplementation. Applied externally, PABA is commonly used to prevent sunburn.

Supplemental doses of PABA fall in the 10–200 mg range. Doses over 1,000 mg can cause nausea and vomiting, which is reversed by lowering intake. Do not take PABA while you are taking sulfa drugs; they cancel each other out.

CHOLINE

Strictly speaking, choline is not a vitamin, because it is synthesized within the body from the amino acids methionine and serine. The body's production of choline is often insufficient for our needs, however, so additional supplies must be obtained from diet or supplements.

Because choline is needed for the synthesis of lecithin, it is an important factor in the metabolism and regulation of fats and cholesterol. And it is needed for the proper function of the liver, gallbladder, and kidneys. The integrity of cell membranes depends on choline. Choline converts to acetylcholine, an important neurotransmitter, and thus it is important in the transmission of nerve impulses and in memory. It is needed in the formation of so-called methyl groups, biochemical compounds that help the body in detoxification processes. It is essential for the health of the myelin sheath, the protective coating of the nervous system, and it prevents abnormal platelet aggregation, thus helping to keep artery walls from becoming clogged with fats and plaque.

Cardiovascular disease, high blood pressure, abnormal blood clotting, and elevated cholesterol are helped by choline in combination with other supplements. With essential fatty acids and B6, it has proved effective in the treatment of tardive dyskinesia, often a drug-induced disorder resulting from long-term tranquilizer abuse, and research indicates its possible therapeutic use with memory improvement. Other known applications are in the treatment of alcoholism and liver disease.

There is no established RDA for choline, although it is estimated that the average American consumes about 400–900 mg a day. Our recommended dosage range of choline is 300–1,000 mg. In doses over 2,000 mg, it can cause diarrhea (the body's natural detoxifying mechanism) and perhaps a fishy body odor as it is broken down in the intestines.

INOSITOL

Like choline, inositol is not considered a true vitamin, because it is synthesized in the body from glucose; because of this relationship, it is sometimes referred to as muscle sugar. Inositol stores are concentrated in the brain and in heart muscle, skeletal muscle, and other tissues.

At least five inositol functions have been identified: Along with choline, it is essential for the synthesis of lecithin and is therefore a factor in the metabolism of fats and cholesterol and in the proper function of the liver and kidneys. It may help keep artery walls free of fat and plaque deposits. Because it may be converted to glucose, it contributes to energy metabolism. Under laboratory conditions in animal studies, it has been helpful in enhancing brain function. And it is needed for hair growth.

Taken in concert with other B vitamins, it may be important in the treatment of heart disease, abnormal platelet aggregation, and premature (nongenetic) hair loss. There are no known side effects of inositol. Dosages of 100–1,000 mg are recommended.

VITAMIN C

In 1749 a surgeon in the Royal Navy discovered that scurvy could be prevented by supplementing sailors' diets with limes, lemons, and oranges. But more than 150 years passed before the magic component of citrus was identified as ascorbic acid, or Vitamin C. And it wasn't until the 1970s, when Linus Pauling published his so-called wild ideas about the role of megadoses of Vitamin C in the prevention and cure of disease, that Vitamin C came into its own. So much has now been written about the powers of this incredible vitamin that even the skeptical have been known to pop Vitamin C when they feel a cold coming on.

What Does It Do?

In one way or another, Vitamin C seems to be involved in almost all bodily functions. It is needed for the formation of collagen, a protein connective tissue that acts as the biological cement that holds cells together. It is needed for the replacement of old tissue and the generation of new, making it invaluable for wound healing. Healthy teeth and bones depend on its presence for strength and flexibility, as do the walls of capillaries and veins.

Vitamin C's capabilities are not limited to structural functions, however. It plays an essential role in the synthesis of several proteins, including those that play a role in many enzymatic and hormonal processes. It helps metabolize calcium and folic acid and aids in the use and absorption of iron, and is critical in the formation of the health-promoting prostaglandins PGE1 and PGE3. It can also greatly lower elevated blood levels of cholesterol and uric acid.

Its most profound effects, however, are in the overall strength of the immune system. Vitamin C is instrumental in the production of interferon, the body's own antiviral agent. And it stimulates the body's anti-infection white blood cells, the phagocytes, to seek out and devour bacteria and viruses.

It is a natural antihistamine. Vitamin C seems to stabilize mast cells (which normally release symptom-causing histamines in the airways and GI tract in the presence of allergens), thus preventing allergic reactions. It also enhances the action of the enzyme histaminase, which quickly metabolizes histamine. Asthmatics, especially those suffering from exercise-induced asthma, hay fever sufferers, arthritics, and those suffering from viral infections can all benefit from the immune support provided by Vitamin C.

Vitamin C also acts as a powerful antioxidant, detoxifying many harmful free-radical substances, both those in the environment and those produced by the body.

Therapeutic Applications of Vitamin C

We regularly use large therapeutic doses of Vitamin C to help our patients stabilize allergic reactions and to help them through the uncomfortable first few days of withdrawal, when they give up their allergic/addictive foods. This Vitamin C therapy is discussed on page 262.

But there are many other therapeutic uses for C:

- Linus Pauling found that, for many people, daily doses of 250–1,000 mg of Vitamin C would make the immune system strong enough to fend off cold viruses. And he demonstrated in his studies that in the early stages of a cold, 10–15 grams of C daily would in some instances stimulate interferon production and strengthen antiviral cells to fight off the cold.
- Extra C is even more vital in the case of serious infection, for the body's C is mobilized to fight the infection and drained away from other areas of the body where it is needed. This depletion can make us more vulnerable than ever to allergies, rheumatoid arthritis, depression, elevated cholesterol, and other problems.
- Because of its role in maintaining healthy tissue and as a powerful anti-inflammatory antioxidant, supplemental doses of C are important in the prevention and treatment of most degenerative diseases.
- Cancer is both an immune system disease and a disease of the cells. Vitamin C's dual action in stimulating the thymus, promoting interferon production and healthy leukocytes, its role in maintaining a proper prostaglandin balance through control of fatty-acid metabolism, and its role in collagen tissue formation make it a potentially valuable cancer-fighting nutrient.
- Studies at the University of Washington have demonstrated that Vitamin C prevents the gums from being permeated by the microorganisms that cause periodontal disease.
- There is increasing evidence that Vitamin C's restorative powers promote recovery from heart attack and in some cases strengthen the walls of veins and arteries. Serum cholesterol levels also decrease when an appropriate supplemental source of C is added to the diet. An Australian study demonstrated that C-deficient lab monkeys had elevated cholesterol, but quickly recovered when C was added to their food. In an English study, the total blood cholesterol level of elderly patients decreased in just six weeks through the addition of just one gram of C daily to their regular diets. At our California clinics, we routinely use supplemental Vitamin C as part of our program to reduce elevated serum cholesterol.

Vitamin C Supplementation

How much C should you take? *Plenty*—at least 3 grams a day as a maintenance dose and up to 90 percent bowel tolerance. If you are taking more Vitamin C than you need, you will develop a slight diarrhea; this will go away as soon as you cut back 10 percent or so on the amount you're taking. I recommend that you test yourself to determine your own optimal dosage by taking C until the onset of diarrhea. Your correct dose will then be about 90 percent of the amount that induced diarrhea. This is what "90 percent bowel tolerance" means.

One reported side effect (one not proved in my clinical experience with thousands of Vitamin C-supplemented patients) is that large doses of Vitamin C can promote calcium oxalate kidney stones in those with a previously diagnosed tendency for them, especially in conjunction with deficiencies of magnesium and B6. Others are loss of tooth enamel and gastrointestinal irritation when C is taken in acidic form. But it's my feeling that, in conjunction with overall good nutrition, hefty daily doses of C can do you nothing but good, especially when it comes to protection from viral infections and allergic reactions.

Research at our clinical lab has shown that Vitamin C in crystal form is preferable to powder, which in turn is preferable to capsules, which in turn are better than tablets. Buffered C, as it is called, contains calcium ascorbate, magnesium, potassium, and zinc bicarbonates. In this nonacidic form, it apparently works to neutralize mast-cell-mediated allergic responses in the gastrointestinal tract and is more completely absorbed into the blood, so that serum levels of C are increased dramatically. It also helps prevent the loose-bowel response that some people suffer at high doses. Finally, because it is nonacidic, buffered C diminishes the tooth enamel loss and gastrointestinal irritation.

VITAMIN E—TOCOPHEROL

With the possible exception of Vitamin C, no other vitamin has been as controversial and has had so many provocative claims made about it as Vitamin E. Known as tocopherol, from the Greek meaning "to give birth" or "bring forth," it was so named in 1922 by its discoverers Evans and Bishop, who found that rats deprived of this new nutrient became sterile. This led to claims that it would improve virility and enhance sexual prowess, though the connection between these particular functions and infertility are pretty slim. But thus the reputation of E as the "sex vitamin" was off and running.

On the other hand, the medical community has stuck to its role of archconservative regarding Vitamin E and actually reduced the RDA originally set in 1968. This of course goes back to the head-in-the-sand attitude that equates the absence of a severe deficiency state with good health.

Functions of Vitamin E

Research has shown that while Vitamin E is unlikely to improve your sex life directly, it has extremely valuable applications. For one thing, it is a powerful antioxidant, protecting the body, the cellular membranes, the genetic material within cells, and many of the nutrients you take in, from oxidation and free-radical damage. This, and its role in essential-fatty-acid metabolism and prostaglandin balance, account for many of its powers, as follows:

- Protects fatty acids from breaking down and becoming rancid.
- Maintains the effectiveness of Vitamin C and the B vitamins by protecting them from oxidation.
- Increases the efficiency of muscles, especially the heart muscle, by reducing oxygen requirements.
- Protects hormones, particularly the pituitary and adrenal gland hormones.
- Protects the genetic material DNA from free-radical oxidation, which may work to prevent cancer.
- Protects the myelin nerve sheaths.
- Alleviates arthritis pain. In a recent medical study from Israel, Vitamin E offered 52 percent of osteoarthritics significant pain relief (as opposed to 12 percent with placebo alone).
- Performs several extraordinarily important cardiovascular functions. Vitamin E prevents abnormal blood clotting by slowing clotting time, decreasing and controlling platelet aggregation or stickiness, and slowing activity of the clot-inducing prostanoid thromboxane A2. It is also needed for the manufacture of another prostaglandin called PGI2 or prostacyclin, the body's natural anticlotting hormone. And it functions to strengthen capillaries and to guard against their increased permeability.
- Performs several immune-system functions. *The Journal of the American Geriatric Society* reported that lab mice gained immune strength from supplemental doses of E. This probably occurs because of Vitamin E's role in prostaglandin formation and inhibition of free radicals. This has implications not only for viral and bacterial infections, but for cancer, heart disease, strokes, allergies, aging, and wound healing. Under test condi-

tions, autoimmune diseases such as lupus erythematosus have shown improvement. (Autoimmune diseases are those caused by antibodies that attack the body that produces them, as though the tissues were allergic to themselves.)

- Acts as a detoxifier. The common air pollutants ozone and nitrous oxide do their damage by promoting oxidation of fats in cells and membranes. Researchers at Duke University have demonstrated that Vitamin E's antioxidant effect protects lung tissue from air pollutants—when taken in doses six times greater than the RDAs.

Therapeutic Applications of Vitamin E

Many of Vitamin E's uses have to do with its antioxidant powers and its role in promoting a balance of prostaglandins.

- Cystic breast disease. Vitamin E increases adrenal hormone production, which is directly linked to the reduction of noncancerous cystic breast disease. A Baltimore study, conducted by Dr. Robert London of Sinai Hospital, found that 600 IUs daily eliminated or reduced these painful cysts. The problem returned when supplementation was discontinued.
- Abnormal blood clotting. E's ability to reduce abnormal blood clotting has implications for those suffering from atherosclerosis, diabetes, thrombophlebitis, strokes, perhaps cancer, and for anyone taking oral contraceptives. Women on the pill have lowered levels of Vitamin E and a higher risk of abnormal blood clots. Supplementary E (up to 1,200 IU a day) may reverse this.
- Thrombophlebitis. World-renowned cardiovascular surgeon Dr. Michael DeBakey and a group of New Orleans doctors have successfully used intravenous Vitamin E for patients with inflamed thrombosis of the veins.
- Atherosclerosis. Vitamin E not only reduces abnormal platelet clumping, but also lowers elevated serum cholesterol and raises the level of beneficial HDL cholesterol.
- PMS. Because of its role in the production of prostaglandins, E is helpful in controlling premenstrual syndrome. In connection with his Baltimore study of cystic breast disease, Dr. London asked subjects to rate their PMS symptoms. The Vitamin E therapy, intended for cystic breast treatment, unexpectedly brought dramatic improvements in PMS.
- The bends. Vitamin E is now routinely used to prevent seizures in hyperbaric oxygen therapy, traditionally used to treat deep-sea divers for the bends.

Other areas of Vitamin E therapy include adrenal and pituitary insufficiencies, general allergy control, migraines, liver disease, ulcers, anemia, and prevention of infant blindness.

Vitamin E Supplementation

I hope I've convinced you that you should disregard the minuscule RDA of 12–15 IU of E daily. Depending on its therapeutic application, 50–1,200 IU are recommended. Be sure you are not hypersensitive or allergic to the oil in which your brand of E is suspended and that it is stored properly to prevent rancidity. To combine the vitamin with synergistic selenium, there are brands of "dry" E that contain no carrier oil. Those who have problems with fat digestion and absorption should go out of their way to obtain Vitamin E in the more easily absorbable micellized liquid form.

Vitamin E should not be taken in conjunction with heart medications, blood pressure medications, or anticoagulants, or by diabetics, without a doctor's advice. Since some people—very few—have reported a temporary rise in blood pressure from taking E, dosage should begin at 100 IU and be increased gradually, with daily monitoring of one's blood pressure.

Do not be put off by the many variations under which you may find E sold—alpha, dl alpha, tocopherol acetate, or succinate. The differences are minimal and the distinctions not important enough to bother about here.

9

Minerals

Vitamins seem to steal the spotlight when it comes to supplementation. But minerals, along with amino acids and essential fatty acids, also play powerful roles in our body chemistry. Minerals go hand in hand with vitamins in building healthy bones, teeth, tissue, and blood, and in regulating the activities of hormones, chemical mediators, and enzymes that affect everything from digestion to emotions to immune protection to thought. Unlike some vitamins, minerals cannot be synthesized from various chemicals. They are not manufactured in the body and must be obtained, in complete form, through diet or supplementation.

The eighteen essential minerals are classified as either bulk or trace minerals. Bulk minerals are those needed in relatively large quantities on a regular basis: calcium, potassium, magnesium, chloride, sodium, phosphorus, and silicon. Trace minerals are needed only in minute quantities: iron, chromium, fluoride, copper, cobalt, iodine, vanadium, manganese, selenium, molybdenum, and zinc.

The presence of minerals in our diet is affected not only by what we choose to eat, but by the conditions under which our food is grown or brought to market. Sun, soil, harvest, and transport conditions affect our fruit, vegetables, nuts, seeds, and grains. Overfarming our lands purportedly depletes them of valuable minerals like iron, zinc, and selenium. Many animals raised for meat eat chemical-laden diets and live their lives without benefit of sun or fresh air. Processing, refining, and perhaps "enriching" our food further adds to the unpredictability of its mineral content. Even if we had a reliable way of measuring the mineral content of our food, we still have the problem of determining how much of our mineral intake is actually being absorbed into the bloodstream where it can be put to use.

A deficiency in any one of these minerals can lead to serious medical problems, from the regulation of cellular activity, to the integrity of our teeth and bones, to the ability of the blood to transport oxygen. I have seen too many patients whose health problems could be traced back to a single mineral deficiency. A teenager whose raging acne cleared up entirely after zinc supplementation. A case of high blood pressure and cardiac arrhythmias completely reversed after severe magnesium deficiency was diagnosed by a simple blood test. And it would be impossible to count the tired, worn-out people who just needed more iron.

A routine blood-chemistry test can detect some, though by no means all, mineral deficiencies. It is useful more as an indication of further testing, as a barometer of potential problems. This basic blood chemistry is part of a complete blood work-up available from your doctor or a major lab. Because at Optimum Health Labs we are interested not just in average but *optimum* blood levels of all nutrients, our blood mineral analysis approaches the problem a bit more critically. Each of ten minerals is tested separately, using procedures developed specifically for that mineral. Some of these procedures are mentioned under the individual mineral discussions that follow.

While a low blood level of a particular mineral may point to a dietary lack, it may also indicate other problems. A potassium deficiency, for example, is rarely a problem of dietary intake. Rather, it often reflects careless use of diuretics or laxatives, overconsumption of sodium, or kidney, intestinal, or stomach problems. A deficiency in sodium or chloride, the major salts in your body (called electrolytes), often indicate trouble with the regulation of the kidneys or adrenals. Calcium and inorganic phosphorus are also controlled not only by diet, but also by the bioavailability of Vitamin D, by the consumption of magnesium, or by the kidneys and the parathyroid. Found predominantly in the bones, calcium and phosphorus also play an important role in the blood chemistry. Low serum iron or magnesium levels can point to all kinds of chronic health problems, from gastrointestinal bleeding to malabsorption or diuretic abuse.

As with vitamins, there is such a thing as too much—or too little—of a given mineral. The bell-shaped curve (Figure 2, page 32) applies to trace minerals as well. As usual, the optimal amount is in the middle, while the marginal states fall on either side of the optimum amount. The danger falls at either end of the curve—deficiency on the low end and toxicity on the high end.

For this reason, minerals should not be taken indiscriminately. The desirable supplemental amount for each mineral varies considerably—from a suggested 1 mg a day of copper to 1,000 mg of calcium.

As might be expected, these amounts differ considerably from the RDAs (recommended daily allowances). While the RDA is higher than ours in a couple of cases, the powers that be seem to find no use at all for some minerals that we more clinically experienced nutritionists feel are sorely lacking in most diets. Vitamins and minerals, by the way, should not be packaged together, because some vitamins and minerals (e.g., iron and Vitamin E) negatively affect each other in storage. They can be taken together, however, assuming there is the buffering effect of food consumed at the same time.

Those minerals most central to the Optimum Health Program are discussed below. Complete tables for these and the remaining minerals begin on page 174.

IRON

Though only a trace mineral, iron has far more than a trace of influence on our health. Absorbed through the gastrointestinal mucosa, bound and carried to storage by the protein transferrin, it combines with another protein in the body to form hemoglobin, the red-colored material inside red blood cells needed to carry life-sustaining oxygen to all cells.

Iron serves other bodily functions as well. It stimulates the thymus gland and thus is important to the immune system. It is needed in sufficient amounts to allow Vitamin B12 and folic acid to do their job. It also plays a critical role in the formation of the active form of thyroid hormone and an essential muscle protein, myoglobin. Studies on humans conducted by Tucker and colleagues at the University of North Dakota concluded that iron plays a role in attention span, ability to concentrate, verbal fluency, analytic thought, and abstract cognitive performance.

Iron deficiency is thought to be the single most common nutritional deficiency in the world today. Infant anemia is common. Many children and teenagers, many men, and 30–50 percent of all women are suboptimal or deficient in iron. The average American woman, consuming 1,500–2,000 calories a day, gets only 9 mg of iron—50 percent of the RDA. Athletes, who tend to put strenuous demands on their system without thinking about nutritional compensation, are often laid low by inadequate iron (more about this on page 395).

There are many instances in which increased iron intake is indicated: pregnancy, breast-feeding, vegetarianism, competitive and endurance sports, and the rapid growth periods of infancy and adolescence. Food allergies can lead to iron deficiency via chronic bowel irritation and a small but constant loss of blood. Iron is also depleted by caffeine, antacids, the antibiotic tetracycline, Vitamin C deficiency, excess menstrual flow, or competition from certain other minerals (such as calcium and magnesium) for absorption.

Anemia is not the only manifestation of iron deficiency. As Table 5 below shows, there are two stages of iron deficiency that precede anemia. And while standard blood chemistry tests and blood counts can easily pick up on iron-deficiency anemia, they often fail to detect the two levels of iron deficiency that lead up to full-blown anemia. But even at the lowest level, iron deficiency can have us walking around feeling subpar, suffering from fatigue, muscle weakness or spasms, insomnia, proneness to recurring infections, or general mental lethargy. The diagnostic techniques and the symptomology of all three levels of iron depletion are shown in the table.

Occasionally, toxic levels of iron are a problem. Alcoholism and oversupplementation with iron can lead to a disease of iron metabolism known as hemosiderosis, characterized by excess body stores of iron, especially in the liver. Hemosiderosis is associated with cirrhosis (scar-

Table 5—The Three Stages of Iron Deficiency

Stage	Method of Detection	Physiological Consequence
I. Total body iron depletion	Serum ferritin	Depletion of iron store in liver, spleen, and bone marrow.
II. Iron deficiency (red blood cell formation)	Serum iron Total iron-building capacity Transferrin saturation	Iron stores have been depleted, and levels of iron carried in the plasma decrease, and transferrin formation in the liver increases. Total iron-binding capacity increases to levels of 400–500 mg/100 ml. Percentage of saturation of transferrin with iron falls from a mean of 30 percent to about 15–18 percent.
III. Iron-deficiency anemia	Hemoglobin RBC count Hematocrit Mean cell hemoglobin concentration	Hemoglobin concentration falls below 12 gm/100 ml. The degree of iron-deficiency anemia can be evaluated with additional blood data.

ring) of the liver, increased incidence of liver cancer, sepsis (severe bacterial infection), diabetes, and heart disease. The transferrin-transporting protein becomes saturated with iron and unable to handle yet more. The untransported excess iron deposits itself in the lungs, pancreas, and heart, as well as the liver.

A serum ferritin test will catch iron deficiency (or excess) at all levels, before red blood cells become affected. Ferritin is a protein that aids in the storage of iron (as transferrin does in the transporting of iron). Its level in the blood serum accurately reflects the body's total iron stores, and correlates well with iron levels in the bone marrow, spleen, heart, kidneys, intestinal mucosa, and liver.

CALCIUM

Calcium is the most abundant mineral in the body. The average adult is carrying around 3 to 4 pounds of calcium, 97 percent of it in the teeth and bones. But calcium is needed for more than healthy teeth and bones. It also plays a role in nerve transmission, cell permeability, and blood pressure regulation.

Women in the prime of life are especially susceptible to calcium malutilization and deficiency; deficiency is found in as many as 30 percent of American women over the age of nine. In addition, over 40 percent of *postmenopausal* women suffer from osteoporosis—a weakness and brittleness of the bones as the result of calcium loss. Until recently, osteoporosis was considered an inevitable condition of aging ("brittle old bones"). But evidence indicates that the incidence of osteoporosis is much higher in those with a low calcium intake and that the condition can be improved dramatically with proper calcium supplementation, along with daily weight-bearing exercise and additional Vitamin D. Please note that premenopausal women who exercise to a level resulting in amenorrhea (no periods) experienced osteoporosis of the vertebral bodies (backbone). Again, the bell-shaped curve—too much *or* too little (in this case, exercise) is no good.

Deficiencies of calcium can also lead to childhood rickets, stunted growth, muscle cramping, abnormally heavy menstruation, hypertension (high blood pressure), nervousness, insomnia, irritability, and perhaps immune-system suppression.

Now, don't run to the refrigerator and drink a quart of milk. It is a big mistake to consider milk the best source of calcium. Milk does contain lots of calcium; in fact it accounts for 75 percent of all the calcium Americans imbibe. But the *great majority of people worldwide* are allergic to milk, and/or are lactose intolerant, meaning that they lack the enzyme necessary to digest the milk sugar, lactose. In fact, in some cases the digestive problems associated with milk may lead to intestinal inflammation or bleeding and actually *cause* calcium deficiency. (More about lactose intolerance on page 243).

Since absorbable calcium is in plentiful supply in many vegetables, beans, nuts, seeds, and fish, it is certainly preferable to get our calcium from these sources (and from supplements) than to load up on the artery-clogging fats of whole milk and leave ourselves open to serious allergies and bowel disturbances. Sufficient quantities of dietary magnesium, sunshine-induced Vitamin D, and gastric hydrochloric acid are necessary for the assimilation of calcium. Iron, on the other hand, competes with calcium and magnesium for absorption and should be taken separately. A list of calcium-rich nondairy foods appears on page 441.

MAGNESIUM

Magnesium is the second most abundant mineral in the human body, working closely with calcium to regulate heart and muscles. Research has shown that magnesium—often called the antistress mineral—has a calming effect, resembling that of a natural sedative. Along with B6, it prevents the formation of calcium oxalate stones, the common form of kidney stones, gallstones, and calcium deposits. Like phosphorus, it is a constituent of bone and soft tissue. A cofactor of essential-fatty-acid metabolism, it plays a significant role in the prevention and treatment of various forms of cardiovascular disease. In fact, all the functions of essential fatty acids and prostaglandins are influenced by magnesium deficiency—abnormal blood clotting, elevated cholesterol, premenstrual syndrome, high blood pressure, lowered body metabolism and temperature, asthma, obesity, and hyperactivity.

A sufficient intake of magnesium may be extremely important in the treatment of hypertension, alcoholism, tooth decay, and overweight. A recent study reported in *Science* shows that low magnesium levels are common with a condition of pregnancy called preeclampsia. Preeclampsia is associated with high blood pressure, fluid retention, proteinuria, coagulation defects, and inadequate oxygen supply to the uterus, placenta, and fetus during pregnancy. Over 5 million pregnant women and fetuses die from preeclampsia each year. Supplementation with magnesium reduces blood pressure, improves blood coagulation, and prevents oxygen deprivation, thus adding strong nondrug support to other treatment the patient may require.

Although magnesium is in plentiful supply in the food chain, deficiencies can nevertheless result from the chronic use of oral contraceptives, the abuse of diuretics, a diet too high in saturated and trans fats and processed foods, or an excess of dietary calcium and oxalic acid and vegetables containing the mineral-binding phytate (or phytic acid).

Standard blood chemistry tests for serum levels of magnesium do not reveal actual deficiencies because intracellular magnesium concentrations are not always reflected in blood concentration levels. At our laboratory we prefer that red-blood-cell magnesium levels be checked.

Magnesium is most beneficial when taken in a multimineral supplement containing 3 parts calcium to 2 parts magnesium, along with betaine HCl to enhance assimilation.

ZINC

Zinc turns out to be far more influential in our body chemistry than had been realized. Though the RDA for zinc is only 15 mg per day, supplemental levels of 20–50 and in some cases even 100 mg have had remarkable effects on acne, acrodermatitis, eczema, and psoriasis, and even with hyperactivity, learning disabilities, and (in lozenge form) the common cold. It plays an important role in alcoholism (zinc deficiency is strongly connected to the fetal alcohol syndrome) and in cardiovascular health. It is a vital cofactor of essential-fatty-acid metabolism, especially in the conversions of DHGLA (dihomo/gamma linolenic acid) to PGE1 (see Figure 5, page 146). Also, along with niacin, it is important in hydrochloric acid production in the stomach.

Zinc is thus a powerful immune-system stimulant. It activates the thymus gland, which in turn produces the immune-cell-stimulating hormone thymosin. Thymosin differentiates the various lymphocytes of the immune system, including T-lymphocytes and cancer-destroying "natural killer" cells. Zinc is known to aid in the restoration of the integrity, and thus the permeability, of the skin and mucosal linings of the air passages and the gastrointestinal tract. It increases the levels of the protective secretory immunoglobin A (IgA) in the saliva and in the intestinal tract and also is needed for IgM and IgG production.

Zinc may even be a simple remedy for the common cold, preferable to aspirin. While aspirin alleviates cold symptoms, it does not alter the course of disease and may interfere with the beneficial healing effects of fever. One double-blind study showed that patients whose colds were treated with zinc were sick for only 3.7 days, as opposed to 10.8 days for the placebo-treated patients. (This most likely occurs as a result of zinc's ability to enhance the immune system.)

Indications of a zinc deficiency are injuries and fractures that don't heal, chronic inflammatory skin conditions, retarded growth in a child, abnormal cravings for sweets, impaired taste or smell, *excessive tooth decay,* frequent infections, hair splitting, poor appetite and circulation, and high cholesterol levels.

Zinc deficiency is perhaps best detected by an RBC (red blood cell) zinc determination and atomic spectrophotometry, *not* by serum zinc levels.

SELENIUM

Selenium is a relatively hard-to-obtain but vital mineral that has only recently been recognized as playing an important part in human biochemistry. Though animals that produce milk, wool, and meat have been given selenium supplements for decades, the RDAs for selenium in humans were not even established before 1978.

Working closely with Vitamin E, selenium is a major antioxidant, protecting the body against free-radical damage to cell membranes and intracellular genetic material. It influences essential-fatty-acid metabolism, protein synthesis, the immune system, and the maintenance of normal growth and fertility. It also strengthens the retina of the eye by causing proliferation of retinal blood vessels and improves retinal light reception. It may play a role in the prevention of cataracts. In addition, it regulates certain prostaglandin functions and is essential to the optimal effect of Vitamin E. In conjunction with Vitamin E, its therapeutic value has been asserted in the treatment of cancer, Osgood-Schlatter disease (inflammation of the bone growth center just below the knees), and heart disease. It is involved with healing wounds and in combating the toxicity of pollution.

Deficiency symptoms may include the brown aging spots found on the skin, poor hair and skin tone, repeated infections, cataracts, hemolytic problems, heart disease, male sterility, cardiac drug toxicity, and perhaps propensity toward cancers.

The optimal selenium intake is 50–400 mcg a day. Overdose—in the unlikely event of continuous selenium intake over 1,000 mcg daily—can cause nausea, skin lesions, headaches, hair loss, fatigue, and lack of appetite. The cure for this is simply to cut back on the dosage.

10

Amino Acids

While fats and carbohydrates in the diet are needed to provide energy, only protein can build cells and repair tissue. And protein is made up entirely of amino acids, joined together in various sequences and configurations. Linked in long polypeptide chains, they form the proteins that make up much of muscle fibers, bone, hair, and collagen and other connective tissue. Grouped in round clusters, they form proteins that are the basis of the oxygen-carrying hemoglobin in our blood and of hormones such as insulin, thyroid, growth hormone, and all immune globulins (antibodies). In yet different patterns, amino acids act as the building blocks of the natural narcoticlike substances of the brain and body, enkephalin and beta endorphin. There is no cell in the body that does not depend on amino acids to fulfill literally thousands of complex biochemical functions. Whether joined to form antibodies, acting as components of digestive enzymes and hormones, working in the liver to form transport proteins to carry other dietary proteins, or giving their support to oxygen transport and muscle, they are needed for our equilibrium and well-being.

Amino acids are necessary for the transmission of nerve impulses (and consequently muscular contractions, heartbeats, thoughts, and feelings) across the synapses between nerve endings in the spinal cord, brain, and peripherally in the body. This "spark" they help create, sending electric impulses through the brain's neurological circuits, is involved with our moods, emotions, memory, arousal, and sleep. No wonder amino acids are sometimes called brain food.

Proteins and thus amino acids are involved in the formation of the basic genetic materials DNA and RNA. DNA and RNA are in turn instrumental in instructing amino acids on how to link together to form the proteins we call genes and chromosomes. It is a closed, interdependent, and delicate system. Thrown out of kilter by even a single amino-acid deficiency, the body's immune system can turn against its own genetic material, failing to recognize it and labeling it "foreign invader." This may lead to trouble known as autoimmune disease, susceptibility to viral and bacterial infection, and to degenerative disease processes. As mentioned above, antibody production, another immune system function, is also dependent on the amino acids.

The list of known amino-acid functions gets longer all the time. They can be used as a natural sleep aid, an antidepressant, an analgesic, or an appetite suppressant. They have been used to stimulate the thymus gland, to improve memory, to build muscle, to burn fat, to treat baldness, to stimulate the release of hormones, and to control weight. Because they guard against the breakdown of nerve and tissue, they are considered "anti-aging" nutrients.

Twenty dietary amino acids have been identified. Eight—and in some people nine—of these are considered essential because they must come from dietary or supplement sources. But even the "nonessential" ones, the ones we can make from other nutrients, are often *necessary* —when dietary sources are inadequate, or we lack the ability to manufacture them in adequate amounts.

The amino acids classified as essential are lysine, leucine, isoleucine, methionine, phenylalanine, histidine, threonine, tryptophan, and valine. Cysteine and tyrosine might as well be considered essential, since they are dependent on the others for their existence. Arginine may fit into this category as well, since it cannot be synthesized in quantity. The other "nonessential but necessary" amino acids are alanine, cystine, glutamine, glycine, hydroxyproline, proline, serine, and aspartic acid.

Inadequate intake of amino acids can lead to breakdowns in the system. A balance of amino acids can be obtained from a diet containing a continuous supply of quality protein (assuming complete digestion and absorption) or a supplement containing all the amino acids in correct balance. Most important, specific biochemical and physiological functions can be improved and optimized with therapeutic doses of individual amino acids.

DIETARY AND SUPPLEMENTARY SOURCES OF AMINO ACIDS

For years the medical profession operated on the "eat a steak" plan as the preferred method of getting an adequate supply of amino acids. What folly! Not only did this load the body up with proinflammatory saturated fats and hard-to-digest animal protein (potentially highly allergenic), but it overlooked the special uses of the individual amino acids.

The best source of amino acids is quality protein—protein food that contains an amino-acid ratio similar to that found in our own bodies.

Foods with the highest ratios are mother's milk (rated 100, a perfect score), whole egg protein (94), and cow's milk (85). Meat and fish rate between 86 and 76.

This does not mean that you have to eat a high-saturated-fat, high-cholesterol, highly allergenic diet to get the aminos you need. Fish and chicken are as good a source of essential amino acids as red meat. Rice is ranked 80, potatoes 78. As all vegetarians know, it is possible to get complete dietary proteins by combining certain vegetable protein foods in the same meal. Rice and kidney beans, for example, form a complete protein. The chart on page 445 will show you many ways to combine foods to get complete proteins.

A *variety* of quality protein in the diet is important, for the aminos function together in a delicate balance. A deficiency of one amino can lead not only to a breakdown in the functions it controls, but to a buildup of others and thus an imbalance.

To ensure an optimal amino-acid supply, you can take them in supplement form. Amino acids taken as supplements are "free form" amino acids, meaning that they are already completely digested into individual amino acids; in this form, they are much more easily and quickly absorbed from the GI tract, and, as a result, much less apt to be associated with digestive and allergic problems.

Amino acids are generally supplemented in one of two ways: one, a supplement containing all the amino acids in proper balance (recommended for those who have problems with the digestion of protein, for athletes, so that they don't "cannibalize" needed body protein in the course of strenuous training, and for people trying to lose weight); two, individual amino acids, singly or in combinations (taken therapeutically to treat special health conditions or problems).

It is these specialized uses of individual amino acids with which we are concerned here. An increasing number of competitive athletes, for example, take a combination of individual amino acids, which are reported in animal studies to stimulate the natural release of growth hormone, which in turn builds muscles, burns fat, stimulates the immune system, accelerates healing. This is a safe and legal practice, unlike the use of steroids. DL-phenylalanine is relieving chronic pain of arthritis, back pain, and migraine, with reported high success in relieving chronic depression as well. Lysine is proving effective for herpes sufferers, glutamine for alcoholics.

The reason for taking single amino acids is partly because it's impossible to eat enough individual amino-acid-rich food to provide a therapeutic dose. But, more important, it gives the individual amino acid a "head start." It is thought that different amino acids compete with one another to pass through the blood-brain barrier and enter the brain; under normal circumstances, an insufficient quantity of the desired amino acid gets through. Taken individually, it avoids the competition.

GUIDELINES FOR AMINO-ACID SUPPLEMENTATION

A discussion of six amino acids that we frequently use at Optimum Health Labs follows. But first a few guidelines for amino-acid supplementation:

- Individual amino acids should be taken on an empty stomach, between meals or before bed, with water or diluted fruit juice. *They should not be taken in conjunction and in competition with protein foods.*
- Be sure you are also following the routine Optimum Health Program supplementation schedule. All amino acids are dependent on certain vitamins, minerals, and essential fatty acids to do their job.
- Amino acids should not be taken indefinitely. They are meant to solve problems; when the problem is solved, therapy should be modified or discontinued. We do not as yet know the long-term impact of individual amino-acid supplementation. Be conservative and play it safe.
- Don't be in a rush. It may take one to three months to feel the full effect of amino-acid therapy.
- Take amino acids only in consultation with a nutritionally oriented physician. Many amino acids may have potentially harmful effects if taken in ignorance of correct dosages and combinations.

TRYPTOPHAN

L-tryptophan is often a big loser to other amino acids in competing for transportation through the brain barrier into brain tissue, where it can do its thing.

Through a fairly complex biochemical pathway, L-tryptophan in the brain is converted into the neurotransmitter serotonin. Serotonin has the power to stimulate or inhibit the transmission of nerve impulses—those "sparks" we talked about earlier—across the synapses.

Serotonin is sometimes called the sleep chemical. Scientists believe that serotonin is responsible for the normal sleep state, decreasing the electrical activity in the brain. In addition to promoting longer, more restful sleep, supplementary tryptophan can also reduce the time it takes to fall asleep by about 50 percent. And unlike sedative-induced sleep, tryptophan (in 1–5 gram dosages) does not produce sleep distortions (such as change in rapid eye movement, or REM, sleep) as measured by EEG recordings. In fact, sleep changes were not detected even after long-term tryptophan therapy, nor during the month after withdrawal.

Did you ever know anyone who needed a glass of warm milk or a cheese sandwich before bedtime? There's a logical explanation: These foods are both high in tryptophan. Incidentally, because tryptophan not only becomes serotonin but also becomes niacin (B3), supplementation with niacin results in increased serotonin from tryptophan and consequently the same benefits.

While large amounts of serotonin have a sedative effect—it can also reduce anxiety and depression in some people—moderate amounts improve memory, concentration, and the ability to make judgments. A deficiency of serotonin can lead to depression, restlessness, and lower pain and stress tolerance.

Tests done here and in Europe showed that commonly prescribed antidepressant drugs such as Elavil and Tofranil were no more effective than tryptophan in treating chronic depression. And tryptophan is not only far less toxic, but also seems to have longer, more sustained effectiveness.

Still other uses for tryptophan are now being explored. It has been observed that migraine sufferers seem to have lower blood serotonin levels than most people. In one study, 50 percent of migraine sufferers tested felt marked improvement while taking tryptophan. In another study, L-tryptophan at 3 grams daily significantly reduced pain associated with dental surgery. Its use in the treatment of alcoholism is also being studied. And yet another important function is its role in the formation of antibody-producing immune cells known as B-lymphocytes.

One last note about tryptophan. It is essential for the production of niacin, and niacin aids in the metabolism of tryptophan as well as the metabolism of essential fatty acids to health-regulating prostaglandins. So be sure you are taking your other supplements while taking tryptophan.

Note: For amino-acid supplementation tables, see page 186.

DL-PHENYLALANINE

Almost all protein derived from animal, nut, and vegetable sources contains the L- form of phenylalanine. L-phenylalanine is rapidly absorbed by the digestive tract and used as a building block for the body's protein tissues, brain neurotransmitters, hormones, and structural material. A few plants and bacteria produce the rarer D-phenylalanine. D-phenylalanine is then very slowly converted to L-phenylalanine. But during that interval before it is converted, the D-form works to enhance the production—and at the same time prevent the rapid breakdown—of a group of natural powerful painkillers, the endorphins. Thus D-phenylalanine has been shown to have remarkable natural, nontoxic pain-relieving effect in such chronic ailments as arthritis, bursitis, lower back pain, myalgias, neuralgias, migraine, PMS cramps, headaches, and sports- and work-related injuries.

This is a remarkable discovery, because chronic pain is the most disabling, expensive, and common medical disorder in America today. But although it physically and emotionally cripples tens of millions of people and robs them of their ability to lead happy and productive lives, most doctors and victims are lamentably unaware of the wide variety of nondrug, nonsurgical therapies for chronic pain, particularly in the areas of food-allergy control and nutrition.

The DL-Phenylalanine Breakthrough

The amino acid DL-phenylalanine, a fifty-fifty mixture of the two forms, is a major pain-management breakthrough. It is a powerful painkiller. Preliminary clinical reports show good to excellent relief of chronic pain syndromes in 70–80 percent of the subjects studied, with only 5–10 percent showing no relief. For example, 84 percent of the subjects with rheumatoid arthritis, 81 percent of those with osteoarthritis, 67 percent of those with migraines, and 73 percent of those with low back pain reported good to excellent results. Keep in mind here that the primary treatment of choice is elimination of food allergens from the diet.

DL-phenylalanine appears to enhance the effectiveness of acupuncture and reduce the need for other painkilling drugs by as much as 50 percent, and acts as an effective analgesic even when other painkillers have been of no help.

There have been no reported significant side effects or toxic reactions to therapeutic doses of DLP. This is an extremely exciting and unexpected discovery for a substance of such potent pain-reducing ability. Although two subjects experienced mild jitteriness from DLP, this symptom disappeared when the dosage was taken with meals. DLP seems even less toxic than many vitamins, which themselves have a wide range of safety. Nevertheless, DL-phenylalanine should not be taken by those who are pregnant, diabetic, or have high blood pressure, without a physician's recommendation and supervision. Also, infants or children with a condition called phenylketonuria should avoid it entirely.

To add to its luster, DLP is not addictive, and it is not tolerance-developing. In fact, the longer it is taken, the more effective it becomes in reducing pain. No other analgesic can make this claim.

Since the FDA reluctantly must classify DLP as a nutrient and amino acid, and not as a drug, it is presently available without prescription and at a reasonable cost. Again, this does not mean that chronic pain sufferers should attempt to diagnose and treat their condition on their own.

The pain-relief powers of DL-phenylalanine sometimes overshadow a couple of its other capabilities, which should be mentioned. It is essential in producing another amino acid, tyrosine, a direct precursor to another of the brain's mood-elevating neurotransmitters, norepinephrine. This hormone seems to counter depression, increase mental alertness and memory, and encourage the ability to make judgments. This hints at its usefulness in the treatment of learning disorders and psychological problems. Finally, L-phenylalanine is also converted to another transmitter, phenethylamine (PEA). PEA is chemically very similar to a known appetite suppressant and antidepressant, amphetamine, but without amphetamine's potential for serious toxicity.

Dosages

The effective pain-relief dosage for most people seems to be two 375 mg capsules three times a day (2,250 mg daily), preferably 20–30 minutes before each meal. Since test subjects taking 12,000 mg a day suffered no noticeable side effects, this is an extremely safe intake level for most people.

The above daily dose takes between two and fourteen days to begin working and about one to three weeks before significant pain relief occurs. Because it is slow-acting, it is not effective in acute, short-term kinds of pain. It can be taken in anticipation of pain, however. For instance, by taking it well in advance of the menstrual flow, you can often reduce or eliminate the monthly pain associated with it.

Some people find that they can cut back on the amount taken after the first pain relief is experienced. A number have even reported enjoying a pain-free month by taking DLP just one week out of the four.

ARGININE AND ORNITHINE

Arginine and ornithine are manufactured within human cells during normal body metabolism. Though considered nonessential, they are often in shorter supply than is optimally needed.

These two amino acids work together along with other nutrients to stimulate the release from the pituitary of human growth hormone (HGH). HGH is what allows children to reach adult size and to develop adult physical traits. HGH also appears to stimulate the immune system (thymus), accelerate wound healing, strengthen bones and connective tissue, prevent abnormal blood clotting, increase white fat metabolism, and increase muscle size and strength.

By the age of thirty, there is little HGH release, and most authorities agree that the blood level falls to near zero by the age of fifty. Nevertheless, biochemists have found that it is still stored in the pituitary and that therapeutic doses of arginine and ornithine (and to a lesser extent tyrosine and tryptophan) can stimulate HGH release, which in turn stimulates the immune system, increases protein synthesis, and alters the metabolism to burn fat instead of protein.

For this reason, arginine and ornithine have become the latest gimmick in the body-building and weight-loss industries. Amino-acid combinations sold as "fat blockers" and "fat fighters" have turned up on the market with big claims made for their weight-loss powers. But judging by our four-month-long clinical studies at OHL, with few exceptions they *do not promote overall weight loss.* However, in athletes they do seem to increase body leanness, muscle strength, and aerobic endurance.

This makes arginine and ornithine a very useful addition to the training regimens of men and women athletes looking for a safe, effective (nonsteroid) way to increase muscle mass and endurance. Two of our 1984 Olympic track-and-field athletes, who are also clients of OHL, John Powell and Carol Cady, swear by it. In fact, our studies show that it does this very effectively, though in some cases, since muscle weighs more than fat, the gain in muscle mass results in a slight overall weight gain. In other words, as the percentage of body fat goes down, weight goes up.

The availability of arginine/ornithine supplementation allows athletes (many of whom have been taking costly and dangerous injectable HGH) to switch to a safer and more humane procedure. But, more important, it frees up the limited supply of HGH for children suffering from pituitary dwarfism. Such children need HGH extracts in order to mature to adulthood, but the high demand for it among athletes makes a scarce commodity even scarcer—needlessly, as we have seen, since arginine/ornithine provides all the development athletes require.

Again, arginine/ornithine supplementation should be taken only in consultation with a nutrition- and sports-minded physician. For one thing, because arginine suppresses the utilization of lysine, it may bring on herpes flare-ups.

L-CARNITINE

Manufactured in the body from two other amino acids, lysine and methionine, L-carnitine is a nonessential amino acid. However, it can be produced only when there is a sufficient supply of these aminos, plus Vitamins C and B6 and iron.

L-carnitine has been demonstrated to play an important part in improving fat metabolism in the heart (as well as other organs and tissues), thus lowering cholesterol and triglycerides in the blood, raising HDL cholesterol, and perhaps preventing cardiovascular disease. It performs an additional cardiovascular function as a vasodilator, strengthening the heart and relieving angina and certain cardiac arrythmias.

L-carnitine finds its therapeutic use in its role as an efficient transporter of fatty acids through the cell membranes into the power plants of the cell, the mitochondria. This may be a boon to athletes, since a major function of fat is its use by the muscles as a secondary energy source. During exercise, the muscles burn a combination of fatty acids, glucose, and amino acids. If the muscles are able to burn fatty acids more efficiently, glucose stores last longer. Thus endurance-exercise time may be prolonged, muscle fatigue lessened, and oxygen uptake increased. Because of this, the athlete may be able to train and compete harder, without a buildup of fatigue- and exhaustion-inducing lactic acid. L-carnitine may give athletes an endurance edge.

L-LYSINE

L-lysine (in collaboration with Vitamin C and another amino acid, proline) is important in the formation of collagen, and thus it plays a major role in growth and repair of bone, cartilage, and connective tissue. And, like so many other amino acids, it is needed for the production of certain hormones, enzymes, and antibodies.

L-lysine is abundant in animal sources of protein—fish, chicken, eggs, milk—but deficient in grains, nuts, vegetables, etc. So unless vegetable proteins are properly combined (page 445), L-lysine is often inadequate in the diets of vegetarians or those who eat little meat.

The exciting news is that *L-lysine is proving extremely effective in treating the herpes simplex virus.* Since it is conservatively estimated that 50–75 percent of both adults and children (and 90 percent of the elderly) harbor this virus in either active or inactive form, that is good news indeed. Therapeutic doses of L-lysine are effective because they improve the balance of amino acids favorably, reducing viral growth. Most important in this balance of herpes-inhibiting amino acids is the ratio of L-lysine to arginine: the greater the ratio, the better for the suppression of the herpes virus. In tests at the University of Indiana, L-lysine supplementation was 96 percent effective in suppressing herpes symptoms; you couldn't do much better than that.

The suggested dose of L-lysine during an eruption of herpes simplex is two 500-mg capsules two to four times a day, until the infection has cleared. To keep the virus under control, a 500 mg capsule daily is recommended. More information about herpes treatment begins on page 383. One word of caution: Some scientific reports indicate that lysine can lead to elevated serum cholesterol in some people.

L-GLUTAMINE

L-glutamine is the form of glutamic acid that readily crosses the blood-brain barrier, where it is used by brain cells (in addition to glucose) as a fuel for their metabolism.

L-glutamine finds its therapeutic use in the treatment of alcoholism. The theory is that alcoholics, due either to a metabolic or a genetic imbalance in the brain, are unable to get enough glutamic acid through the brain barrier. Alcohol has been seen to improve the transport of glutamic acid across the brain barrier and may thus explain in part the alcoholic's craving. Therapeutic doses of the easily transportable L-glutamine appear to make it much easier for an alcoholic to nourish the brain cells and to stop drinking and to prevent mental deterioration. (Please keep in mind that—in addition to avoidance of alcohol—elimination of allergic and addictive foods and supplementation with essential fatty acids are the nutritional foundation of successful alcohol management.)

By extension, L-glutamine may prove effective with all forms of addiction, especially sugar/carbohydrate cravings. Too, because of its connection to brain-cell metabolism, it is being studied for possible use with psychiatric impairment and intelligence improvement. Therapy in connection with alcohol and tobacco addiction is discussed in Part V, under ADDICTION.

11

Essential Fatty Acids: The Missing Piece of the Nutrition Puzzle

Every so often a discovery is made that, like the importance of food allergy/addiction, seems to shed light on the whole picture of what constitutes good health. Such a discovery is the role of essential fatty acids (EFAs). As researcher Dr. Donald O. Rudin remarks, "They are the last major nutrient family to be recognized. In more ways than one, they are our nutritional missing link."

This breakthrough has opened up yet another major avenue of approach to optimum health—an avenue as important as the elimination of food allergies or the rotation diet or exercise, or vitamin and mineral supplementation. I am so convinced of the importance of the essential fats that they have become part of the suggested *routine* supplementation on the Optimum Health Program.

As research continues, the evidence piles up that the essential fats—specifically, a proper balance of essential fats—is a vital factor in many health disorders. The following is just a partial list of the problems that have a demonstrated connection to essential-fatty-acid deficiency or imbalance. It is the feeling of most people in the nutrition field that this list will continue to grow.

Brittle nails · Tinnitus, or ringing in the ears · Cold intolerance · Dry skin · Dandruff · Depression (especially the depressions of childhood, alcoholism, and PMS) · Alcoholism, hangover, and depression · PMS (premenstrual syndrome) · Cystic fibrosis · Cystic mastitis · Hyperactivity (with family history of hereditary allergy) · Genetic obesity (10–15 percent of all obese people) · Reactive hypoglycemia · Diabetes · Hypochlorhydria · Chronic pain or increased sensitivity to pain · Asthma · Eczema (atopic dermatitis) · Hypertension · Hypercholesterolemia · Low HDL cholesterol · Acute and chronic/relapsing schizophrenia · Multiple sclerosis · Irritable bowel syndrome/spastic colon · Abnormal platelet aggregation · Heart disease · Cancer · Agoraphobia · Infertility · Extreme thirst/tendency toward dehydration · Migraines · Arthritis.

The role of essential fats in the above disorders is discussed later in this chapter in the section beginning on page 147. But first let's see what the essential fats are and how they work.

UNDERSTANDING THE ESSENTIAL FATS

The nonessential and essential fatty acids occurring in nature fall into three classifications:

- Saturated fats, which are found abundantly in such commonly consumed foods as meat, milk products, eggs, and certain warm-seawater fish and shellfish—like shrimp, spiny lobster (sea crawfish), and crab.
- Mono- and polyunsaturated fats, found in many warm-weather vegetable and seed oils such as sunflower oil, corn oil, safflower oil, cottonseed oil, olive oil, and palm oil.
- Partially hydrogenated (partially saturated) fats, such as those found in many shortenings and margarines.

In recent decades it has become common knowledge that the high consumption of saturated fats in the American diet is directly implicated in the high rate of atherosclerosis in this country, as well as in the high cancer rate. Knowing this, many people are drastically cutting back on their consumption of fats in the interest of preventing these devastating diseases.

This is fine up to a point, but a reduction in saturated fats addresses only one aspect of the problem and misses a couple of crucial facts. It is now known that there are "good" fats, dietary fats essential for health, and that these are sorely lacking in the typical diet. And it is also known that the partially hydrogenated "essential" fats found in cholesterol-free margarine and to a lesser degree in certain oils—which many people consume in the interest of avoiding the saturated fats—are equally devastating to our health.

What all this boils down to is that we need a *balance* of dietary fats for optimum health. It is true that we should cut down on our consumption of saturated fats. We also need to *eliminate* unnatural partially hydrogenated fats, which can literally act as metabolic poisons in the body. Most important, there are certain fats that our body absolutely needs but cannot produce from other dietary fats, and these fats need to be *increased* in our diets.

STALKING THE ESSENTIAL FATS

The fats that have generated such excitement and interest among nutritional biochemists and nutritionally oriented physicians in recent years are a small group of polyunsaturated fatty acids: cis-linoleic acid (cLA), alpha linolenic acid (ALA), gamma linolenic acid (GLA), eicosapentaenoic acid (EPA), docosahexaenoic acid (DHA), and arachidonic acid (AA). Because cis-linoleic acid and alpha linolenic acid cannot be synthesized in the body and must be gotten from food sources or supplements, they are classified as *essential fatty acids.* In a healthy, biochemically sound individual, the remaining fatty acids on the above list can be synthesized from the first two—cis-linoleic and alpha linolenic acids. So, because it is not absolutely necessary to get these other essential fats from dietary sources as well, they are not technically classified as essential fatty acids.

But they might as well be, for with the exception of arachidonic acid, most people do not get a sufficient supply of these other fatty acids in their diets, nor are they able to convert sufficient amounts of them from cis-linoleic and alpha linolenic acid, even if consumption of these two essential fats appears to be sufficient. In other words, most of us are not healthy and biochemically sound enough to do the job. The result: a deficiency in some of the fats, an excess of arachidonic acid from an excess of saturated fat in our diet, and an overall imbalance in the types of fats consumed.

THE PROSTAGLANDIN CONNECTION

There are three major reasons why EFAs are so important. One is that they are a major source of energy (calories). Secondly, they are a crucial ingredient of the membranes in all body tissues and thus an important factor in determining the biological properties of those tissues. A deficiency of essential fatty acids, therefore, can cause serious problems. One of these may well be an increase in the permeability of the mucosal membrane of the digestive tract, leading to the increased ability of incompletely digested food and other toxins to enter the bloodstream, eventually as immune complexes causing inflammatory reactions anywhere in the body. But the impermeability of all membranes—the skin, the airways—may be compromised by EFA deficiency or metabolic defects, leading to an array of complications from dehydration to decreased immunity. In one experiment reported by Dr. David Horrobin, the acknowledged leader in EFA research, severely EFA-deficient rats were submerged up to their necks in a tank of water for twenty minutes, during which time their body weight increased by an average of *50 percent*! When they were removed from the water, the weight quickly disappeared into thin air. Their EFA deficiency had made them highly vulnerable to anything that wanted to get in—or out—of their systems.

The third, and I believe the most important, reason that essential fatty acids are so critical to health and well-being is that *at the end of their biochemical pathway through our body they become prostaglandins* (PGs). The particular essential fats we're discussing here are the precursors—the metabolic starting point—for prostaglandins of three separate categories, the 1, 2, and 3 series, and related substances called prostanoids. Here are a few of the established effects of the prostaglandins:

- They can raise or lower your blood pressure.
- They can stimulate or inhibit your immune system.
- They can act as a "happiness chemical" in the brain.
- They can increase or decrease the formation of blood clots.
- They can constrict or dilate your blood vessels and airways.
- They can cause fever.
- They can cause excess mucus production in the nose, airways, and digestive-tract lining.
- They can help protect the stomach and duodenal lining from the potentially destructive effect of hydrochloric acid.
- They can shrink swollen nasal passages.
- They can cause or control inflammation, including the inflammation of an allergic reaction.
- They can stimulate or relax the uterine muscles.
- They can cause headaches, such as migraines.
- They can increase fluid pressure inside the eye.
- They can induce labor of pregnancy.
- They can stimulate steroid production.
- They can suppress pancreatic bicarbonate (antacid) secretion into the small intestine.
- They can suppress your natural appetite and hunger control.
- They can adversely affect pancreatic control of blood sugar.
- They may control the deposition of fat and its metabolism in the body.

Supplies of the three different prostaglandin (PG) series—PGE1, PGE2, and PGE3—are needed in balance. This is so because each of the prostaglandins has different functions, some of which contradict, counteract, and hold in check the functions of others. Generally, PGE1 and PGE3 have beneficial synergistic effects, while PGE2 and related prostanoids, depending on the circumstances, can be either helpful or extraordinarily harmful. For example, PGE1 and PGE3 (specifically PGI3) both decrease platelet aggregation, which is important in the prevention of abnormal blood clotting. PGE2 and a related prostanoid, thromboxane A2, *increase* platelet aggregation. PGE1 and PGE3 are anti-inflammatory; PGE2 *causes* inflammation. PGE2 has been demonstrated to increase tumor growth in rats; PGE1 has been shown to stop or reverse tumor growth. PGE1 can act as a diuretic, while PGE2 can cause water retention. *Unfortunately, most of us produce too much of the often troublesome PGE2 and related prostanoids, and not enough of PGE1 and PGE3.*

And there's another problem with PG production. The hormonelike PGs are short-lived; they are degraded and inactivated during a single passage through the lungs. Because of this, and because they do not come fully formed as prostaglandins from dietary sources, a continuous supply of them is needed to perform their hundreds of health-enhancing metabolic functions. That supply must come from essential fats in the diet.

HOW ESSENTIAL FATTY ACIDS GROW UP TO BECOME PROSTAGLANDINS

This is the tricky part. Why is it that we don't get a balance of essential fats in our diets or that we are unable to convert them successfully into PGs? Why is it that we produce too much PGE2 and not enough PGE1 and PGE3? The answer can be found in two places: our diets and the metabolic obstacle course that dietary fats must travel to become PGs. As background to a discussion of these two factors, take a look at Figure 4, which shows the path that cis-LA (cis-linoleic acid) and ALA (alpha linolenic acid) take to become PGs. Note that cis-LA *must* be converted to GLA en route to becoming PGE1 and ALA *must* be converted to EPA en route to becoming PGE3 and PGI3. This conversion is accomplished through the activity of an enzyme called delta-6-desaturase (DDS).

Problem 1. Getting Essential Fatty Acids from Our Diets

A look at the food sources for the various essential fatty acids (Table 6, page 143) reveals the first problem with getting a proper balance of

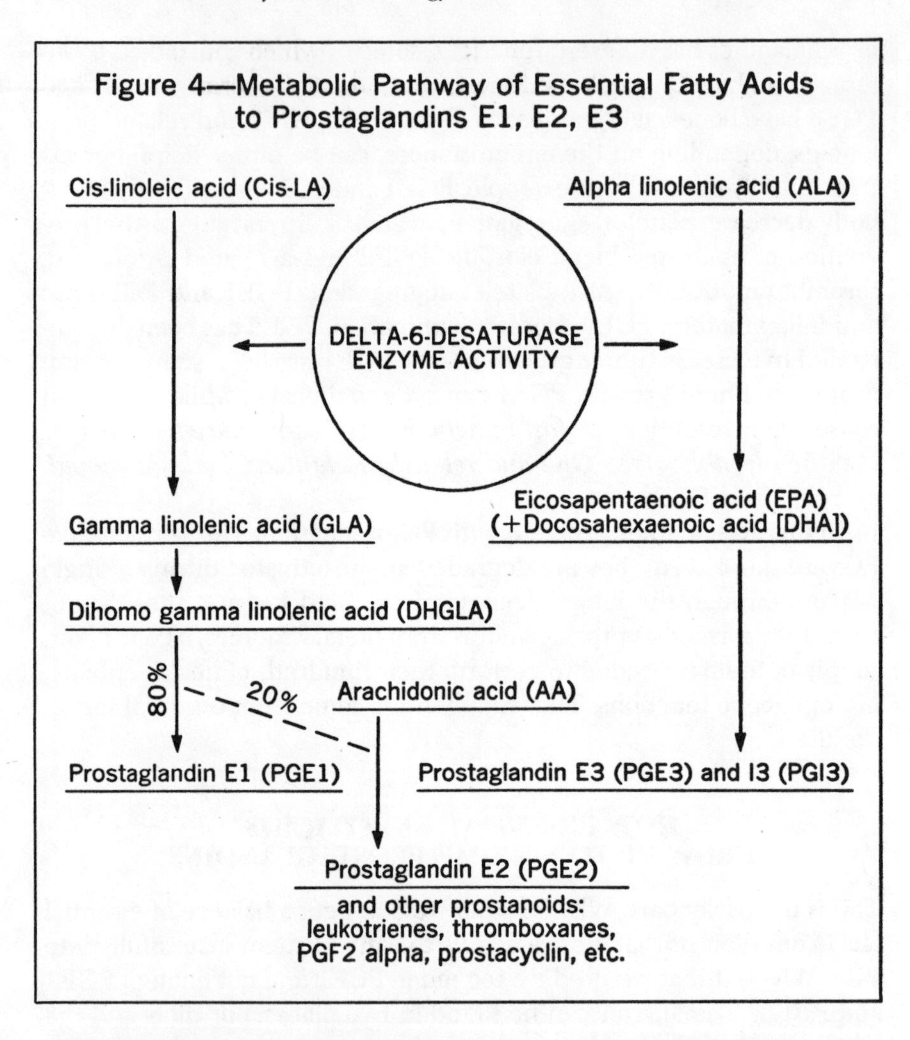

essential fats. The typical American diet, with its high intake of red meat, dairy products, eggs, and warm-water seafood, is high in arachidonic acid and low in many of the other essential fats, especially oily fish, cold-weather plant oil, and unprocessed "cis" vegetable and seed oils. No wonder our PG production is so heavily weighted in favor of the prostaglandins of the 2 series!

But, you're saying, I get plenty of these oils in salads, and I cook with these oils all the time. Well, what you see is not always what you get. It's true that many vegetable and seed oils contain plentiful amounts of polyunsaturated fats in what is called the *cis* (same side) form, which refers to the arrangement of atoms in their molecular structure. However, in the processing of these oils to improve stability, taste, and odor,

Table 6—Food Sources of Fatty Acids

PGE Series	Fatty Acid	Food Sources
1	Cis-linoleic acid (cis-LA)	Warm-weather vegetables and seeds, such as corn oil, safflower oil, sunflower oil.
1	Gamma linolenic acid (GLA)	Human mother's breast milk, evening primrose oil, borage.
1	Dihomo gamma linolenic acid (DHGLA)	Rare—in small amounts in certain organs, e.g., spleen, kidney.
2	Arachidonic acid (AA)	Meat from warm-weather animals, most freshwater fish, warm-seawater fish, and marine life, eggs, milk products.
3	Alpha linolenic acid (ALA)	Primarily linseed (flaxseed) oil; to a lesser degree soybean oil, walnut oil, chestnut oil, some dark green leafy vegetables, some beans and other cold-weather plants.
3	Eicosapentaenoic acid (EPA) Docosahexaenoic acid (DHA)	Cold-seawater fish and marine life (salmon, cod, mackerel, sardine, haddock cold-water halibut, sea bass), and at least two freshwater fish, crappie and trout.

a substantial amount of their cis form is converted to the *trans* (opposite side) form. This small change in molecular structure means that they are no longer functional essential fats and cannot be converted to prostaglandins. Moreover, these fats in the trans form can actually *block* the conversion of cis-linoleic acid into GLA and of alpha linolenic acid into EPA.

The process of hydrogenation—to which many oils, especially in margarine and shortenings, are subjected to improve stability and consistency—converts much of the essential cis form into trans fatty acids (and incidentally to saturated fats). Heating an oil at moderate to high temperatures (above 300 degrees F) has the same effect.

As a result of all this refining, heating, and processing, vegetable and seed oils are the major source of destructive trans fatty acids in our diets. Unfortunately, many doctors are unaware of the existence of the trans fatty acids and recommend that their patients switch from butter to cholesterol-free margarine—which may contain 25–35 percent or more trans fats and thus actually increase the ratio of potentially harmful fats to beneficial ones. To avoid the overconsumption of these trans fats, we have to go out of our way to be sure that the oils in our diet are only *cold-pressed* vegetable and seed oils, consumed in very moderate amounts. (Check the label. If the container does not say "unprocessed" or "cold-pressed," it's the wrong kind of oil.) *Margarine should be totally avoided.*

Table 7 lists the essential-fatty-acid content of various oils. The percentages shown in the diagram refer to the oils *in their unprocessed or cold-processed form.* The same oil in its refined state will have lost much of its EFA content. You can see from this chart that certain oils have a significant essential-fatty-acid content and so are much to be preferred as a dietary source.

Table 7—Oils High in Essential Fatty Acids (in their unprocessed or cold-pressed state)

Northern, Cold-Weather (Omega-3) Oils			Southern, Warm-Weather (Omega-6) Oils		
	%omega-3	%omega-6		%omega-3	%omega-6
Linseed	50%	20%	Safflower	0.5%	70%
Walnut	10%	20%	Sunflower	0.5%	60%
Soy	7%	40%	Corn	0.5%	60%
Wheat germ	5%	40%	Cottonseed	0.5%	50%
Chestnut	5%	40%	Cashew	0.5%	20%
Beechnut	3%	40%	Peanut	0.5%	20%
Soybean	30%	15%	Olive	0.5%	10%
Fish oil*	30% (EPA)	4% (AA)	Coconut	0.5%	10%
			Evening primrose oil		60% (GLA and cis-LA)

*Salmon, mackerel, cod, sardine, haddock, cold-water halibut, cold-water sea bass (few freshwater fish are high in EPA fatty acids [exceptions: crappie and trout]).

Problem 2. Surviving the Metabolic Obstacle Course

Now we come to the second problem in achieving a balanced and adequate supply of PGs: completing their biochemical transformation from cis-LA and ALA into the three types of prostaglandins.

Easier said than done. Take a look at Figure 5 (page 146), which is a revised version of Figure 4, showing the various factors that can block or enhance the metabolic process. That crucial first step, the conversion of cis-LA to gamma linolenic acid and ALA to eicosapentaenoic acid, is a veritable minefield.

The enzyme delta-6-desaturase, which is located in cellular membranes throughout the body, is necessary for these conversions to take place. However, there are many factors that can block the activity of this enzyme, not the least of which is the aging process. Delta-6-desaturase activity begins its peak activity about three to six months after birth, but declines sharply by about eighteen months of age and is sluggish or almost nonexistent by the age of forty. As you might expect (and as Figure 6, page 226, illustrates), many of our more entertaining dietary and life-style habits actually block this all-important conversion —from our high consumption of saturated and trans fats to smoking and drinking, stress and obesity. And those nutritional factors that would stimulate the essential-fatty-acid conversion, such as adequate protein and certain vitamins and minerals, are often lacking or suboptimal in our diets.

So, lacking the active delta-6-desaturase enzyme necessary to make the conversion to GLA and EPA in our systems, the next option would seem to be to skip over the cis-LA- and ALA-rich foods and go directly to foods containing GLA and EPA. But if you glance back at Table 7, you see that the only food sources of gamma linolenic acid are human mothers' breast milk, borage, and evening primrose oil—not likely to be staples of your diet. Dietary sources of EPA and DHA are a bit easier to come by—cold-water marine fish such as salmon, cod, sardine, mackerel, halibut, sea bass, herring, and the freshwater fish crappie—but one would have to eat *one to two pounds per day* to get all the EPA and DHA one optimally needs.

The Solution: GLA and EPA Supplements

By now you can see that getting the right essential fats from your diet is not an easy job, unless you're prepared to make numerous and forceful changes in your life-style and eat a lot of oily fish. By far the easiest

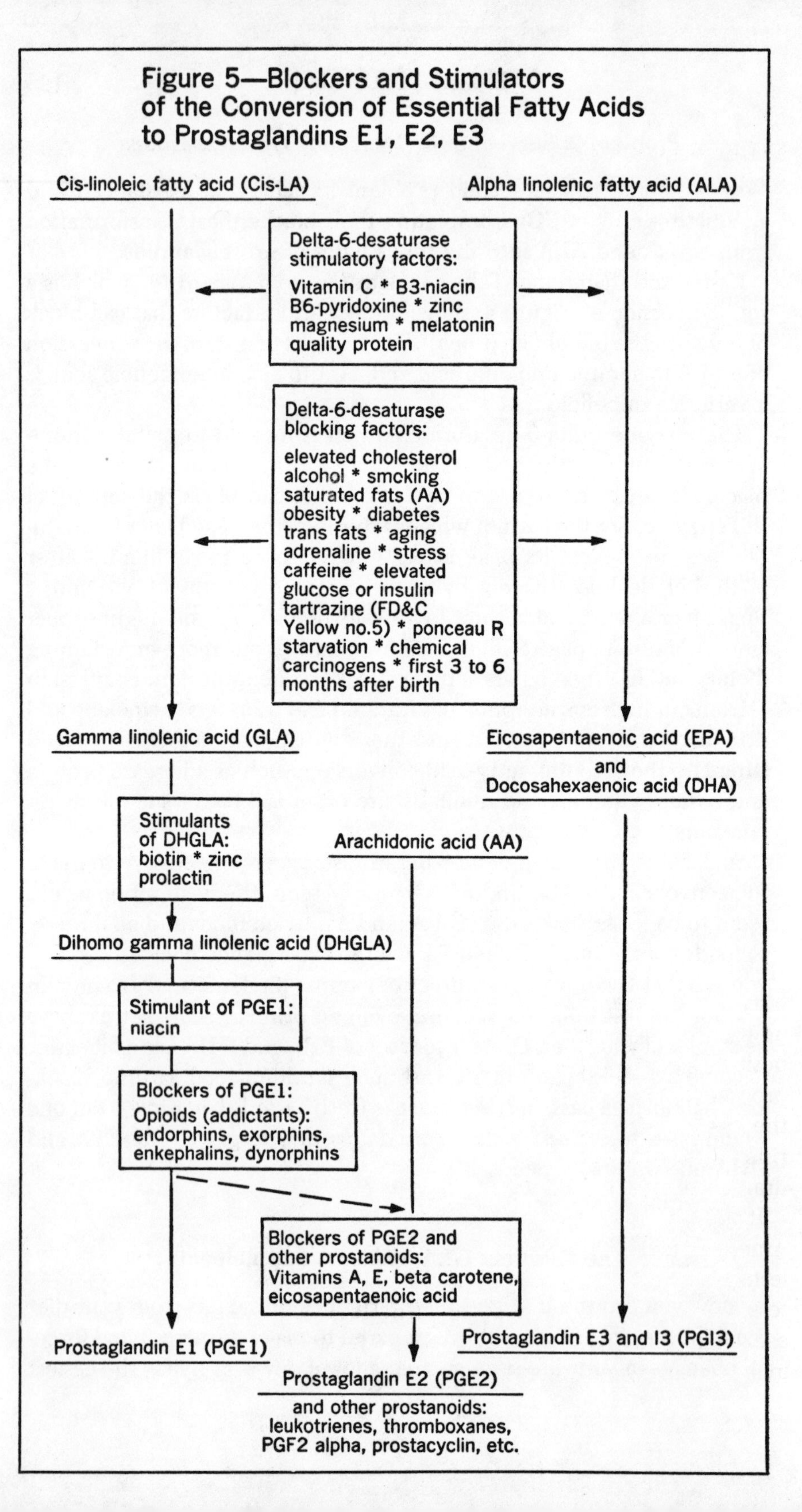
Figure 5—Blockers and Stimulators of the Conversion of Essential Fatty Acids to Prostaglandins E1, E2, E3
Cis-linoleic fatty acid (Cis-LA)
Alpha linolenic fatty acid (ALA)
Delta-6-desaturase stimulatory factors:
Vitamin C * B3-niacin
B6-pyridoxine * zinc
magnesium * melatonin
quality protein
Delta-6-desaturase blocking factors:
elevated cholesterol
alcohol * smcking
saturated fats (AA)
obesity * diabetes
trans fats * aging
adrenaline * stress
caffeine * elevated
glucose or insulin
tartrazine (FD&C
Yellow no.5) * ponceau R
starvation * chemical
carcinogens * first 3 to 6
months after birth
Gamma linolenic acid (GLA)
Eicosapentaenoic acid (EPA)
and
Docosahexaenoic acid (DHA)
Stimulants of DHGLA:
biotin * zinc
prolactin
Arachidonic acid (AA)
Dihomo gamma linolenic acid (DHGLA)
Stimulant of PGE1:
niacin
Blockers of PGE1:
Opioids (addictants):
endorphins, exorphins,
enkephalins, dynorphins
Blockers of PGE2 and other prostanoids:
Vitamins A, E, beta carotene,
eicosapentaenoic acid
Prostaglandin E1 (PGE1)
Prostaglandin E3 and I3 (PGI3)
Prostaglandin E2 (PGE2)
and other prostanoids:
leukotrienes, thromboxanes,
PGF2 alpha, prostacyclin, etc.

and most dependable way to get your daily fix of GLA and EPA is to take them as supplements in capsule form—GLA in the form of evening primrose oil and EPA in the form of MaxEPA.

The evening-primrose plant grows in temperate climate at all altitudes—from sea level to 9,000 feet. The oil of the evening primrose is the only substantial source of gamma linolenic acid. Evening primrose oil is 8 to 9 percent GLA.

Eicosapentaenoic acid and the closely related docosahexaenoic acid both come from the same source: cold-seawater fatty fish. The supplementary form, MaxEPA, comes directly from the oil of such fish. If it seems illogical that fatty fish could help to prevent such ailments as heart disease, high blood pressure, diabetes, and stroke, when recent emphasis has been on the reduction of fats, one has only to look at studies of Greenland Eskimo populations and of northern Japanese fishing communities. The fact is that these people, whose consumption of oily fish accounts for as much as 60–80 percent of the diet, have a very low incidence of these ailments.

Dosages of these supplements and a fuller discussion of essential-fatty-acid therapy begins on page 193. First, let's look at some of the rather miraculous ways in which those essential fats operate.

THE REMARKABLE HEALTH BENEFITS OF ESSENTIAL FATTY ACIDS

Coronary Disorders

Heart disease was almost unknown until the turn of this century, when fatty fish started losing ground to the leaner fish that most Americans now favor, and when Vitamins E and B6, along with the mineral magnesium, began to disappear from our food supply as a result of refining processes. When in the 1920s the processing of vegetable oils and thus the introduction of man-made trans fats (e.g., shortenings and margarines) came along, heart disease statistics began to climb inexorably and dramatically.

It's well known that the high saturated lipid (fat) content of the American diet—45 percent by some counts—leads to a buildup of cholesterol in the plaque of the artery walls. Estimates are that atherosclerosis is responsible for about 50 percent of the deaths in this country each year. Another way of looking at this is to realize that a mere 12 inches of diseased coronary arteries supplying the heart muscle are responsible for 600,000 heart attack deaths annually and some 177,000 bypass surgeries.

But not all cholesterol is bad; in fact, there's a "good" cholesterol, a kind called high-density lipoprotein (HDL), which can be increased by consuming more of the fatty fish common to the Eskimo diet. However, an equally important consideration in the management of cholesterol is the *ratio* of HDL to LDL (low-density lipoprotein). LDL cholesterol is the kind we generate in part from eating so much red meat, egg yolks, and dairy products.

GLA and EPA have several effects that improve that ratio. Evening primrose oil, with its high gamma linolenic acid content, has been shown to produce a dramatic decrease in LDL cholesterol (average decrease of 51 mg in humans with elevated serum LDL cholesterol) without affecting HDL cholesterol. And EPA, in the form of MaxEPA, increases the level of the good HDL cholesterol. Eskimo studies and other clinical investigations have also shown that EPA is associated with low triglycerides in the blood, further decreasing the risk of heart disease. Blood glucose, a minor risk factor in heart disease as well as diabetes, was also low in those people with diets high in EPA.

The tendency of the blood to clot has both desirable and undesirable effects. It's good when it stops the bleeding of a wound, bad when it leads to heart attack or stroke. People with arteries damaged by smoking, cholesterol, and high blood pressure have an abnormally high tendency for the blood to clot. This is because the typical diet—high in saturated fats, high in arachidonic acid, low in cis-linoleic and alpha linolenic acids—leads to high production of the proinflammatory prostaglandins of the 2 series, which promote platelet aggregation. PGE1 and PGE3 both *decrease* platelet clumping—another reason to rectify the balance of PGs.

The phenomenon of coronary artery vasospasm, leading to death from heart attacks, is getting increasing attention, because it often strikes those with no previously diagnosed tendency of heart disease and no evidence upon autopsy of diseased, atherosclerotic arteries. Vasospasm was once thought rare, but it is now believed that 30 percent or more of heart attacks may be the result of the smooth muscles in the walls of the coronary arteries going into muscular spasm. These attacks may be caused by a multiple of factors that cause sudden and severe constriction of the arteries to the heart, cutting off oxygen supply. If the oxygen loss is temporary, heart tissue will survive. If oxygen cutoff is not severe, the artery will relax after the initial spasm. But for those with arteries already partially blocked by atherosclerotic plaques or for those with an already reduced oxygen supply (smokers, for example), oxygen cutoff is likely to be severe and prolonged, further increasing muscle spasm. PGE1, derived from cis-linoleic and gamma linolenic acids, dilates the blood vessels, rendering them less vulnerable to spasm. PGE2, and the related PGD2, which are often released during heart spasm, *constrict* blood vessels.

What are some other heart benefits of balanced EFA-derived PGs? Because PGE1 and PGE3 dilate the blood vessels, they are factors in lowering blood pressure. They reduce angina pectoris, both because of their role as vasodilators and because of their role in decreased platelet aggregation and cholesterol buildup. Irregularities of the heartbeat are less likely to develop. In lab animals fed essential fatty acids and/or injected with PGE1, the extent of damage to heart muscle was reduced after a heart attack.

Obesity

Studies have shown that aggressive essential-fatty-acid supplementation (with evening primrose oil) in genetically obese people will result in gradual but substantial weight loss for about half of the test subjects *without dieting.* This has proved to be especially effective for people with chronic, seemingly intractable obesity—people with some metabolic abnormality. For a long time the inability of certain genetically predisposed people to burn calories efficiently was surmised to be caused by a faulty lowered basal metabolism.

But now research that began as a study of the brown bear's ability to hibernate and yet maintain an elevated body temperature has uncovered the existence of a second type of fat—brown fat. This fat tissue, which accounts for about 10 percent of one's total body fat, is located mostly in the thoracic cavity attached to large blood vessels, along certain ribs, in the nape of the neck, in the armpits, and between and below the shoulder blades. This brown fat contains a high percentage of fat-burning units called mitochondria. The big difference between white fat (the kind you can see on a steak or on your tummy) and brown fat is that *brown fat, when properly nourished and stimulated, burns up excess calories as heat and prevents the excess calories from being deposited as unsightly white fat.* The actual metabolic abnormality in almost all obese and overweight people seems to be that they lack the ability to "trigger" or stimulate brown fat cells to maintain a high heat-producing rate of metabolism. As a result, on the same or fewer calories, they gain weight, while their leaner counterparts lose or maintain weight.

Gamma linolenic acid, in the form of evening primrose oil, by producing PGE1 has been implicated as a stimulant of brown fat cells and acts perhaps to increase caloric heat release and decrease energy-storing white fat. Essential fatty acids are themselves polyunsaturated fats, and obese people have a lower percentage of polyunsaturated fat in their cellular membranes than do thin people. So far EFA supplementation has not proved effective for those with the usual problem of losing a few extra pounds—those less than 20 percent overweight.

Arthritis and Other Immune-Related Disorders

At one time it was thought that all prostaglandins caused inflammation. But it turns out that certain PGs, especially PGE1, PGE3, and prostacyclin, or PGI2, are actually *anti-inflammatory.* Both PGE1 and PGE3 increase the production of an anti-inflammatory chemical called cyclic AMP (or cAMP). Both inhibit the release of inflammatory arachidonic acid (which converts to PGE2), and block the production of highly inflammatory leukotrienes. They reduce the release into inflamed tissues of certain digestive (or lysomal) enzymes from neutrophils and macrophages, the so-called scavenger cells, thereby reducing inflammation. And they increase the action of T-lymphocytes, a primary immune cell, which has been found to be functionally deficient in many diseases, including rheumatoid arthritis, lupus erythematosis, scleroderma, and other autoimmune diseases. One of the major effects of PGE1 and PGE3 is to offset the painful, inflammatory effects of arachidonic acid and the resulting PGE2 and leukotrienes.

The anti-inflammatory drugs—aspirin, Naprosin, Indocin, Motrin, Advil, and certain steroids—attack prostaglandin production from fatty acids. This made sense when it was thought that all prostaglandins were implicated in inflammatory diseases. But now that the effects of the prostaglandins are better understood, it becomes apparent that while these drugs can relieve pain, fever, swelling, and tenderness, they also inhibit the effects of the beneficial PGE1 and PGE3. This explains the mystery of why steroid drugs are effective in blocking inflammation but may actually prevent healing and appear to have no long-term effect on the course of disease. PGE1 and PGE3, on the other hand, may work far more effectively than these drugs, because of their ability to block the release of arachidonic acid and its by-products (prostaglandins of the 2 series) and thus halt the course of disease and allow healing to occur.

Here are some of the potential anti-inflammatory, immune-system benefits of essential fatty acids:

- In rheumatoid arthritis, which an increasing number of health professionals feel is partially the result of food-immune complexes becoming deposited in and around joints, initiating the inflammatory response, both MaxEPA and evening primrose oil supplementation have proved effective in reducing the overall degree of stiffness and the number of joints affected.
- Multiple sclerosis, which seems to involve an abnormality in immune-system function, correlates as well with a deficiency of essential fatty acids. A diet low in saturated fats seems to benefit many of those with MS, especially if it is started soon after diagnosis. EFA therapy is not a cure, but it seems in many cases to significantly slow the progression of MS.
- Eczema, psoriasis, and acne have responded in scientific studies to supplementation with evening primrose oil and MaxEPA, particularly in combination with therapeutic doses of zinc and Vitamin A. Earlier studies, which tried to treat the essential-fat deficiency with linoleic acid alone, were less successful.

  Breast-fed infants often develop cradle cap (eczema of the scalp) and other skin disorders when they switch from the breast to bottle feeding. Breast milk contains high levels of gamma linolenic acid. Cow's milk and formulas do not. The fact that eczema develops during this transition seems to confirm that the delta-6-desaturase enzyme is inadequate at the time of weaning and that evening primrose oil supplementation may be necessary from infancy in bottle-fed babies. One of the big pluses of breast-feeding (see page 293) is the high GLA content of breast milk.
- Sjögren's syndrome—dry eyes and mouth—which can have far-reaching complications, has been shown to respond to evening primrose oil supplementation. PGE1 is known to stimulate both the tear glands and salivary glands.
- Cancer's best defense is a strong immune system, and we have already noted that PGE1 and PGE3 restore sluggish T-lymphocyte cells, primary immune cells, to normal. PGE1 appears necessary for interferon and fever production, both powerful immune mechanisms. In test-tube experiments, prostaglandins made from gamma linolenic acid actually caused human cancer cells to revert back to normal. I strongly feel that we are on the wrong track in trying to destroy cancer cells through immune-system suppression—i.e., radiation and chemotherapy—because of the damage they do simultaneously to healthy immune cells. A more effective approach, it seems to me, is to attempt to normalize cancer cells while *stimulating* immune cells. Since cancer cells are often associated with abnormal amounts of PGE2 and other inflammatory prostanoids, and with low levels of PGE1 and PGE3,

improving levels of PGE1 and PGE3 through aggressive supplementation may help stop and even reverse cancer growth.

Female Problems: PMS, Cystic Mastitis, and Brittle Nails

Increased water retention, which, as we've seen, is often an effect of the prostanoids, can lead to the abdominal swelling, fluid retention, pain, depression, and other manifestations of premenstrual syndrome, long considered a mostly psychological "female trouble." Taken on a regular basis, evening primrose oil and MaxEPA (along with the elimination of allergic foods) have relieved PMS symptoms in a remarkable 90–95 percent of cases. Heavy, prolonged bleeding is also cut down considerably with EFA therapy.

Evening primrose oil and MaxEPA supplementation, in conjunction with Vitamin E, also prevents cyst development and reduces existing cysts in cystic mastitis, a very common disorder that results in painful, if benign, breast cysts.

An almost universal result of essential-fatty-acid supplementation is the strengthening of once-brittle nails. Brittle nails are not a life-threatening health problem, but this discovery can be extremely useful in diagnosing EFA deficiency and in determining the effects of EFA therapy.

Diabetes

Diabetes may be connected to a deficiency of essential fats, and/or an imbalance in prostaglandins. Early attempts to treat diabetes mellitus by rectifying this deficiency with cis-linoleic acid alone had limited success, with some marginal reduction in the cardiovascular and retinal complications of diabetes. Because an inhibition of the delta-6-desaturase enzyme necessary for the conversion of the essential fats may be at the heart of the problem, it is thought that therapy with evening primrose oil and MaxEPA, both of which bypass the delta-6 inhibition problem, will bring about a higher degree of success. It is also believed that increasing the levels of PGE1 and PGE3, along with zinc and chromium, would reduce the diabetic's resistance to effective insulin action and reduce the complications of long-term insulin therapy. Several recent studies show that insulin therapy accelerates the long-term complications of diabetes (abnormal platelet aggregation, blindness, and perhaps heart disease).

Brain-related Disorders

Many seemingly unrelated mental and psychiatric disorders—from depression to hyperactivity to schizophrenia to alcoholism—seem to respond to EFA therapy. This is not so surprising, since essential fatty acids comprise a good percentage of the lipids in the nervous system, thus providing a source for the production of PGs and the strengthening of nerve-cell membranes. A deficiency of essential fatty acids seems to be common to many of the brain disorders studied. So it is logical that supplementary GLA and EPA, which bypass the conversion process, are effective in treating these disorders.

Alcoholism

Drinking alcohol seems to increase brain levels of PGE1, but after drinking stops, PGE1 levels drop drastically, causing the syndrome we label hangover. And since alcohol inhibits delta-6-desaturase activity, DHGLA stores from which PGE1 is derived are not adequately replenished, leading over time to a chronic PGE1 deficiency. It is possible that one explanation for excessive drinking is that it is an attempt to normalize PGE1 levels. Replacing PGE1 levels through supplementation can reduce alcohol withdrawal symptoms (irritability, depression, malaise, headache, etc.).

Hyperactivity

Hyperactive children often go on to become alcoholics. Given the similar pattern of EFA deficiency and delta-6 inhibition, this makes a lot of sense. Supplementation with essential fatty acids and their cofactors has been very effective, often producing dramatic reversals, in nearly 80 percent of hyperactive children. Researcher Dr. David Horrobin theorizes that one reason for the success of other food-allergy-related therapies for hyperactivity has to do with the fact that certain foods and additives inhibit the formation of prostaglandins, especially when essential-fatty-acid levels are already low. Many hyperactive children also have eczema, asthma, migraines, and other disorders indicating a malfunctioning immune system—again connected to PGE1 and PGE3 deficiencies. Even further, two thirds of hyperactive children report abnormal thirst, which may be closely related to problems of permeability of the skin in connection with the role of fatty acids in the strengthening of tissue membranes. Here again the role of essential amino acids, C, zinc, B6, and magnesium is important, since low levels inhibit the production of prostaglandins. Many hyperactive children have low levels of these nutrients.

There is one more very interesting point to be made about hyperactive children: Hyperactive males outnumber females by about three to one. Put this together with the fact that males require an EFA intake about three times higher than that of females to prevent deficiency, and you may have an explanation as to why males are more susceptible not only to hyperactivity, but to alcoholism, diabetes, and heart disease. And it indicates that supplementation for males should perhaps be considerably higher than that for females.

Schizophrenia

Finally, though it is not a concern for people on the Optimum Health Program, schizophrenics have been shown to be deficient in PGE1 and PGE3 and to improve in many cases with aggressive EFA supplementation (and cofactors of EFA—Vitamin C, B3, B6, zinc, and magnesium). In anecdotal reports, EFA therapy has in some cases proved superior to that of drugs, which tend to flatten emotions and promote social withdrawal. A key to treatment of schizophrenia may be the normalization of PGE1 and PGE3 production, leading to the stabilization of nerve-impulse transmission.

ESSENTIAL-FATTY-ACID THERAPY ON THE OPTIMUM HEALTH PROGRAM

The story of the essential fatty acids is a fascinating, if complicated, one. Their presence seems to be felt in every nook and cranny of our systems. I hope you are convinced, as I am, of the importance of achieving an adequate and balanced supply of essential fats.

There are three angles of approach to optimizing essential fats:

1. Adjust the diet. Since most American diets are high in the foods that contain saturated fats or arachidonic acid, which produce the "bad" prostaglandins, and low in the foods that produce the "good" prostaglandins, there is plenty of room to improve the PG balance through diet. Also, diets high in saturated fats and trans fats also block the activity of the delta-6-desaturase enzyme needed for the conversion of cis-LA and ALA to PGE1 and PGE3, so reforming one's diet has a twofold purpose.

2. Change one's life-style. Cutting down on smoking, drinking, and coffee, while learning to relax, takes time and willpower. But that's what is needed to decrease the blocking factors that inhibit the delta-6-desaturase enzyme. Alcohol, particularly, plays a role in depleting brain stores of DHGLA and hence PGE1 (see Figure 6, page 226), so reducing alcohol intake is important even if you are taking GLA supplements.

3. Bolster the diet with supplements. Supplementation with gamma linolenic acid in the form of evening primrose oil, and EPA/DHA in the form of MaxEPA is by far the fastest, easiest, most effective way of correcting EFA deficiencies and imbalances. There are so many things that can interfere with delta-6-desaturase activity that even a sharp reduction in saturated fats coupled with an increase in cis-LA and ALA, along with the life-style changes suggested, are usually not enough to do the trick, especially after the age of forty.

Supplementation should include the cofactors of essential-fatty-acid metabolism—the vitamins C, E, A, beta carotene, biotin, B3, and B6, plus the minerals zinc and magnesium. If you refer again to Figure 6, you'll see that these cofactors (particularly zinc) are especially important in enhancing the mobilization of DHGLA stores.

Protocol for Essential-Fatty-Acid Therapy

Dietary Manipulation

1. Reduce the consumption of saturated fats/arachidonic acid.
   - (a) Rotate meats—red meat should not be eaten more than once every five days.
   - (b) Rotate eggs and milk products—not more than once every five days.
   - (c) Rotate warm-seawater shellfish and crustaceans (crab, shrimp, lobster)—not more than once every five days.
   - (d) Eliminate fried foods.
2. Increase the consumption of polyunsaturated fats.
   - (a) Reduce consumption of trans fats. Avoid all margarines, refined salad and cooking oils, partially hydrogenated vegetable and seed oils. Be careful—these turn up in hundreds of processed and packaged food products.
   - (b) Increase the intake of both cis-linoleic acid and alpha linolenic acid. Buy and consume in moderation only cold-pressed vegetable and seed oils, especially linseed oil, which is an excellent source of ALA. (Refer to Table 7, page 144, which lists the essen-

tial fat content of oils.) Eat more fatty fish—cod, salmon, sardine, mackerel, haddock, herring, etc.

3. Avoid foods containing tartrazine and other chemical additives and preservatives.
4. Get adequate quality protein daily. (See page 445.)

Life-style Changes

1. Exercise aerobically regularly to control excessive cortisol and adrenaline/catecholamine production, leading to excessive psychological and physiological stress. See Chapter 18.
2. Eliminate alcohol for the first ninety days on the Optimum Health Program and reduce it to only occasional use thereafter.
3. Give up smoking, if necessary with the assistance either of Vitamin C-to-bowel-tolerance (page 262) or intravenous Vitamin C therapy.
4. Cut way back on or eliminate caffeine.

Supplementation

1. Evening primrose oil: 4–6 capsules twice a day before meals. Once improvement is achieved, decrease to 3 twice daily.
2. MaxEPA: 2–3 capsules twice a day before meals.
3. Be sure you are also supplementing with the cofactors of essential-fatty-acid metabolism:*
   (a) The vitamins C, E, A, B3, B6, biotin, and beta carotene.
   (b) The minerals zinc and magnesium.

Note: A couple of additional notes regarding EFA supplements:

Suggested dosages for specific disorders appear under their individual headings in Part V.

There is some evidence that men need more EFAs than women to prevent deficiencies, and so intake for men should be on the high side of the suggested dosages.

When supplementing with EFA, extra Vitamin E supplementation may be required to prevent fatty-acid oxidation and free-radical formation. Perhaps 800 IU of Vitamin E may be indicated at the high end of the recommended EFA supplement doses.

It is uncommon, but there have been reports of side effects from evening primrose oil: dandruff, flushing, loose stools, and perhaps mild

*The routine supplementation suggested on the Optimum Health Program (see Table 4, page 87) assures adequate levels of these cofactors.

headaches. Reduce dosage if this occurs. Very high doses of Vitamin A —over 100,000 IU daily—should not be taken in combination with EFA supplementation.

Beware of fraudulent brands of evening primrose oil. Be sure that the label clearly states that there is a least an 8 percent gamma linolenic content. OHL's brand is reliable, as are any of the brands packaged under the Efamol trademark.

While some change will be noticed in a very short time—stronger fingernails, thicker hair, improved complexion and skin texture, alleviated depression—since you are altering basic body chemistry, you should allow one to three months for the benefits of EFA supplements to take full effect.

Vitamin Tables

Table 8 — Vitamin A	
Function	
Tissue repair and maintenance, especially mucous membrane; eyes; hair; and skin; important in immune-system vigilance, especially secretory IgA and prostaglandin balance; potent antioxidant.	
Food Sources	
Fish, liver, green and yellow fruits and vegetables, dairy products, apricots, prunes, avocado, alfalfa, broccoli, carrots, cheese, eggs, and kale.	
Daily Adult Dosage Range	**When Taken**
10–25,000 IU*	After meals
Combinations	
To Be Encouraged	To Be Avoided
Vitamin C, zinc, calcium, magnesium, Vitamin E, B-complex, choline, phosphorus, essential fatty acids.	Alcohol, coffee, excess iron supplementation, laxatives, sugar, tobacco, mineral oil.
Possible Adverse Reaction or Toxicity	
Toxicity may occur with prolonged excessive use and results in dry skin, headaches, irritability, hair loss, cracks at the corner of the mouth, and pain in long bones; in vast majority of cases, toxicity symptoms disappear rapidly after supplementation is discontinued.	
Parts of Body Primarily Affected	
Eyes, hair, skin, mucous membranes, teeth, bones, immune function.	
Health Disorders That May Respond to Supplemental Therapy	
Many skin disorders, including acne, eczema, psoriasis; inflammatory bowel disease; alcoholism; infections; gum disorders; most diseases (because Vitamin A enhances immune function and has an anti-inflammatory, antioxidant impact).	

*To relieve certain undesirable conditions, it may be beneficial to exceed this dose, but *only* under a doctor's supervision.

<table>
<tr><th colspan="2">Table 9—Beta Carotene</th></tr>
<tr><th colspan="2">Function</th></tr>
<tr><td colspan="2">Converted to Vitamin A when needed; independent of Vitamin A, serves as an important antioxidant and may help prevent certain types of cancer; may function as internal sun screen.</td></tr>
<tr><th colspan="2">Food Sources</th></tr>
<tr><td colspan="2">Orange and yellow fruits and vegetables, green leafy vegetables.</td></tr>
<tr><th>Daily Adult Dosage Range</th><th>When Taken</th></tr>
<tr><td>20–50,000 IU
(The best supplemental source is carrot juice.)</td><td>With meals</td></tr>
<tr><th colspan="2">Combinations</th></tr>
<tr><td>To Be Encouraged</td><td>To Be Avoided</td></tr>
<tr><td>Vitamin E.</td><td>Alcohol, coffee.</td></tr>
<tr><th colspan="2">Possible Adverse Reaction or Toxicity</th></tr>
<tr><td colspan="2">Excessive amounts of beta carotene can cause a noticeable yellowing of the skin, especially the palms of the hands and bottoms of the feet; this is not dangerous and quickly normalizes upon discontinuation or reduction of beta carotene intake.</td></tr>
<tr><th colspan="2">Parts of Body Primarily Affected</th></tr>
<tr><td colspan="2">Lung tissue, areas of high free-radical formation, skin.</td></tr>
<tr><th colspan="2">Health Disorders That May Respond to Supplemental Therapy</th></tr>
<tr><td colspan="2">Perhaps lung cancer; sunburn; perhaps all inflammatory diseases associated with the formation of excess free radicals and inflammatory prostaglandins.</td></tr>
</table>

Table 10—Vitamin B1 (Thiamine)

Function	
Carbohydrate, fat, and protein metabolism; digestion (production of HCL); growth; nervous system function.	
Food Sources	
Whole grains (especially brown rice), brewer's yeast, fish, meat, nuts, poultry, wheat germ, sunflower seeds, black strap molasses.	
Daily Adult Dosage Range	**When Taken**
10–75 mg	With meals
Combinations	
To Be Encouraged	To Be Avoided
All other B-complex vitamins, Vitamin C, E, manganese.	Alcohol, coffee, tea, excess sugar and refined carbohydrates, antacids.
Possible Adverse Reaction or Toxicity	
None known if balanced with other members of B complex.	
Parts of Body Primarily Affected	
Nervous system, carbohydrate metabolism, circulation, gastrointestinal system.	
Health Disorders That May Respond to Supplemental Therapy	
Alcoholism; beriberi; indigestion; bowel regularity; possibly some mental illness; excessive psychological stress; anemia.	

Table 11 — Vitamin B2 (Riboflavin)	
Function	
Carbohydrate, fat, and protein metabolism; immune-system functions.	
Food Sources	
Eggs, green leafy vegetables, most nuts and beans, poultry, whole grains, brown rice, dairy products, black strap molasses, brewer's yeast, organ meats.	
Daily Adult Dosage Range	**When Taken**
10–75 mg	With meals
Combinations	
To Be Encouraged	To Be Avoided
All other B-complex vitamins, especially B6, B3, Vitamin C, and phosphorus.	Alcohol, coffee, bicarbonate of soda, excess sugar, antibiotics, tranquilizers, tobacco.
Possible Adverse Reaction or Toxicity	
No adverse reactions have been reported within the supplemental range (B2 will often produce a bright yellow urine, which has no clinical consequence).	
Parts of Body Primarily Affected	
Eyes, hair, skin, nails, nervous system, digestive tract, antibody and red-blood-cell formation, metabolism.	
Health Disorders That May Respond to Supplemental Therapy	
Maldigestion; excess stress; chronic diarrhea; alcoholism; slow healing; possibly certain mental disorders; acne; irritable bowel syndrome; elevated cholesterol.	

Table 12—Vitamin B3 (Niacin)	
Function	
Production of glucose from protein and fats; energy metabolism; metabolism of carbos, fats, and proteins; circulation; digestion (production of HCl in stomach); regulation of serum cholesterol; regulation of platelet aggregation; regulation of PGE1 and PGE3 (and indirectly prostaglandins of the 2 series).	
Food Sources	
Lean meats, fish, poultry, milk products, most beans, eggs, green leafy vegetables, whole grains, peanuts.	
Daily Adult Dosage Range	**When Taken**
25–200 mg	With meals
Combinations	
To Be Encouraged	To Be Avoided
B-complex, especially B1, B2, and B6; Vitamin C, magnesium, phosphorus, zinc, protein, essential fatty acids.	Alcohol, coffee, excess sugar, antibiotics, steroids.
Possible Adverse Reaction or Toxicity	
High doses (over 50 mg) of niacin may cause a temporary flush due to release of histamine and dilation of blood vessels, including tingling and itching of skin; niacin flushing is harmless; increase dosage slowly to build tolerance to flushing, and supplement under direction of nutritionally oriented physician or health-care professional. (Some people also notice a slight elevation in liver enzymes. Long-term observation of these mild elevations demonstrate no long-term serious side effects—i.e., as with flushing, they apparently are of no clinical significance.) It also adversely affects glucose tolerance tests and may change insulin requirements.	
Parts of Body Primarily Affected	
Brain, nervous system, circulatory system, skin, digestion, blood chemistry, liver.	
Health Disorders That May Respond to Supplemental Therapy	
Hypercholesterolemia (elevated cholesterol); acne; arthritis; leg cramps; headache (migraine); poor circulation; fatigue; sleep disorders; anxiety; abnormal platelet stickiness; hypochlorhydria and other digestive problems.	

Table 13—Vitamin B5 (Pantothenic Acid)	
Function	
Essential for cellular metabolism; energy cycle; formation of antibodies; nervous system function; support of adrenal gland function; anti-inflammatory function; antioxidant.	
Food Sources	
Organ meats, poultry, egg yolk, most beans, whole grains, wheat germ, most fish (especially salmon), sunflower seeds, most nuts and dark green vegetables, avocado.	
Daily Adult Dosage Range	**When Taken**
50–1,000 mg	With meals
Combinations	
To Be Encouraged	To Be Avoided
B-complex, especially B6, B12, biotin, folic acid, Vitamin C.	Alcohol, coffee, excess stress.
Possible Adverse Reaction or Toxicity	
Excessive intake (greater than 1000 mg all at once) can result in stomachache and may have a laxative effect.	
Parts of Body Primarily Affected	
Adrenal glands, digestive tract, immune system, nervous system, skin; also plays vital role in energy metabolism of all cells.	
Health Disorders That May Respond to Supplemental Therapy	
Excess stress; allergies; inflammatory digestive disorders; chronic fatigue; constipation; adrenal gland insufficiency; eczema; healing of wounds, including surgical wounds.	

Table 14—Vitamin B6 (Pyridoxine)	
Function	
Immune-system activation (antibody formation); thymus stimulation; essential fatty-acid and prostaglandin metabolism; digestion (HCl production); synthesis of RNA and DNA, required for metabolism of amino acids; formation of hemoglobin; cellular energy metabolism; brain neurotransmitter production.	
Food Sources	
Organ meats, whole grains, most beans, dairy products, avocados, bananas, most fish, egg yolk.	
Daily Adult Dosage Range	**When Taken**
10–500mg	With meals
Combinations	
To Be Encouraged	To Be Avoided
All other B-complex vitamins, Vitamin C, magnesium, potassium, zinc, quality protein.	Alcohol, birth control pills, coffee, exposure to radiation, excess exercise, excess psychological stress.
Possible Adverse Reaction or Toxicity	
There have been reported cases of peripheral neuropathy (poor muscle coordination, numbness, and near paralysis) when seven individuals were supplementing with daily dosages *above* 2,000 mg for extended periods of time (note that the B6 was being taken independent of the other B complex group); when supplementation was discontinued, symptoms gradually disappeared.	
Parts of Body Primarily Affected	
Central nervous system, skin, prostaglandin production, blood formation, endocrine glands, thymus and immune cells, cardiovascular system.	
Health Disorders That May Respond to Supplemental Therapy	
Hypertension; hyperactivity; psychological depression; abnormal platelet stickiness; premenstrual syndrome; possibly schizophrenia; possibly some forms of mental retardation especially in children; nausea in pregnancy; excess stress; calcium oxalate; kidney stones; overuse injuries, allergic reactions, and infections associated with endurance sports; elevated cholesterol; inflammatory fluid retention; atherosclerosis; counteracts effects of MSG sensitivity.	

Table 15 — Vitamin B12 (Cobalamin)	
Function	
Blood-cell formation; nervous system functions; essential for metabolism of iron and folic acid; digestion of carbohydrates, fats, and proteins; formation of RNA and DNA.	
Food Sources	
Beef, fish, eggs, milk products, pork (animal foods only).	
Daily Adult Dosage Range	**When Taken**
100–1,000 mcg	With meals
Combinations	
To Be Encouraged	To Be Avoided
B-complex, especially folic acid and B6; Vitamin C, iron potassium, sodium, and calcium.	Alcohol, coffee, laxatives, smoking.
Possible Adverse Reaction or Toxicity	
None known.	
Parts of Body Primarily Affected	
Nervous system, red blood cells, energy metabolism, iron and folic acid utilization.	
Health Disorders That May Respond to Supplemental Therapy	
Metasulfite/sulfite hypersensitivity; perhaps asthma; B12 deficient anemia; bursitis; chronic fatigue; insomnia; excess stress; alcoholism; calcium bone spurs.	

<table>
<tr><th colspan="2">Table 16 — Biotin</th></tr>
<tr><th colspan="2">Function</th></tr>
<tr><td colspan="2">Synthesis of essential fatty acids; production of anti-inflammatory prostaglandins; metabolism of fats, carbohydrates, and proteins.</td></tr>
<tr><th colspan="2">Food Sources</th></tr>
<tr><td colspan="2">Egg yolk, brewer's yeast, most beans, most fish (especially sardines), whole grains (especially brown rice), liver.</td></tr>
<tr><th>Daily Adult Dosage Range</th><th>When Taken</th></tr>
<tr><td>50–300 mcg</td><td>With meals</td></tr>
<tr><th colspan="2">Combinations</th></tr>
<tr><td>To Be Encouraged</td><td>To Be Avoided</td></tr>
<tr><td>B-complex, especially B12, folic acid and B5; Vitamin C, zinc, magnesium, and quality protein.</td><td>Alcohol, coffee, antibiotics, raw egg white.</td></tr>
<tr><th colspan="2">Possible Adverse Reaction or Toxicity</th></tr>
<tr><td colspan="2">None known.</td></tr>
<tr><th colspan="2">Parts of Body Primarily Affected</th></tr>
<tr><td colspan="2">Hair, skin, muscles, cell growth, metabolism.</td></tr>
<tr><th colspan="2">Health Disorders That May Respond to Supplemental Therapy</th></tr>
<tr><td colspan="2">Prostaglandin-dependent depression and other mental disorders; dermatitis, including eczema; perhaps metabolic obesity; in conjunction with essential fatty acids and related nutritional cofactors: dry skin, brittle nails, thinning hair; premenstrual syndrome.</td></tr>
</table>

Table 17—(Phosphatidyl) Choline

Function

Synthesis of lecithin; metabolism of fats and cholesterol; proper function of liver, gall bladder, and kidney; important neurotransmitter (as acetylcholine).

Food Sources

Egg yolk, organ meats (especially liver), whole grains, beans (especially soybeans), wheat germ, lecithin, brewer's yeast, fish.

Daily Adult Dosage Range	When Taken
50–2,000 mg	With meals

Combinations

To Be Encouraged	To Be Avoided
B-complex, Vitamin A, B12, folic acid, inositol, quality protein, linoleic acid foods.	Alcohol, coffee, excess sugar.

Possible Adverse Reaction or Toxicity

High doses of choline bitartrate have caused diarrhea (over 2,000 mg); high doses of choline chloride may produce a fishy body odor.

Parts of Body Primarily Affected

Gall bladder, kidneys, brain, liver.

Health Disorders That May Respond to Supplemental Therapy

High serum cholesterol; memory loss; angina; abnormal platelet aggregation; perhaps certain cases of Alzheimer's disease.

Table 18—Folic Acid	
Function	
Synthesis of RNA and DNA; blood cell formation; metabolism of all amino acids; formation of hemoglobin; formation of hydrochloric acid in the stomach; formation of collagen; regulation of iron and B12 utilization.	
Food Sources	
Beets, cabbage, eggs, milk products, whole grains, dark green leafy vegetables, citrus fruits, organ meats, most fish. Note: Most folic acid is destroyed by cooking, but enough remains to make the above foods nutritionally valuable.	
Daily Adult Dosage Range	**When Taken**
500–5,000 mcg	With meals
Combinations	
To Be Encouraged	To Be Avoided
B-complex, especially B12; biotin and B5, Vitamin C.	Alcohol, coffee, fever, oral contraceptives, certain drugs, cigarettes.
Possible Adverse Reaction or Toxicity	
Great care must be taken not to supplement with folic acid alone in the presence of B12 deficiency and pernicious anemia, folic acid supplementation will mask the symptoms of pernicious anemia, but ultimately result in serious repercussions, including death.	
Parts of Body Primarily Affected	
Blood cells, liver, endocrine system, digestive tract, connective tissue, central nervous system.	
Health Disorders That May Respond to Supplemental Therapy	
Folic-acid deficiency; anemia; chronic fatigue; excess stress; alcoholism; cigarette smoking; prevention of neurological birth defects, such as spina bifida; iron and B12 deficiency anemia.	

Table 19—Inositol	
Function	
Synthesis of lecithin; metabolism of fats and cholesterol; proper function of liver and kidney; energy metabolism.	
Food Sources	
Most fruit (especially citrus), whole grains, most meat (especially liver), raw dairy products, egg yolk; beans (especially soybeans), most vegetables.	
Daily Adult Dosage Range	**When Taken**
100–1,000 mg	With meals
Combinations	
To Be Encouraged	To Be Avoided
B-complex, B12, phosphatidyl choline.	Alcohol, coffee.
Possible Adverse Reaction or Toxicity	
None known.	
Parts of Body Primarily Affected	
Heart, brain, kidneys, liver, muscles, hair, platelets.	
Health Disorders That May Respond to Supplemental Therapy	
Possibly helpful in abnormal blood clotting and atherosclerosis; high cholesterol; fatigue; excess stress.	

Table 20—PABA (Para-aminobenzoic Acid)

Function	
Blood cell formation; stimulation of intestinal bacteria; metabolism of protein; natural sunscreening skin.	
Food Sources	
Organ meats, whole grains, eggs, most raw dairy foods (especially yogurt), dark green vegetables, bran, black strap molasses.	
Daily Adult Dosage Range	**When Taken**
40–400 mg	With meals
Combinations	
To Be Encouraged	To Be Avoided
B-complex, folic acid, Vitamin C.	Alcohol, coffee, sulfa drugs, antibiotics.
Possible Adverse Reaction or Toxicity	
Extremely high levels (greater than 1,000 mg) may cause nausea and vomiting; also, PABA supplementation should be avoided when taking sulfa drugs.	
Parts of Body Primarily Affected	
Hair, intestine, skin, blood cells.	
Health Disorders That May Respond to Supplemental Therapy	
Possibly some forms of baldness; some parasitic diseases; excess stress; skin (applied topically to burns, dry skin, sunburn); also effective as a sun-blocking agent when applied topically in a cream.	

Table 21 — Vitamin C

Function

Essential for production of collagen and elastin; potent antiaddictive therapy (helps prevent withdrawal symptoms); digestion; proper immune function; formation of red blood cells; healing; the body's primary antioxidant; adrenal function; metabolism of other vitamins and minerals, especially folic acid, calcium, and absorption of iron; metabolism of carbohydrates, fats, and proteins; synthesis of RNA and DNA; production of interferon; stimulation of thymus gland and white blood cells of immune system; natural antihistamine; stimulation of PGE1 and PGE3 production.

Food Sources

Fresh, uncooked fruits (especially citrus) and vegetables, dark green vegetables.

Daily Adult Dosage Range	When Taken
250 mg–90 percent bowel tolerance	With meals

Combinations

To Be Encouraged	To Be Avoided
All vitamins, minerals, and essential fatty acids, especially bioflavonoids.	Antibiotics, antihistamines, steroid drugs, birth control pills, tobacco, high fever, stress, aspirin and other anti-inflammatory medications, chlorine.

Possible Adverse Reaction or Toxicity

Too much Vitamin C will cause loose stools (slight diarrhea), remedied by decreasing intake to normalize the bowel movement. (The procedure of determining the highest supplemental dose that does *not* cause diarrhea is called Vitamin C to bowel tolerance therapy and should be done with the guidance of a nutritionally oriented M.D.—see page 262.) Possible loss of tooth enamel with chronic ascorbic-acid supplementation; theoretically with Vitamin B6 and/or magnesium deficiency, increased risk of calcium oxalate kidney stones.

Parts of Body Primarily Affected

Adrenal glands, blood vessels, all connective tissue (especially collagen), gums, heart, immune system, serum cholesterol, serum uric acid, digestive system, and absorption.

Health Disorders That May Respond to Supplemental Therapy

Stress; most diseases including viral diseases; alcoholism; allergies; high cholesterol; high uric acid (gout); sinus congestion; hay fever; possibly cancer and heart disease; abnormal platelet aggregation (abnormal blood clotting); exercise-induced asthma; addictions (to prevent withdrawal symptoms).

Table 22—Vitamin D	
Function	
Essential for metabolism of calcium and phosphorus, therefore bone formation; nervous system; skin.	
Food Sources	
Egg yolk, organ meats, fortified dairy products.	
Daily Adult Dosage Range	**When Taken**
100–400 IU (rarely supplemented)—best source is direct sunlight.	With meals
Combinations	
To Be Encouraged	To Be Avoided
Vitamin A, Vitamin C, calcium, magnesium, phosphorus, choline.	Mineral oil, phenobarbital, laxatives.
Possible Adverse Reaction or Toxicity	
Excessive Vitamin D intake can cause hypercalcification of the bones, joints, and other tissues, also diarrhea, muscular weakness, nausea, and vomiting—perhaps irreversible damage to the blood-vessel walls.	
Parts of Body Primarily Affected	
Bones, teeth, nervous system, skin, thyroid, heart, blood clotting.	
Health Disorders That May Respond to Vitamin D	
Osteoporosis; acne and other skin disorders; stress; abnormal blood clotting; perhaps immune system, perhaps cancer of the large intestine.	

Table 23—Vitamin E	
Function	
The body's very best natural anticoagulant and primary fat-soluble antioxidant; immune-system protector and stimulator; reproduction system; maintenance of all tissues; circulation.	
Food Sources	
Eggs, organ meats, wheat germ, soybeans, dark green vegetables, some fruits, nuts, brown rice, butter.	
Daily Adult Dosage Range	**When Taken**
50–1,200 IU	With meals
Combinations	
To Be Encouraged	To Be Avoided
Vitamin A, B-complex, Vitamin C, magnesium, manganese, selenium, inositol, essential fatty acids.	Excessive fat intake, birth control pills, some forms of iron supplements, mineral oil chronically used as laxative.
Possible Adverse Reaction or Toxicity	
Initial supplementation at higher doses (over 400 IU) may cause transient increase in blood pressure; doses in excess of 2,000 IU may suppress the immune system.	
Parts of Body Primarily Affected	
Blood vessels, heart, blood-clotting mechanism, lungs, skin, immune system, reproductive organs.	
Health Disorders That May Respond to Supplemental Therapy	
Vascular difficulties, including thrombophlebitis; abnormal platelet stickiness (abnormal blood clotting) and intermittent claudication (off and on lameness associated with arterial diseases of the limbs); fibrocystic breast disease; menopause; heavy metal poisoning; atherosclerosis; high cholesterol; some forms of impotency and infertility; vascular headaches; angina pectoris; eczema; dry skin. *Topically:* burns, scars, wounds, and eczema.	

Mineral Tables

Table 24 — Calcium	
Function	
Bone and tooth formation; blood clotting; nervous system; heart rhythm; muscle function; cellular metabolism	
Food Sources	
Dark green vegetables, most nuts and seeds (especially sesame), liver, root vegetables (especially carrots), milk products, sardines, salmon.	
Daily Adult Dosage Range	**When Taken**
1,000–1,500 mg	With meals
Combinations	
To Be Encouraged	To Be Avoided
Sunshine (Vitamin D), Vitamin A, Vitamin C, magnesium, protein, adequate hydrochloric acid.	Excess phosphorus, lack of exercise, excess-saturated fat, oxalic, phytic acids, and excess iron.
Possible Adverse Reaction or Toxicity	
Excessive intake (above 2,500 mg) may cause imbalance with metabolism of magnesium, phosphorus, and iron.	
Parts of Body Primarily Affected	
Blood, bones, heart, skin, teeth, arteries, muscles, nerves.	
Health Disorders That May Respond to Supplemental Therapy	
Osteoarthritis; insomnia; osteoporosis; muscle cramps; bone healing; fatigue; menstrual cramps; premenstrual syndrome.	

Table 25 — Chromium	
Function	
Carbohydrate metabolism (energy); metabolism of fatty acids and cholesterol; protein synthesis.	
Food Sources	
Brewer's yeast, milk products, whole grains, corn oil, black pepper, mushrooms.	
Daily Adult Dosage Range	**When Taken**
100–600 mcg	With meals
Combinations	
To Be Encouraged	To Be Avoided
Selenium, Vitamin E, essential amino acids.	Excess iron.
Possible Adverse Reaction or Toxicity	
None known.	
Parts of Body Primarily Affected	
Blood, circulation, glucose metabolism.	
Health Disorders That May Respond to Supplemental Therapy	
Diabetes; hypoglycemia.	

Table 26—Copper	
Function	
Formation of bone and red blood cells; skin and immune function; nervous system; synthesis of RNA. Perhaps conversion of beta carotene to Vitamin A.	
Food Sources	
Liver, whole grains, green leafy vegetables, almonds, most fish, most beans, avocado, cauliflower, raisins, oysters.	
Daily Adult Dosage Range	**When Taken**
1–2 mg	With meals
Combinations	
To Be Encouraged	To Be Avoided
Zinc, iron, Vitamin C.	Excess zinc, excess iron, cadmium.
Possible Adverse Reaction or Toxicity	
Excess intake (over 20 mg) may cause imbalance in zinc and iron metabolism, and lead to headache, confusion, and anxiety.	
Parts of Body Primarily Affected	
Blood, bones, circulatory system, hair, skin.	
Health Disorders That May Respond to Supplemental Therapy	
Certain forms of anemia; may help rheumatoid arthritis in some people.	

Table 27 — Iodine	
Function	
Thyroid function, and therefore energy metabolism, growth and repair of all tissues; regulation of fat stores, protein synthesis, metabolism of cholesterol.	
Food Sources	
Seafood (fish) and sea vegetables such as kelp and dulse, iodized salt.	
Daily Adult Dosage Range	**When Taken**
50–200 mcg	With meals
Combinations	
To Be Encouraged	To Be Avoided
Vitamin C.	Fluorine, chlorine.
Possible Adverse Reaction or Toxicity	
It may be possible to create hyperactive thyroid with excess intake of iodine.	
Parts of Body Primarily Affected	
Hair, nails, skin, teeth, thyroid gland.	
Health Disorders That May Respond to Supplemental Therapy	
Goiter; hypothyroidism; fatigue.	

Table 28—Iron	
Function	
Formation of hemoglobin, therefore oxygen use and energy production; muscle function; thyroid function; immune system; protein metabolism; normal growth; cognition; attention span; verbal fluency.	
Food Sources	
Liver, oysters, red meat, green leafy vegetables, eggs, fish, wheat germ, legumes, poultry, whole grains.	
Daily Adult Dosage Range	**When Taken**
18–30 mg	Between meals with a nondairy snack (no calcium or magnesium taken at same time)
Combinations	
To Be Encouraged	To Be Avoided
Copper, Vitamin C, B12, folic acid, phosphorus, Vitamin E, essential amino acids.	Excess magnesium, calcium, copper, chromium, phosphorus phytate-containing vegetables.
Possible Adverse Reaction or Toxicity	
Excess iron intake can lead to iron toxicity resulting in immune-system suppression, liver, heart, lung, and kidney problems; also will throw off normal mineral balance and produce a condition called hemosiderosis associated with an increased incidence of liver cirrhosis, liver cancer, diabetes, serious bacterial infections, and heart disease.	
Parts of Body Primarily Affected	
Blood, bones, hair, nails, skin, tongue, teeth, immune system, brain.	
Health Disorders That May Respond to Supplemental Therapy	
Iron-deficiency anemia; blood loss; iron-deficiency-related suboptimal athletic performance; recurring infections; attention and cognitive defects.	

<table>
<tr><th colspan="2">Table 29 —Magnesium</th></tr>
<tr><th colspan="2">Function</th></tr>
<tr><td colspan="2">Maintains PH balance of blood and tissue, metabolism of carbohydrates, metabolism of calcium and Vitamin D; synthesis of RNA and DNA; bone formation; amino-acid metabolism; muscle function; regulation of blood pressure; important cofactor in enhancing essential fatty acid metabolism to anti-inflammatory prostaglandins PGE1, PGE3, and PGI3.</td></tr>
<tr><th colspan="2">Food Sources</th></tr>
<tr><td colspan="2">Most nuts, most fish, green vegetables, honey, whole grains, brown rice.</td></tr>
<tr><th>Daily Adult Dosage Range</th><th>When Taken</th></tr>
<tr><td>300–1,000 mg</td><td>With meals</td></tr>
<tr><th colspan="2">Combinations</th></tr>
<tr><td>To Be Encouraged</td><td>To Be Avoided</td></tr>
<tr><td>B-complex, especially B6, Vitamin D, Vitamin C, calcium, phosphorus, essential fatty acids, essential amino acids.</td><td>Excess intake of calcium, iron, phosphorus, or Vitamin D, excess fat in diet, diuretics, excess stress, alcohol, smoking, steroids, diabetes, excess sugar.</td></tr>
<tr><th colspan="2">Possible Adverse Reaction or Toxicity</th></tr>
<tr><td colspan="2">Excess intake (over 3,000 mg) may have laxative effect, and in amounts over 5,000 mg, may cause nausea and calcium/phosphorus imbalance.</td></tr>
<tr><th colspan="2">Parts of Body Primarily Affected</th></tr>
<tr><td colspan="2">Muscles, teeth, bones, arteries, nerves, heart, blood, immune system, placenta/fetus during pregnancy.</td></tr>
<tr><th colspan="2">Health Disorders That May Respond to Supplemental Therapy</th></tr>
<tr><td colspan="2">Premenstrual syndrome; hypercholesterolemia; calcium oxalate kidney stones; stress; alcoholism; fatigue; hypertension; hyperactivity; preeclampsia, abnormal platelet aggregation; magnesium depletion secondary to long-term diuretic use; chronic diarrhea and excess perspiration.</td></tr>
</table>

Table 30—Manganese	
Function	
Metabolism of choline, biotin, B1, Vitamin C, carbohydrates, fats, proteins, and cholesterol, bone formation, blood formation, nervous system, antioxidant system.	
Food Sources	
Whole grains, egg yolk, green vegetables, bananas, most beans, celery, pineapple.	
Daily Adult Dosage Range	**When Taken**
5–50 mg	With meals
Combinations	
To Be Encouraged	To Be Avoided
B6, Vitamin C, calcium, Vitamin E.	Excess calcium, phosphorus, or iron
Possible Adverse Reaction or Toxicity	
Excess intake (over 100 mg) may cause disturbance in mineral metabolism, especially iron, but symptoms are not well defined.	
Parts of Body Primarily Affected	
Brain, muscles, nervous system.	
Health Disorders That May Respond to Supplemental Therapy	
Muscle repair (after injuring a muscle); diabetes; fatigue; chronic inflammatory conditions associated with excess free-radical formation.	

Table 31 — Phosphorus	
Function	
Bone and tooth formation; tissue growth and repair; energy production; muscle function, especially heart; metabolism of calcium; nervous system; metabolism of vitamins, carbohydrates, fats, and proteins.	
Food Sources	
Meat, fish, poultry, eggs, whole grains, nuts and seeds, legumes, yellow cheeses.	
Daily Adult Dosage Range	**When Taken**
500–800 mg (rarely supplemented)	With meals
Combinations	
To Be Encouraged	To Be Avoided
Vitamin A, D, calcium, magnesium, 3 ml manganese, iron.	Excess sugar, excess iron, calcium, or magnesium.
Possible Adverse Reaction or Toxicity	
None known. Excess phosphorus, supplemental or dietary, can cause imbalance in calcium metabolism associated with osteoporosis.	
Parts of Body Primarily Affected	
Bones, brain, nerves, teeth, energy metabolism.	
Health Disorders That May Respond to Supplemental Therapy	
Arthritis; stress; tooth and gum disorders; recent study indicates that sodium phosphate supplement may increase VO_2max and delay lactic acid buildup, resulting in a substantial improvement in athletic performance, especially endurance sports.	

Table 32—Potassium	
Function	
Regulates sodium and water balance in body, nervous system, muscle function, amino-acid metabolism, heart rhythm.	
Food Sources	
Most vegetables (especially green leafy vegetables), oranges, bananas, whole grains, sunflower seeds, potatoes (especially the skin), dates, figs, apricots, lima beans, red meat, seafood.	
Daily Adult Dosage Range	**When Taken**
50–300 mg	With meals
Combinations	
To Be Encouraged	To Be Avoided
Sodium, Vitamin B6, calcium, magnesium, essential fatty acids.	Excess sodium, excess sugar, stress, alcohol, coffee, steroid drugs, diuretics, laxatives, excess phosphates.
Possible Adverse Reaction or Toxicity	
Excess intake (over 3,000 mg) may cause imbalance in calcium/magnesium/phosphorus metabolism, resulting in cardiac arrythmia and/or hypertension.	
Parts of Body Primarily Affected	
Blood, heart, kidneys, muscles, nerves, cell membranes.	
Health Disorders That May Respond to Supplemental Therapy	
Heart arrythmias; alcoholism; allergies; burns; hypertension; stress; muscle weakness; chronic fatigue; potassium depletion secondary to long-term inflammatory bowel disease; chronic diarrhea; chronic diuretic use.	

Table 33—Selenium	
Function	
Essential for normal growth and fertility—a primary antioxidant and therefore protects cells from damage by free radicals.	
Food Sources	
Depends on selenium content of soil in which food was grown: *whole* grains, wheat germ, broccoli, onion, tomatoes, tuna, some meats, eggs.	
Daily Adult Dosage Range	**When Taken**
50–400 mcg	With meals
Combinations	
To Be Encouraged	To Be Avoided
Vitamin E, other antioxidants, essential fatty acids, iron.	Mercury, rancid fats, cadmium, excess iron, sulfates, excess saturated and trans fats, smoking, alcohol, stress.
Possible Adverse Reaction or Toxicity	
Excess selenium intake, especially as the inorganic salt sodium selenite (over 1,000 mg) can result in toxicity—nausea, skin lesions, headache, loss of appetite, hair loss, fatigue.	
Parts of Body Primarily Affected	
Pancreas, immune system, soft tissues, cell membranes, cardiovascular system.	
Health Disorders That May Respond to Supplemental Therapy	
Possibly cancer; heart disease; cataracts; Osgood-Schlatter disease and other degenerative diseases; wound healing; toxicity from pollution.	

Table 34 — Sodium	
Function	
Regulates water balance in body; regulates osmotic transfer of all material through cell membranes; muscle function; nerve coordination; digestion (production of HCl).	
Food Sources	
Salt, seafood, carrots, beets, poultry, celery, meat, cheese, processed foods.	
Daily Adult Dosage Range	**When Taken**
Hardly ever supplemented, as dietary sources are so numerous	With meals (in foods)
Combinations	
To Be Encouraged	To Be Avoided
Vitamin C, potassium, magnesium, calcium.	
Possible Adverse Reaction or Toxicity	
Excess sodium intake causes potassium loss, kidney problems, high blood pressure, edema, fatigue, anxiety.	
Parts of Body Primarily Affected	
Blood, muscles, kidneys, nervous system.	
Health Disorders That May Respond to Supplemental Therapy	
Sodium depletion states (rare).	

Table 35 — Zinc	
Function	
Metabolism of B-complex vitamins; production of digestive enzymes; production of insulin; formation of RNA and DNA; cavity prevention; immune function; proper healing; blood-pressure regulation; essential fatty acid and prostaglandin metabolism.	
Food Sources	
Whole grains, most seafoods (especially oysters), sunflower seeds, liver, soybeans, onions.	
Daily Adult Dosage Range	**When Taken**
10–50 mg	With meals
Combinations	
To Be Encouraged	To Be Avoided
Vitamins A, B3, B6, C, calcium, copper, magnesium, essential fatty acids, essential amino acids.	Alcohol, oral contraceptives, excess copper or calcium, excess stress, excess saturated and trans fats, steroids, obesity, diabetes, radiation, smoking.
Possible Adverse Reaction or Toxicity	
None known, however excess intake of zinc may interfere with absorption and metabolism of other minerals, e.g., iron and copper.	
Parts of Body Primarily Affected	
Thymus gland, T-lymphocytes, NK cells, blood coagulation, red blood cells, heart, prostate gland.	
Health Disorders That May Respond to Supplemental Therapy	
Alcoholism; diabetes; wound healing; hypercholesterolemia; some types of infertility; prostate problems; hypertension; abnormal platelet aggregation; hyperactivity; premenstrual syndrome; inflammatory bowel disease; hypochlorhydria; secretory IgA deficiency, dental caries, common cold (if taken in lozenge form).	

*Note: Because they are so rarely supplemented, there are no charts for fluoride, vanadium, molybdenum, and cobalt.

Amino-Acid Tables

Table 36—Arginine	
Function	
An essential amino acid involved with immune system stimulation, growth hormone release, tissue repair and formation, perhaps increased muscle size and strength, increased fat metabolism; also involved in urea-cycle metabolism.	
Food Sources	
Most protein foods, especially nuts, seeds, beans, peanuts, chocolate.	
Daily Adult Dosage Range	**When Taken**
500–6,000 mg	Between meals, in divided doses
Combinations	
To Be Encouraged	To Be Avoided
Carbohydrate beverages, such as diluted fruit juice.	Lysine, or high lysine foods, such as brewer's yeast, dairy products, or eggs.
Possible Adverse Reaction or Toxicity	
Arginine, for some unknown reason, may cause the proliferation of herpes virus; growth hormone release may have adverse effects on diabetes and pregnant women, perhaps causing abnormal growth pattern in children.	
Parts of Body Primarily Affected	
Liver, kidney, pituitary gland, immune system	
Health Disorders That May Respond to Supplemental Therapy	
Promotes increased muscle mass and strength through stimulation of human growth hormone release; aids suboptimal thymus function; increases rate of tissue repair; enhances development of stronger support tissues (muscles, tendons, ligaments), perhaps increased fat metabolism; may aid in certain cases of growth retardation in children.	

Table 37 — DL-Phenylalanine	
Function	
Increases production and prolongs life of body's own analgesic and mood elevating chemicals called endorphins, enkephalins, and dynorphins; useful in all chronic pain conditions such as arthritis, bursitis, lower back pain, migraine, premenstrual cramps, whiplash, etc. (The only exception is the chronic pain of terminal visceral cancers.)	
Food Sources	
Most animal protein (L-phenylalanine), few plants, and bacteria (D-phenylalanine).	
Daily Adult Dosage Range	**When Taken**
1,000–3,000 mg	Between meals only
Combinations	
To Be Encouraged	To Be Avoided
Carbohydrate liquids, such as diluted fruit juice.	Other protein foods or beverages consumed at the same time.
Possible Adverse Reaction or Toxicity	
Theoretically, in some individuals, may result in an increase in blood pressure; in some rare individuals, may cause slight nervousness or shakiness.	
Parts of Body Primarily Affected	
Brain with increased levels of PEA, noradrenaline and endorphin levels; all of body, leading to decreased pain and decreased sensitivity to pain.	
Health Disorders That May Respond to Supplemental Therapy	
Chronic pain syndromes; psychological (nonpsychotic) depression; excessive hunger; food bingeing; mental fatigue; mental dullness.	

Table 38 — L-Carnitine	
Function	
Assists in transport of free fatty acids into mitochondria of cells for energy production; important regulatory effect upon fat metabolism in heart and skeletal muscle. We use carnitine in individuals with high triglycerides; since it aids in fatty acid metabolism, it can help lower triglycerides dramatically and at the same time provide energy.	
Food Sources	
There are no vegetable sources of carnitine; food sources include muscle and organ meats; it is, however, manufactured in the body from two other amino acids, lysine and methionine.	
Daily Adult Dosage Range	**When Taken**
500–3,000 mg	Between meals
Combinations	
To Be Encouraged	To Be Avoided
Vitamin C, B6, B3, zinc, magnesium, and the amino acids lysine and methionine.	Other protein foods or beverages consumed at the same time.
Possible Adverse Reaction or Toxicity	
None known.	
Parts of Body Primarily Affected	
Mitochondria of heart cells, blood, blood lipids.	
Health Disorders That May Respond to Supplemental Therapy	
Angina pectoris; hypertriglyceridemia; hypercholesterolemia; easy fatiguability; poor athletic endurance.	

Table 39 — L-Glutamine

Function	
As an "excitory" neurotransmitter, it assists in the firing of neurons in the brain.	
Food Sources	
There are no food sources of glutamine, only glutamic acid, from which it is formed; glutamic acid has little of glutamine's beneficial properties; it is a common amino acid found in many protein foods.	
Daily Adult Dosage Range	**When Taken**
500–2,000 mg	Between meals, in divided doses
Combinations	
To Be Encouraged	To Be Avoided
Vitamin C, Vitamin A, B-complex.	Other proteins consumed at the same time.
Possible Adverse Reaction or Toxicity	
None reported.	
Parts of Body Primarily Affected	
Primarily brain.	
Health Disorders That May Respond to Supplemental Therapy	
Alcoholism; hypoglycemia.	

Table 40 — L-Tryptophan	
Function	
Converted to neurotransmitter called serotonin in the brain; serotonin is an inhibitory neurotransmitter and assists in sleeping and relaxation—L-tryptophan is therefore helpful in insomnia, stress, depression, and increased tolerance of pain.	
Food Sources	
Milk, some cheeses (e.g., Cheddar), bananas, turkey.	
Daily Adult Dosage Range	**When Taken**
500–3,000 mg	Between meals or at bedtime
Combinations	
To Be Encouraged	To Be Avoided
Carbohydrate beverages, such as diluted fruit juice.	Other competing protein in foods or beverages consumed at the same time.
Possible Adverse Reaction or Toxicity	
May cause headaches in some individuals at dosages above 2,000 mg daily; may, on rare occasions, exacerbate bipolar depression (like manic depressive states).	
Parts of Body Primarily Affected	
Brain neurotransmission, liver, kidney, brain, essential fatty-acid metabolism to prostaglandins—hence, every cell or tissue of the body.	
Health Disorders That May Respond to Supplemental Therapy	
Chronic (nonpsychotic) depression; anxiety; insomnia and other sleep disorders; postoperative chronic pain; perhaps immune-system suppression (immune deficiency syndromes).	

Table 41 — Lysine	
Function	
Suppresses herpes virus; tissue repair and formation.	
Food Sources	
Milk products, eggs, meat, fish, fowl, brewer's yeast.	
Daily Adult Dosage Range	**When Taken**
500–3,000 mg	Between meals
Combinations	
To Be Encouraged	To Be Avoided
Carbohydrate beverages, such as diluted fruit juice.	Other protein food or beverages; arginine or high arginine foods.
Possible Adverse Reaction or Toxicity	
May cause elevation of cholesterol in high dosages.	
Parts of Body Primarily Affected	
Liver, kidney, pituitary gland, immune system.	
Health Disorders That May Respond to Supplemental Therapy	
Herpes zoster (shingles) and herpes simplex, I and II.	

<table>
<tr><th colspan="2">Table 42—Ornithine</th></tr>
<tr><th colspan="2">Function</th></tr>
<tr><td colspan="2">Human growth hormone release; immune system stimulant.</td></tr>
<tr><th colspan="2">Food Sources</th></tr>
<tr><td colspan="2">None.</td></tr>
<tr><th>Daily Adult Dosage Range</th><th>When Taken</th></tr>
<tr><td>500 mg–3,000 mg</td><td>Between meals</td></tr>
<tr><th colspan="2">Combinations</th></tr>
<tr><td>To Be Encouraged</td><td>To Be Avoided</td></tr>
<tr><td>Arginine, B6, C, exercise</td><td>Lysine, other protein foods or beverages consumed at same time</td></tr>
<tr><th colspan="2">Possible Adverse Reaction or Toxicity</th></tr>
<tr><td colspan="2">Suppressed lysine activity; should not be taken by children; can cause sleep disturbances; can cause elevated liver function; do not take in cases of pregnancy; chronic or acute hepatic (liver) illness, high blood pressure, diabetes.</td></tr>
<tr><th colspan="2">Parts of Body Primarily Affected</th></tr>
<tr><td colspan="2">Thymus, hence all the immune system and theoretically all immune functions; skeletal muscles, connective tissues, platelets, liver, kidney, pituitary gland.</td></tr>
<tr><th colspan="2">Health Disorders That May Respond to Supplemental Therapy</th></tr>
<tr><td colspan="2">Aids pituitary, by stimulating production and release of growth hormone; promotes increased muscle mass, through stimulation of human growth hormone, underactive thymus.</td></tr>
</table>

Essential-Fatty-Acid Tables

Table 43—Eicosapentaenoic Acid	
Function	
Production of prostaglandins E3 and I3, essential for proper functioning of all tissue; hormone production; anti-inflammatory; works synergistically with PGE1; helps prevent formation of leukotrienes and other inflammatory prostanoids from arachidonic acid; prevents abnormal platelet aggregation; lowers LDL cholesterol; raises HDL cholesterol.	
Food Sources	
Direct Fish oil concentrate (brand name: MaxEPA); fatty fish such as salmon, mackerel, sardines, cod, herring, haddock. *Indirect* Linseed (flaxseed) oil, chestnut oil, soybean oil, walnut oil.	
Daily Adult Dosage Range	**When Taken**
120–1,800 mg	Just before meals
Combinations	
To Be Encouraged	To Be Avoided
Vitamin A, Vitamin E, B6, B3, magnesium, zinc, Vitamin C, biotin, essential amino acids, beta carotene.	Rancid fats, processed or heated fats; excessive consumption of meat, eggs, dairy products; tobacco, excess alcohol, aspirin, FD&C yellow #5.
Possible Adverse Reaction or Toxicity	
Loose stools, mild nosebleeds, dandruff, anemia.	
Parts of Body Primarily Affected	
Skin, hair, nails cardiovascular system, liver, central nervous system, platelets, arteries, airways, etc.	
Health Disorders That May Respond to Supplemental Therapy	
Hyperlipidemia; premenstrual syndrome; acne, eczema, and other skin disorders; brittle nails; coronary heart disease; high blood pressure; asthma; inflammatory bowel disease; "leaky gut" syndrome; abnormal platelet aggregation; cystic mastitis; rheumatoid arthritis; dysmennorhea (painful menstrual flow); perhaps cancer.	

Table 44—Gamma Linolenic Acid	
Function	
Production of prostaglandin E1, which is essential for the proper functioning of every cell in the body, especially skin; hormone production; anti-inflammatory agent.	
Food Sources	
Direct Evening primrose oil, mother's milk. *Indirect* Cold-pressed unrefined warm-weather vegetable and seed oils.	
Daily Adult Dosage Range	**When Taken**
80–400 mg	Just before meals
Combinations	
To Be Encouraged	To Be Avoided
Vitamin A, Vitamin E, B6, B3, magnesium, zinc, Vitamin C, MaxEPA, essential amino acids, beta carotene.	Rancid fats, processed or heated fats; excessive consumption of meat, eggs, dairy products, tobacco, excess alcohol, aspirin, FD&C yellow #5.
Possible Adverse Reaction or Toxicity	
In high doses, *may* cause slight flushing and transient elevation of temperature; this passes, and will not recur if dose is decreased; possible flare-up of manic/depressive symptoms.	
Parts of Body Primarily Affected	
Skin, hair, nails, metabolism of all cells, endocrine and exocrine glands, heart, platelets, arteries, airways, digestive tract, brain—literally all body parts.	
Health Disorders That May Respond to Supplemental Therapy	
Premenstrual syndrome; all skin disorders such as eczema and psoriasis; some forms of obesity, especially genetic obesity; hyperactivity in children; fatigue; dry skin; elevated serum cholesterol; abnormal platelet aggregation; brittle nails; extreme thirst; dry eyes; dry mouth; asthma; etc.	

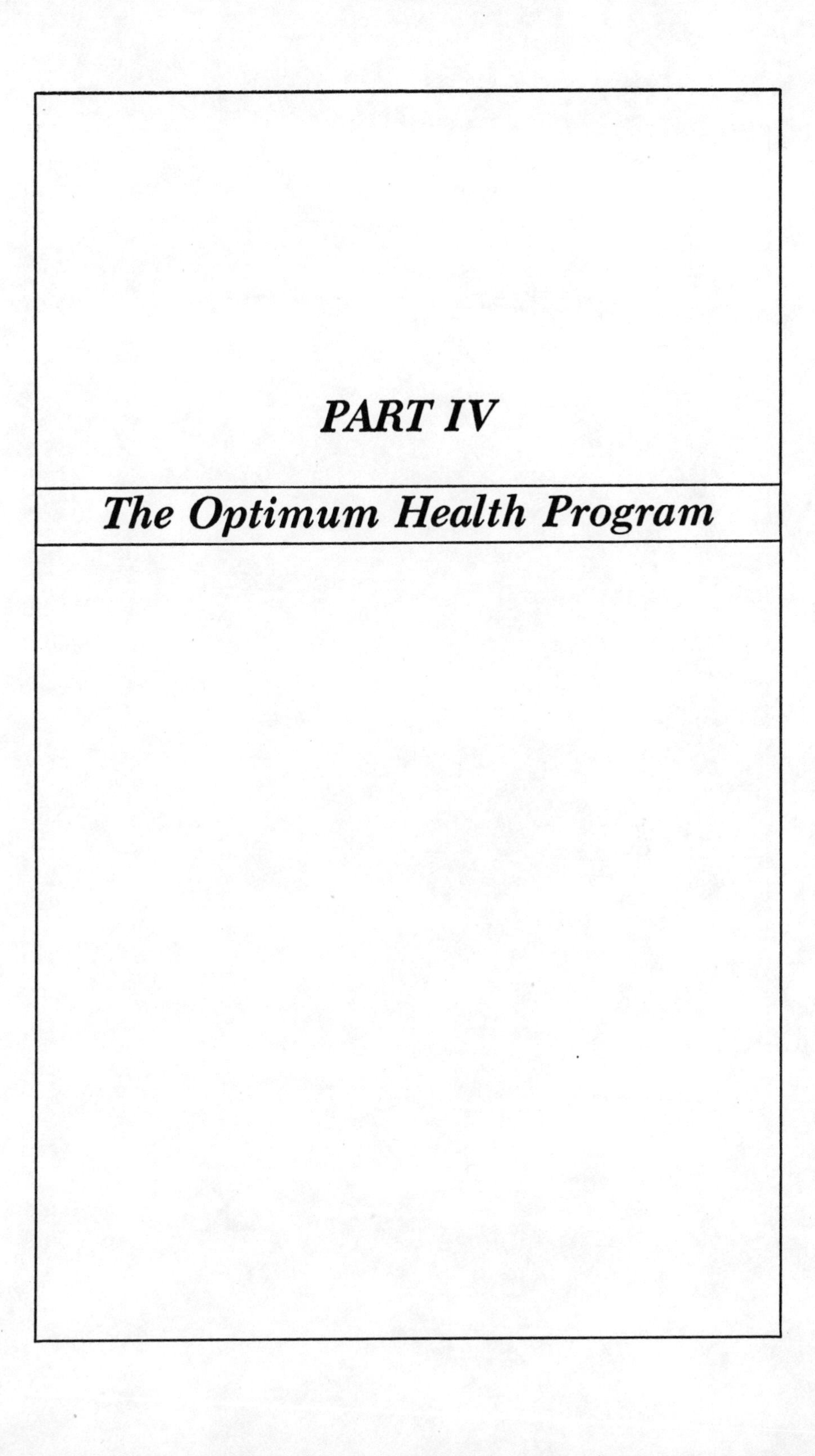

PART IV

The Optimum Health Program

12

Permanent Weight Loss— A Natural By-Product of the Optimum Health Program

A man plagued by cluster headaches and a chronic sinus condition, along with various aches and pains, wrote to tell me how he was doing on our program. "I am one of your strongest advocates," he wrote. "I have never felt better." He went on to describe how he was following the program and how his ailments were disappearing one by one. At the end of his letter, he tagged on a little postscript: "Plus, I lost weight—20 pounds!"

This is not an isolated incident. Time and time again, our patients, who come to us for relief of food allergies (e.g., migraine headaches or rheumatoid arthritis or allergic asthma), report that other problems have solved themselves as well—and often one of these problems is their weight.

Of course, there are many people who come to Optimum Health Labs specifically to lose weight, even though the Optimum Health Program is not directed just toward weight loss. Many of our patients are astounded that after years of periodic crash diets, they are finally able to get rid of those stubborn pounds and keep them off. What's most astonishing to them is that they don't have to go through the usual agony of nearly starving themselves and counting calories.

The Optimum Health Program is not primarily a weight-loss program, but many people come to us primarily to lose weight—often after years of up and down battles with the bulge. For the fact is that the Optimum Health Program is an extremely successful way to lose weight and to keep it off.

Why should this be so? Because the Optimum Health Program addresses overall health, and a lean and stable body weight is just another milestone on the road to optimum health. If you follow this modified program, you don't have to be overweight, and you don't have to measure every mouthful of food you eat. As one of our patients summed it up: "I'm eating more, but I weigh less, and I'm eating food I enjoy without guilt and fear again for the first time in over twenty years."

LOSING WEIGHT: THE WRONG WAY

At any given moment over 40 million Americans are trying to diet themselves skinny on one calorie-restricting crash program or another.

It doesn't help that the ways we choose to go about losing weight often have little lasting effect, and that many of them are counterproductive. What is wrong with most of the weight-loss diets and tactics that most people use to shed weight? The problems can be broken down into three categories:

1. The Health vs. Beauty Factor
2. The Allergy Factor
3. The "Calories In" Factor vs. the "Calories Out" Factor

Let's take a closer look at each one and see how myth and misunderstanding take their toll.

The Health vs. Beauty Factor

Ask a hundred people why they're dieting, and ninety-nine of them will say that they want to look more attractive, they want to fit into their clothes better, they want to look prettier for a boyfriend or wife. They are entirely focused on the cosmetic aspects of weight loss. Rarely is a dieter motivated by the desire to live longer or have more energy or try to prevent cancer, diabetes, or a heart attack. Yet weight is a prime factor in overall good health and is particularly implicated in high blood pressure, heart disease, certain cancers, sugar diabetes, gout, gallbladder disease, high serum cholesterol and triglycerides, vascular inflammation, strokes, and a weakened immune system.

Narrowly focused goals lead to narrowly focused solutions. If all you count is calories, all you get is less to eat. The best way to lose weight is to focus on *all* the causative factors that bear on the problem—eating habits, allergies, metabolism, exercise. Weight loss and long-term weight stabilization should be attacked from every workable angle, as a health problem and not as a beauty problem. Once the problem of overweight is diverted from its obsessive cosmetic focus, and is put in proper perspective as a part of overall health, it can be approached in a rational manner and is much more likely to produce lasting results. *Healthy people aren't fat. The way to get thin is to get healthy.*

The Allergy Factor

Counting calories and trying to feel satisfied and adequately nourished on 800–1,500 calories a day would be a tough struggle for just about anyone. But for those with food allergies—and that's just about all of us—it poses a few additional obstacles.

Restrictive, repetitive, calorie-counting diets are all wrong for people prone to allergies. As we've seen, people with delayed food allergies often *need* to keep eating their allergic foods in order to keep their symptoms under control. They often crave the foods they're allergic to, and when not dieting, they overeat or binge on them. Severely limiting the amount of food they can eat is terribly difficult, especially if they are actually addicted to that food. It requires tremendous commitment and willpower to eat just a small quantity of an addictive food. Too, it is both psychologically and physiologically stressful to the system, for the body is used to being able to get as much of a food as it needs to suppress allergic symptoms and prevent withdrawal symptoms. Too many people think of themselves as somehow morally perverse or weak because they can't seem to stick to a low-calorie diet, when in fact sticking to such a diet under these conditions requires the constitution of a saint.

In addition, because many diets ignore the importance of rotation and variety, they sometimes bring out allergies where none existed before. This is because most restrictive diet plans not only produce malnutrition, but also tend to repeat the same limited low-calorie foods over and over—fertile ground for new allergies to flourish and for weight loss to backfire eventually. Even when you temporarily lose weight, through sheer superhuman effort, you may be adding a couple more allergic foods to your list, making it all the harder to keep the weight off. The way so many people return again and again to their favorite crash diet may also be the way they develop allergies in the first place. Even successful, basically sound diet programs like Pritikin don't work for some patients, because they unwittingly develop allergies to the repetitive menus that too often go undetected.

Chronic water retention, often caused by food allergies, is yet another contributor to excess weight. Losing that last 5–10 pounds on a restrictive calorie diet is nearly impossible if you are still eating allergic foods, even in small amounts. It is a common pattern for many people to gain 2–5 pounds in a day or weekend, and then spend the rest of the week trying to get rid of the weekend bloat and blaming themselves for their overindulgence. In most cases, however, that bloat is simply water that your body is hanging on to, in an effort to dilute the inflammation of tissues caused by the allergic foods. Diuretics can help, though long-term overuse can lead to a dangerous potassium and/or magnesium loss and may trigger potentially lethal cardiac arrhythmias. Even then, the body will fight to hang on to those last few pounds of water. Once delayed food allergies are under control, the body no longer needs that protective cushion of water, and those final stubborn pounds quickly disappear.

Finally, there is reason to believe that delayed food allergies, especially when addictions form, have the impact of slowing or suppressing one's basal metabolism—fewer calories still result in weight (fat) gain. More on this aspect of delayed food allergy below.

Until you get rid of your food allergies, you will find it all but impossible to lose all the weight you want to lose and even harder to keep it off. As long as you are allergic, you will be fighting off the urge to binge on those foods. As long as you are allergic, your metabolism of excess calories will be inefficient and you will be fighting the problem of water retention and perhaps a potentially dangerous related problem: high blood pressure.

Once you eliminate the allergic foods from your diet, the cravings will go away, and you will not always be fighting the urge to raid the refrigerator. Often our patients are astounded that after years of practically having to padlock the pantry, they no longer need to battle with themselves constantly to resist overeating. Said one patient, "The most exciting thing about this program is that for the first time in memory, the compulsion to overeat has simply been eliminated."

Another patient had for years wakened in the middle of the night to raid the refrigerator, always craving the same thing—a glass of milk and a peanut butter sandwich. He thought it must have something to do with his dreams or some forgotten childhood memory. It amused him more than it worried him, since he was only 10 pounds or so overweight, and he'd gotten used to the interrupted sleep. He was not happy when his tests showed that he was allergic to milk *and* wheat *and* peanuts—and as you'd expect, he was miserable for the first three days on the diet. But on the fourth day, the craving was literally *gone.* And by the second month, he had lost 14 pounds, without counting calories, though he had not come to us to lose weight but because of chronic sinusitis and migraines—which had also disappeared. Six months later he was back to eating wheat and peanut butter (on a rotation basis) but not milk, and he always sleeps through the night.

The "Calories In" Factor vs. the "Calories Out" Factor

Here is one of the most persistent and damaging myths about the dynamics of weight loss: the assumption that the fewer calories you consume, the quicker and faster you'll lose weight. It's tragically wrong. *In fact, the longer and more frequently you crash-diet, the harder it is each time to lose weight and the less likely it is that you'll keep that weight off.*

Perhaps you've had the experience of faithfully following a strict diet, losing 2 or 3 pounds the first week, 2 pounds the second week, perhaps a pound the third and fourth week—and then nothing, despite the fact that you were still eating the same foods you ate the first week. Maybe you tried to look back to see if you'd cheated a bit or were careless in your calorie reckonings. And then, to add insult to injury, the minute you went back to your usual diet, even though you were careful, that weight appeared again—almost overnight, it seemed.

Or perhaps you've had a dieting friend complain that even though he's eating only 600 to 800 calories a day, he can't seem to lose weight. Or you've been mystified that your friend who's 50 pounds overweight doesn't really seem to eat any more than you do.

There's a logical explanation for all this, and it isn't that you've been unwittingly cheating on your diet or that your overweight friend dives into the hidden stash of brownies the minute she's alone. At OHL we see cases like this all the time—they are classic victims of ignorance about the real dynamics of weight loss.

It is a myth that obese and overweight people eat more than thin people. And it is a myth, therefore, that obese people eat because of intense neuroses or neurotic anxiety, fear, or depression. Studies show that overweight and obese people are no more neurotic or disturbed than anyone else. And they're not closet gluttons either. More than 170 articles published in the last ten to fifteen years take the position that fat people do not in fact eat any more than thin people. The difference is that for many reasons—malnutrition, food allergies/addictions, excessive saturated fats or sugar in the diet, lack of exercise, heredity, too many set-point-lowering crash diets, a faulty fat-burning "trigger" mechanism, etc.—they just don't have the ability to burn calories efficiently. The problem is not that too many calories come in; it's that too few get out.

The Crash Diet Metabolism Massacre

Because of the way our metabolism actually works, low-calorie diets, especially on a repeated basis, are a sure way to gain weight eventually and to gain it as ugly fat tissue—faster and faster, on fewer and fewer calories, with each diet attempt. The logic of it is so basic that it is incredible that boring, difficult crash diets, with a failure rate exceeding 95 percent, continue to tantalize us with promises of skinny heaven.

Your body, with its estimated 60–70 trillion cells, depends on what you eat to provide enough fuel to keep going. And it is an extraordinarily adaptive organism. When you cut back drastically on the amount of food you normally eat, it slows down the rate at which it burns calories (your metabolic rate) by as much as 20 percent or more, in order to conserve energy and be sure it can keep going. This slowed metabolism may be evidenced by fatigue when dieting, or by intolerance to cooler temperatures you tolerated well before crash dieting. And once that metabolism slows down, you're no longer equipped to burn the number of calories you usually consume when you're not dieting. Once you go back to your usual diet and usual daily caloric intake, those extra calories will quickly end up being stored as you-know-what: fat.

I recall a recent patient, a charming, vivacious cohost for a leading San Francisco TV talk show. I noticed her midmorning oral temperature to be 96.5 degrees F, over two full degrees less than what it should be (a reasonably reliable indicator of suppressed or inhibited metabolism). I immediately asked, since one reason she came to us was to lose 10–15 stubborn pounds, "Have you ever been on a crash diet?" Her response: "Every one ever invented!"

This adaptive ability of the body to speed up or slow down the rate at which it burns calories has been the focus of considerable observation and research in recent years. Attention has centered on the concept of an individual *set point,* a weight level that our body naturally seeks to maintain, even though caloric intake may vary considerably from day to day or week to week. Most dieters can identify with this concept right away. Not only is it true that no matter how hard they diet, the pounds come off only with a titanic struggle, but even when they go on long food binges, consuming incredibly large quantities of foods, they will gain only so many pounds before their weight levels off and "sets" at a particular level.

Every time we crash-diet, as soon as our body catches on to what we're up to, it adjusts our rate of metabolism downward to be sure it has the energy to survive a long siege of deprivation. But we can't diet forever. Eventually we have to return to a "normal" diet. But since it takes the body a while to catch on again, the adaptation response isn't immediate or complete. Although you may go back to eating 2,400 calories a day, your body has reset its thermostat to burn only 1,400. What happens to that extra 1,000 calories? They have no place to go, and the body stores them as "white" fat for a future bout of austerity. Of course, eventually the system catches on to the new higher caloric intake and begins to burn more of those added calories in order to protect itself from impending obesity. But not before you quickly gain back all of those pounds you struggled so hard to lose.

The damage goes even further than that. In the course of temporarily losing weight, especially when it's done without concomitant exercise, you inevitably lose muscle and other vital protein tissue along with the fat. But when those pounds inevitably come back on, they return as fat, not protein tissue, unless you've been exercising regularly.

In one study, over 200 seriously obese people lost a great deal of weight on low-calorie diets in a hospital-controlled setting. Half of them lost more than 62 pounds, 25 percent lost more than 90 pounds, and 38 percent of them came within 30 percent of their ideal weight. But several years later, well over 95 percent of them were back to their original weight. In another study, a group of overweight volunteers reduced their calorie intake by *half* for three months. Even under such drastic conditions, in most cases, weight dropped to only 10–20 percent below normal before it leveled off. That is, even on 50 percent fewer calories, badly needed weight loss stopped. When the diet ended, the test subjects ate voraciously—often more than 5,000 calories a day. But in almost every case, their appetites slowed down, and their weight seemed to stabilize magically as soon as they reached their former poundage. To make a bad situation worse, had a percentage body-fat determination been done, they would have shown an overall increase in body fat at the same former weight.

Brown Fat and Metabolic Inhibitors

It seems that we have two kinds of fat cells. White fat is predominantly the layer just under the skin, which offers insulation and in excess causes those unsightly bulges and cellulite we work so hard to banish. Brown fat is located deep in the body—mostly in the thoracic cavity attached to long vessels, along the back and shoulder bones, in the armpits, and in the nape of the neck. Perhaps 10 to 15 percent of body fat is composed of brown fat cells, while 85 to 90 percent is composed of white fat cells.

The existence of brown fat cells was discovered by scientists investigating the ability of hibernating bears to maintain a persistently high body temperature through the winter. It seems that it is their large store of brown fat, stimulated by the cold temperature to keep the heat production high, that enables them to do this.

The difference between these two kinds of fat cells is that *brown fat burns excess calories to provide for appropriate body heat*—in humans as well as bears—whereas white fat merely stores it. Predictably, overweight people seem to have less activated brown fat than thin people and, as a consequence, lower overall metabolism. A thin person with a good supply of activated, efficiently functioning brown fat can convert his extra calories into body heat and not gain weight when overeating. The fat person on the same or fewer calories gains weight—i.e., stores the extra calories as white fat. Many scientists now believe that the discovery that obesity is mostly a metabolic, not a psychological, disorder solves long-standing mysteries about the nature of obesity and overweight. Insight into the once mystifying brown fat metabolic mechanism teaches us that another way to battle weight is to stimulate brown-fat cell metabolism. As we'll see, a number of dietary and lifestyle factors, including essential fatty acids, may play an important role here.

More Side Effects of Calorie Restriction

By now it should be apparent that restricted calorie intake is, over the long run, a weight-loss disaster. It just doesn't work, because it does not deal with the actual nutritional, biochemical, and metabolic causes of obesity. But that is still not the whole story. Research also tells us of yet other ways that your body's metabolism sabotages weight loss when you try to lose weight simply by cutting down on caloric intake.

When you starve yourself on too few calories, your supply of the cell-membrane enzyme lipoprotein lipase (LPL) increases by a ratio of seven to forty times. This is the ubiquitous enzyme that draws blood fat (triglycerides) from the blood into cells for storage. The more you restrict your calorie intake, the more efficient or "hungrier" it becomes in reponse, helping the body to store the scarce fuel sources much more easily, even on fewer calories. What this means is that the more you restrict calories to lose weight, the easier it is for you to gain the weight back subsequently to the set point—up to forty times easier.

Last, but by no means least, restricted caloric intake also leads to a decrease in immune function and adrenal gland activity and to malnutrition. The body simply cannot get all its nutrients on 600–1,200 calories a day, especially if that diet severely limits the variety of foods you're getting and if you begin the crash diet already suboptimally nourished. Eventually the lack of fiber in the diet, along with vitamin, mineral, amino acid and/or essential-fat deficiencies, will take its toll. Digestion will suffer, the immune system will weaken, and we will become targets for illness. Calorie dieting may be bad for weight loss, but it's worse for your health.

LOSING WEIGHT: THE RIGHT WAY

The rational way to lose weight is not to struggle obsessively to *reduce* the number of calories that come in, but to concentrate on the *quality* of those that come in and *increase* the number that go out. In other words, we must change our diet and life-style and thus our metabolic set point, so that our body *naturally* stabilizes itself at a lower weight. In raising our set point—which is nothing more than the place where our metabolism has decided to park itself until further notice—we raise our ability to lose weight and keep it off permanently.

Everyone's metabolic rate differs. Chances are that people with a low metabolic rate take in more calories than they need, even though their daily calorie consumption is less than that of thinner people. And chances are that they're storing those "excess" calories in white fat cells throughout the body. In people who are more metabolically active, muscles, brains, skin, lungs, and blood require more fuel. They burn their calories faster and more efficiently, and therefore have a higher basal body temperature. Little is left over and stored.

To some extent, a hereditary factor is involved in determining metabolic rate. Mostly, however, our metabolic rate is determined by how we eat and live. Some people eat well and move fast and often; they maintain a high metabolic rate. Others eat poorly, and move as little as necessary; they establish a slow, sluggish metabolism. We have a choice as to whether we fall into the former or the latter group.

So, you're asking, how exactly do I go about falling into that first group? Basically, in the following ways:

1. Eat a nonallergic varied diet and observe good eating habits. The basic Optimum Health Program will go a long way toward solving your weight problem and raising the metabolic rate. This is how you'll get rid of your food allergies and addictions, clear up digestive malfunctions, and lick the problems of food bingeing and water retention.

Small changes in eating habits can make a big difference. Eating slowly, chewing your food well, and eating many small meals rather than three big ones help your body to process what you eat fully and to get rid of excess.

The time at which you eat also has an effect on metabolism. Eating most of one's calories late in the day, or at night when the system has slowed down for rest, is a sure way to guarantee that calories will be stored as fat.

2. Make changes in your life-style and in the composition of your diet, in order to avoid metabolic inhibition and to optimize your intake of metabolic stimulators.

Just as coal burns hotter than wood, so some foods burn faster and more efficiently than others. More precisely, there are certain foods, beverages, and other substances in our diets that act to slow down or suppress the metabolism, leading to fat weight gain despite fewer calories. The basic mechanism seems to be the essential-fatty-acid imbalance caused in part by inhibition of the delta-6-desaturase enzyme, leading to reduced production of PGE1 and PGE3, which many authorities feel are powerful metabolic stimulators.

What are the known inhibitors of the delta-6-desaturase enzyme? Alcohol; saturated fats (meat, dairy products, egg yolks, etc.); trans fats (margarines, shortenings, partially hydrogenated vegetable and seed oils); an excess of refined, simple sugars (candy, pastry, dried fruits, fruit juices, etc.); lack of protein and other essential nutrients in the diet; medications such as steroids and birth control pills.

Excess psychological stress often leads to increased eating, and the adrenaline and cortisol released by the adrenals under stress inhibit delta-6-desaturase activity.

Another factor is deficiencies in those nutrients that stimulate the production and release of PGE1 and PGE3: Vitamins A, beta carotene, B3, B6, biotin, C, and E; the minerals zinc and magnesium; essential amino acids; and, most important, essential fatty acids.

Essential fatty acids seem to play an important role in stimulating the metabolism of brown fat. The brown fat mechanism in weight regulation is still not fully understood, and there is as yet no accurate or precise way to measure the presence of brown fat in the body. As mentioned, what *is* known is that PGE1 and PGE3, the end products of essential-fatty-acid metabolism, may stimulate the mitochondria, or energy-producing units, in brown fat cells, causing them to convert calories into body heat. It is also thought that activated brown fat may itself be composed mostly of essential fats and that the quantity of brown fat can therefore be increased as well as stimulated by the addition of essential-fatty-acid supplements to the diet.

The way to optimize the dietary intake of metabolic stimulators is to eat a diet high in fiber and complex carbohydrates, low in saturated and trans fats, low in alcohol and refined sugars, to reduce stress, and to supplement with essential fatty acids and their cofactors.

3. Exercise in order to burn more calories and to increase the ratio of muscle to fat.

It is wishful thinking, pure and simple, to think that we can keep our weight down without prudent exercise. Calorie-cutting lowers the metabolism. Aerobic exercise is a major factor in raising it.

Obese people need not (and should not) jump into vigorous exercise. In a group of obese women studied, brisk walking for thirty minutes every day for one year *without dietary change of any kind* resulted in a 22 average weight loss.

Fire burns hotter when you add more oxygen to it. The same is true of the body's metabolism. Aerobic exercise increases the body's oxygen intake and raises the temperature of the inner furnace. Exercise also increases the heart rate and the rate of respiration. And it stimulates the production of the hormone noradrenaline, which is activated by the "stress" of exercise, much as adrenaline production is stimulated by psychological stress. And noradrenaline has a highly beneficial effect on the way the body burns fat.

Runners will often tell you that they run in order to be able to eat whatever they want. This is because once their metabolism has increased to compensate for the demands of their exercise, they can burn off far more calories, even when not exercising, far more efficiently than they could if they were sedentary.

Well, you say, I'd rather give up a few cookies than have to sweat for half an hour. But calories consumed vs. calories burned is not an even trade-off. Cutting back calories by 500 a day is not nearly as effective as exercising off 500 calories a day. The runner's metabolic set point has permanently changed, and his weight, regardless of what he eats on a day-to-day basis, is stabilized at a lower level. The metabolism rate is raised to a higher than normal degree during exercise and remains elevated, by as much as 25 percent, for as long as fifteen hours after exercise is discontinued. Even when sitting still or sleeping, the person who exercises is burning calories at a higher rate than the person who sat on his duff all day. His engine is always running.

When you exercise and *how often* you exercise also influence metabolism. If one exercises half an hour to an hour *after* a meal, metabolism of calories is greater than if the exercise precedes the meal. Exercising six times a week triples the weight-loss benefits of exercising three times a week.

Exercise also contributes to raising the set point, because it helps maintain and increase lean muscle mass. Muscle tissue requires more calories for its function and maintenance than dormant white fat tissue. Therefore, the greater your percentage of total lean body mass, or muscle, the more calories you burn simply to keep going. This is another reason that, in the long run, you lose more fat and keep it off by expending 500 calories through exercise than by giving up the triple fudge sundae.

Muscle is energy being used. Fat is energy waiting around to be used. If you are dieting without exercising, you are inevitably losing muscle and connective tissue along with the white fat you're so happy to get rid of. When those pounds return—which they're bound to do unless you're doing something to raise your set point—they'll come back as fat. And each time you diet without exercising regularly, you're giving up more muscle in exchange for fat, increasing your percentage of body fat with each diet. It's been estimated that each year you *don't* exercise, you will lose half a pound of muscle and gain a pound of fat. That means that each decade . . .

All in all, it is reasonable to conclude that successful weight loss is more a matter of the ability to burn calories than it is the willpower to resist them.

THERAPY FOR OPTIMUM WEIGHT

First of All, Are You Really Overweight?

We live in such a crazy world that it is easy to become fixated on images of what constitutes fit and skinny. Blinded by slick magazine covers, we can easily lose sight of our own body, our own history, and of realistic ideas about what constitutes thin and beautiful.

There is no such thing as an ideal weight for everyone of the same height and age. Body type and conditioning (and percentage of body fat) play a much more important part in determining whether you need to slim down. There are plenty of "thin" fat people—those with slight bone structures who are so out of shape that loose flesh is visible on their bones. There are plenty of stocky "hunks" with not an ounce of flab to spare.

Weight charts, which purport to list ideal weight ranges according to age and height, are of little or no use, for they ignore the more important factors that dictate so-called ideal weight: heredity, body type, percentage of muscle and fat, metabolic rate. A small-boned person who is in fact overweight may actually fall below the "ideal" range listed in the rate charts, and a highly fit large-boned individual may weigh much more than the maximum amount listed on the chart. More to the point, these charts are based on national averages—and these days "average" usually means overweight.

You can see that defining obesity is not as simple as it seems. Some say that obesity can be defined as 30 percent above ideal body weight, but we've just seen that ideal body weight is not so easy to determine either, especially when it comes to differentiating the fat heavy person from the fit heavy person. Then there are those who try to classify obesity according to the number of fat cells: 20 billion fat cells equal lean; 40 billion equal average; 50 to 90 billion equal obese. But how do you count fat cells?

Percentage of Body Fat: A Better Test of Optimum Weight

So, if a weight chart can't tell you what you should weigh and if the number of calories you consume is no indication of whether you should be dieting and if fat cell counting is next to impossible, how do you tell if you're overweight or obese? The best indicator, the one that can be determined on an individual basis, is the percentage of body fat. One's percentage of body fat is a reliable measure of health and fitness. Up to a point (the bell-shaped curve functions with percentage of body fat as well), the lower your percentage of body fat, the better. Regardless of your height or bone structure, if your ratio of fat to muscle is high, you could stand to lose weight. But there is also such a thing as too little body fat. Don't get carried away, like those young athletes who, wanting to achieve the same percentage of body fat as their sports heroes, take desperate steps (eating and vomiting, taking laxatives or diuretics, or starving themselves).

Table 45, page 210, gives some statistics about the body fat percentage of the average (meaning unhealthy) male and female, of their athletic counterparts in various sports, and a recommended percentage of body fat for men and women—that is, a percentage that is no longer considered a health risk factor.

A few comments about the figures in the table. Men are leaner and by nature have a lower body fat percentage than women. It is fat tissue that gives women their softness and curves. The percentages listed for athletes are not for world-class athletes but for individuals who regularly work out at the sports facility where these statistics were accumulated. World-class athletes have even lower body fat percentages

Table 45 — Percentage of Body Fat: The True Measure of Overweight

	Male	Female
The average American	20–27%	30–45%
Recommended *maximum* % body fat*	15%	22%
Runners	8.4%	15.2%
Swimmers	8.5%	17.1%
Skiers	14.1%	20.6%
Tennis players	16.3%	20.3%
Racquetball players	8.5%	14.0%
Bodybuilders	8.4%	(Probably less than 15%)

*Above the age of fifty years or so, the percentage of body fat can be slightly higher without representing a health risk.

—as low as 4 percent for men and 10 percent for women. The Romanian Olympic gymnast Nadia Comaneci (according to her coach) had a remarkable 2 percent body fat at her Olympic peak.

Remember, however, that even body fat percentages are not written in stone, and the ideal will vary among individuals. Since each of us has a different bone structure and musculature, ratios will still vary according to body type.

Measuring Body Fat

The two most convenient ways to measure body fat percentage are hydrostatic underwater weighing and skin-fold tests.

Hydrostatic weighing tanks are not available on every street corner, but an increasing number of health clubs and sports training centers provide this service. For a hydrostatic weighing, you sit in a sling and are suspended from a scale into a tank of water. Since fat floats and lean body weight sinks, the scale will weigh only bone, muscle, and other tissue. The underwater measurement is compared to your weight on dry land, along with the volume of water displaced by your body, to determine the percentage of body fat.

Some people still feel that the most accurate measurement of body fat (at least down to 15–20 percent body fat) is skin-fold tests, in which the thickness of fat folds on the skin on various sites of the body are measured with calipers. Though in the past body fat percentage was calculated from the measure of a single fold of skin at the back of the upper arm, it is now deemed important to take measurements from sites on the lower as well as the upper body. Part of the reason for this is that there are differences in the way fat is deposited in males and females—females tending to have more fat in the lower body, men tending to distribute fat more evenly. Specifically, the measuring sites are as follows: the triceps fold (measured vertically at the back of the upper arm); the subscapular fold (a diagonal fold at the base of the shoulder blade); the iliac fold (the "love handle" fold, again a diagonal at the side of the body just above the waist); the abdominal fold (measured vertically just to the side of the navel); and the thigh fold (measured vertically at the center front of the thigh at the midway point between groin and knee).

In lieu of official caliper tests, it is possible at least to see if you're carrying around too much fat by performing "pinch" tests at the skinfold sites. If you can grasp a loose fold of skin at any of the five sites, and if that fold of skin between your fingers appears to be more than 1 inch thick, you are overweight—or, perhaps more accurately, undermuscular.

Cellulite

Before we leave the subject of body fat, I want to say a word about a peculiarly female curse: cellulite. Everyone asks about cellulite, and there is an ongoing controversy about whether it differs from "normal" white fat and about how to get rid of it.

The term "cellulite" is used to refer to the dimpled irregular fat that produces a characteristic "orange peel" or "cottage cheese" appearance and shows up on the hips, buttocks, thighs, and upper arms of 80 percent of American women over the age of fourteen. Though its distinctive appearance may be caused by an increase in the size of fat cells, their spacing, and the breakdown of the connective tissue that works to support the fat deposits, it has been shown in innumerable histological and biochemical tests to be *no different in composition from any other fat.* Therefore getting rid of cellulite is no different from getting rid of any other excess fat: The best solution is the Optimum Health Program.

Second, Why Are You Overweight?

Before you tackle the Optimum Health weight-loss program, it is useful to look at your own case to see exactly why it is that *you* are overweight.

For most people, the answer is pretty simple—they eat metabolically inhibiting foods and beverages and they consume them too repetitively; they have undetected food allergies that cause them to retain water, to digest and absorb their food poorly, and this leads to suboptimal nutrition; and they don't exercise enough, so that their metabolism is perpetually sluggish.

But what about heredity? Well, it seems to play a very important part, but not in the way that you may think. According to *American Family Physician,* obesity is the most common nutritional problem of children in this country. About 45 percent of overweight infants become obese adults. If one parent is obese, a child has a 40 percent chance of being obese also. If both parents are obese, those chances jump to 80 percent. (If neither parent is obese, there is only a 7 percent chance that the child will become overweight.)

Those are pretty devastating statistics, and you might say, "Well, my parents were overweight, so I haven't got a chance to be slim." In a minor way, that is true, for there are clearly some inherited characteristics, such as basic body type, that affect one's physical structure. But what most people "inherit" is a tendency to gain and retain weight. These "inherited" tendencies are genetic only in the sense that the children are predisposed to the same metabolic disorders as their parents *if* they pursue the same nutrition and life-style. You eat what and how your parents ate—that is what you "inherited." This means that your overweight parents—now that you are an independent adult—are no longer the fatalistic/deterministic excuse for being overweight. And it means that if you have children, you have a responsibility to set a nutritional example, especially if you are overweight yourself.

One more metabolic factor that should be investigated early to determine why you are overweight is the possibility that you are suffering from hypothyroidism—an underactive thyroid. Many people who have a hard time dieting feel that they must have an underactive thyroid problem. I believe many people are "clinically hypothyroid"—that is, they look, feel, and appear clearly thyroid hormone-deficient. But when lab-tested via standard blood tests, they are not hypothyroid in the orthodox sense. The symptoms and signs of apparent hypothyroidism still need explanation. I believe the dry skin, low basal temperature, low energy, tendency to become easily fatigued, change in the texture of hair and nails, obesity, etc. are really signs of malnutrition (especially in essential fatty acids). The resulting lowered metabolism is enough to explain the inability to lose weight. Incidentally, repeated crash dieting is often a major culprit here.

What Are YOU Going to Do About Losing Weight?

The system for weight management on the Optimum Health Program appears below. As you can see, there are several components to the program, in addition to the basic dietary and allergy-management guidelines. Ideally, you should follow the entire program. However, not everyone is free to take a walk after breakfast and lunch, and not everyone is willing to give up some of his favorite foods entirely or to abstain from drinking entirely. If you're serious, though, you'll make adjustments, not excuses. One patient who got rid of 26 pounds (and a number of other problems) in two months on the program says he's able to eat in restaurants because he makes the extra effort to carry homemade bread and salad dressing in his briefcase.

It is also possible that not all of the recommendations pertain to you. For example, you may not feel that excess psychological stress is contributing to your weight problem and won't feel it's necessary to practice relaxation techniques. You will get the best results if you follow the program as closely as possible. Each individual factor of the program is a building block in the total approach to weight management.

THE OPTIMUM HEALTH WEIGHT-LOSS PROGRAM

Dietary Management

1. Basic Optimum Health Program: elimination of allergic foods, rotation diet.
2. Consume a diet high in nonallergenic complex carbohydrates and high in fiber.
3. Limit consumption of saturated fats (arachidonic acid): red meat, dairy products, egg yolk, and warm-water shellfish. Eat more poultry, fish, and vegetable protein.
4. Avoid margarines, shortenings, and other sources of partially hydrogenated vegetable and seed oils. Use cold-pressed polyunsaturated oils only.
5. Limit consumption of simple or refined sugars. This includes fruit (especially dried fruit and fruit juices) as well as pastries, sodas, and candy.
6. Eat a substantial breakfast, a hearty lunch, and a light dinner.
7. Eat slowly and chew your food well. Try to allow at least forty-five minutes for a meal.
8. Eat frequent small meals, rather than one large meal at the end of the day.
9. Avoid alcohol, and severely limit caffeine.

Supplementation

Routine Supplementation (page 86) *plus:*

Evening primrose oil: Increase to 8–12 capsules daily
MaxEPA: Increase to 4–6 capsules daily

Note: The vitamin and mineral cofactors needed for optimal metabolism of these essential fatty acids to prostaglandins are included in the routine supplementation.

Multiple amino acid: 2 capsules 20–30 minutes before each meal. (Certain amino acids upon entering the small intestine from the stomach elicit the release of an intestinal appetite suppressant hormone, cholecystokinin (CCK).

DL-phenylalanine: 2 capsules between meals twice a day. L-phenylalanine, which is converted to phenethylamine (PEA) in the body, may act to suppress the appetite.

Additional Recommendations

1. Exercise aerobically five to six days a week. Remember that plain old brisk walking may be an excellent exercise for heavy people. See Chapter 18.
2. Take a brisk thirty-minute walk after breakfast and lunch.
3. Master and practice meditation, biofeedback, yoga, or other deep relaxation techniques daily to reduce the desire for "nervous" eating and to lower the blood levels of adrenaline and cortisol, two potent metabolic inhibitors.

13

Getting Started on the Optimum Health Program: First of All, How's Your Health?

Now we come to the important part: planning and following your own Optimum Health Program. Let's briefly review what you're going to do:

1. Learn about yourself. "I was bowled over," one patient remarked, "when I realized how badly my eating habits have slipped in just the ten months since I got my own apartment. No wonder I've been feeling so lousy lately. I eat about eight foods all the time, and when I added it up, it came to ten cups of coffee a day."

Because everyone has different allergies, digestion patterns, illnesses, symptoms, food preferences, fitness levels, and metabolism, each individual's Optimum Health Program is a unique proposition. Most healthy and near-healthy people don't think too often about how they eat or how often they take an aspirin or when they last had a stomachache. Unless they work out regularly, they don't keep track of how much exercise they get or how sore they were afterward. Many a man or woman hasn't thought for years about his or her childhood illnesses or the summer fourteen years ago when his back went out or she had a long bout with her sinuses. But all of this is very useful information when you decide to take charge of your own health. The purpose of the long questionnaire that makes up the balance of this chapter is to find out about you and your health history and habits.

2. Find out what your allergies are. Chapter 14 explains the methods of testing and diagnosing food allergies—both FICA (Food Immune Complex Assay), an efficient new technique that Optimum Health Labs helped develop, and self-testing.

3. Give up the allergic foods for at least three months. Chapter 15 tells you how to plan a diet that avoids allergic foods. It will also show you how to minimize the uncomfortable withdrawal symptoms that many people experience for a few days when they suddenly abandon their favorite foods. The technique for reintroducing the allergic foods into your diet after the ninety-day period, and monitoring yourself to be sure your body has been cleared of allergic reactors, is also discussed in Chapter 16.

4. Eat a varied diet of nonallergic food on a rotation basis. Chapter 15 outlines the basic principles of good nutrition for optimum health. The rotation diet, an extremely important component in our program, is the subject of Chapter 16. It provides a crash course in food groups and food substitutes (for allergic foods) and record-keeping forms for keeping track of your own diet and symptoms. Because those with food allergies often have digestive problems, digestive support while the body repairs itself is also covered in Chapter 16.

5. Take supplements. Individual essential nutrients and their applications are discussed at length in Part III and under specific symptoms in Part V. A routine supplementation recommendation can be found in Table 3, page 86.

6. Exercise. See Chapter 18 for help in planning and getting started on a regular exercise program.

Note: Although the Optimum Health Program is written so that you can plan and implement your own regimen, be sure, as with any diet, that you consult first with your own physician to be sure there are no restrictions of which you should be aware. Ideally, you should work with a *nutritionally oriented* physician while on the Optimum Health Program. The national headquarters of the following organizations will advise you on finding one in your area: the International Academy of Preventive Medicine, 10409 Town and Country Way, Suite 200, Houston, Texas 77024; Society for Orthomolecular Medicine, 2340 Parker Street, Berkeley, California 95816.

FINDING OUT ABOUT YOU

The purpose of the following long questionnaire is to learn as much as possible about your diet and exercise habits and your general health. This information will be helpful in planning and following your own program. Answer the questions carefully—all that pertain to you—and add any additional useful information that occurs to you as you go along.

General Health

Are you in good health?

How would you rate your energy level?

Do you have any "nagging" symptoms such as headaches, fatigue, recurring colds, sinus problems, or aches and pains?

Are you under a doctor's care?

Do you take any prescription medications?

Do you take any over-the-counter medications?

Have you ever been hospitalized?

List any diseases or health problems you've ever had—headaches, rashes, fainting spells, depression, measles, swollen joints.

Do you have any allergy symptoms that you are aware of?

Do you remember being sick or having health problems as a child?

Personal Diet and Exercise Habits

How do you feel about your eating habits? Are they pretty good, poor, mixed?

Do you eat any differently from the way you did as a child or a teenager?

How have your eating habits changed?

How many meals a day do you eat?

At what hours?

What is your biggest meal?

Your smallest meal?

Breakfast:

Where do you usually eat breakfast?

How much time do you allow?

What do you usually eat?

Does it vary much?

How much coffee, if any, do you drink at breakfast?

Lunch:

Where do you eat lunch?

How much time do you allow?

What do you generally have for lunch?

Does it vary much?

Do you drink coffee with lunch? How much?

Liquor? What kind and how much?

Dinner:

Where do you eat dinner?

How much time do you allow?

What do you usually have for dinner?

How much variation is there from day to day?

Do you snack between meals? How often?

What do you like to snack on and at what hours?

Are there snack foods that you have every day or more than once a day?
What are they?
Do you miss these foods if they're not around, or do you make sure you always have plenty on hand?
Do you ever get up to eat in the middle of the night?
Do you eat just before going to bed or do you keep food near your bed?
Do you have a sweet tooth?
Do you consider yourself a junk-food junkie?
What are your junk-food favorites (doughnuts, soda, Big Macs, potato chips)? How much of them do you eat and how often?
Are you ever aware of cravings for a specific food? What and when?
Have you ever gone on a food binge? Explain.
Do you ever feel bad if you miss having a certain food? What food?
Do you ever notice feeling bad if you skip having coffee or miss a chance to have an expected cigarette or a drink? What happens? What symptoms do you feel?
Do you feel bad (not just hungry) if you miss a meal?
When this happens, are your symptoms relieved after you eat the meal or the food you've been wanting?
Do you ever feel bloated or gassy after a meal?
Do you carry any food in your purse or pocket? What is it?
Is there anything you feel you *must* eat or drink when you get up in the morning?
Before you go to bed?
Did you ever feel upset or irritable and have the feeling go away when you ate something? What was it you ate?
Name your five favorite foods and indicate how often you eat them.
Name another five favorite foods.
Try to list *every* fruit you've eaten in the last year (and indicate how often).
Try to remember *every* vegetable you've eaten in the last year (and indicate how often).
Every kind of bread and pasta or grain eaten in the last year.
Every kind of cereal (e.g., wheat, rye, barley, malt, oats, corn, millet, amaranth, rice).
Every kind of meat or poultry, and how often.
Every kind of fish, and how often.
Cheese.
Cooking and salad oils.
Would you say that you eat a varied diet? Or a repetitive, monotonous diet?
How much coffee do you drink?
Is it regular or decaffeinated?
Do you feel it's too much?
How much milk?
Nonfat milk? Raw milk? Lactase-treated? Lowfat milk?
Pasteurized?
How much water? Tap water or bottled water?
How much alcohol do you drink?

Where do you drink, and how often?
What kind of alcohol do you drink?
Do you think you drink too much?
Do you smoke? How much?
How long have you been a smoker?
Did you ever try to give it up?
How did it feel?
Do you take any supplements (vitamins, minerals, essential fatty acids, amino acids)?
What do you take? Itemize each nutrient and indicate how much you take.
When do you take your supplements?
How long have you been taking supplements?
Do you notice any benefits? Explain.
Do you take any nonprescription medications on a regular basis?
Which ones, for what, and how often? List aspirin, Tylenol, cold medicines, pain medications, sleep tablets, digestive aids, diet pills, skin preparations, etc.
Are you in good physical shape?
How many times per week do you exercise?
How long do you exercise?
What kind of exercise do you do?
How long have you been exercising this way?
And before that?
Do you have any physical disabilities that you feel keep you from exercising? Explain.
Why do you exercise?
What are the benefits you feel (if any) from your exercise program?
Are you happy with the amount of effort you spend exercising?
What is your weight?
Is this a "normal" weight for you?
What would you like to weigh?
Have you ever been at this preferred weight? When?
What is your percentage of body fat?
Do you ever diet? How many times would you say you've been on a diet?
When was the last time?
What kind of diet were you on?
Did you take diet pills while you were on the diet?
Did they help? Any side effects?
Was it difficult to follow? Explain.
Did you lose the weight you wanted to lose?
Did you keep the weight off?
For how long?

Now you have a lot of information about your general health and allergy history, as well as about your eating and exercising habits, probably more than you wanted to know. But this is useful information, especially if you take just a few more minutes and try to analyze it a bit. See what you can learn about yourself and if you can draw some conclusions.

Certainly any past illnesses or present symptoms or illnesses indicate that you should definitely consult with your nutritionally aware physician or health professional before proceeding to the diet.

But the most useful information in planning your own Optimum Health Program is probably what you learned about yourself in Personal Diet and Exercise Habits. You should be able to see—knowing what you know now about the Optimum Health Program—where the problems of less-than-optimum health started and where there is room for improvement. You may not have realized, for example, that you eat such a small number of foods (80 percent of all calories come from only eleven different foods in the typical American diet), or that you drink quite so much soda or that you feel better or worse after you eat certain foods. Perhaps you weren't aware that your exercise time has dropped off to only a couple of days a week, or you weren't tuned in to the frequency and significance of those midnight refrigerator raids. Perhaps the list of favorite foods will help you to test yourself for allergies.

Keep this questionnaire where you can refer to it as you plan your diet and do your allergy self-tests. It will also be good to refer back to six months from now. There may be some big changes.

14

Testing for Food Allergies: Finally, the FICA!

The identification and elimination of food allergies is a crucial first step on the road to optimum health. Yet the accurate diagnosis of food allergies has always been the bane of allergy treatment. This chapter outlines the existing clinical methods for determining your food allergies—including the exciting new automated FICA test that we now use at our licensed clinical laboratory—plus methods for testing yourself for food allergies.

It should come as no surprise that food-allergy testing is fraught with problems, since, as we've seen, allergies are extremely difficult to pin down: Symptoms show up in many forms, in any area of the body; reaction time may vary from immediately to a few days later; many foods may be involved; the symptoms are often masked; an allergic food may even make you temporarily feel better, not worse; and an allergen may not provoke a reaction at every exposure. Patient tales of epic journeys from one doctor to another, from clinic to hospital, are common. "Once I was tested and found I was allergic to oranges, but not to wheat," a patient recalled. "The next month I took another test which said I was allergic to wheat but not to oranges. That's when I gave up."

THE OLD WAY

For years, the test of choice for diagnosing allergies has been the skin test. The scratch test (or prick test or patch test) involves breaking the outer layer of skin and introducing a minute amount of the suspected antigen (food, spore, pollen, mold, dander, dust) that is being tested. Often a patch with the antigen attached is placed over the break in the skin. The theory is that tissue mast cells coated with food-specific (IgE) antibodies just under the skin surface will react to the food allergen, releasing histamine and other chemical mediators, causing wheal formation (swelling), redness, and itching. The skin is later observed for the degree of swelling (the "wheal") and for redness ("erythema"); if it exceeds a certain level, it is judged to be evidence of an allergy to that substance.

It all seems simple enough, except that there are two big problems. Even with airborne allergies, the tests are not always considered accurate. They are practically useless for detecting delayed food allergies, since skin tests presumably measure the presence of IgE antibodies, and as we've learned, only a small percentage of food allergies are IgE-mediated. Our research and new food-allergy tests clearly indicate that the active antibody is more likely to be IgG.

Skin testing, in short, is unreliable. In addition it is costly, painful, and time-consuming. It is pretty dismal that this test has for so many years continued to be the one most often used to diagnose food allergies.

In recent years, a few advances have been made in testing for IgE-mediated allergies. The DMSO test, an improvement on the old skin test, uses the chemical DMSO (dimethyl sulfoxide) to assist in carrying foods through the skin barrier. Preliminary evidence shows that it may help catch some food allergies that go undetected in the standard scratch or prick test. Another allergy test is the intradermal skin test, in which food extracts are injected under the skin to see if a reaction develops. Again though, the DMSO may be somewhat more effective than the old scratch or prick tests, it still catches only that small percentage of IgE-mediated food allergies.

The much heralded IgE RAST test, a radioimmunoassay technique, allows the clinician to identify and to quantify food-specific IgE antibodies in the bloodstream. In this test a patient's blood sample is combined with a specific food and a radioactively labeled anti-IgE (or "anti-antibody") antibody. *If* the patient's IgE antibody molecule corresponds to the particular food extract being tested, the radioactive anti-IgE antibody will then bind with the patient's IgE, and an allergic reaction to that substance has been proved.

This seems to be a big improvement over skin testing, but as with skin tests, doctors keep trying to foist the IgE RAST test on their patients as a way of determining all food allergies. It's a doomed mission for the same reason the skin test is doomed—it's testing IgE-mediated allergies only. Unfortunately, with few exceptions, this is all that many patients suffering with food allergies can look forward to from their personal physician or allergist. What often happens to these patients is that they are misdiagnosed, by these highly inappropriate methods, as having allergies that don't exist; or they are told they haven't any food allergies when they do and that their problems have no discernible physical cause. Their physician then chalks another one up to psychosomatic origins.

THE NEW WAY

Until recently, the cytotoxic test was the only marginally reliable method available to diagnose delayed, *non-IgE*-mediated food allergy. To do the cytotoxic test, a fresh blood sample is taken from the patient and centrifuged, primarily to remove the white blood cells. The white blood cells are then put in contact with a minute amount of a carefully prepared extract of each food or substance being tested. Each tested substance is placed on a separate silicon-coated microscope slide and covered with a plastic cover slip. (Plastic covers are preferable to ordinary glass ones, since glass has the potential to damage white blood cells, causing many false positive reactions.) Between one and two hours later, a laboratory technician examines each slide to determine the degree of damage to the blood cells. It has been reported that foods to which you are allergic are able to change the shape and appearance of these cells, even to cause the rupture and destruction of white blood cells.

This test—when done properly as described above—is an improvement over any previously available laboratory test for food allergy, but it has some persistent and frustrating limitations.

The quality controls necessary are formidable, and they begin with the patient, who must abstain from food and drink, cigarettes, alcohol, mouthwash, and toothpaste for twelve hours before the blood is drawn.

The most frustrating aspect of the cytotoxic test is that many of the people who most need help cannot be helped. Many allergy suffers have come to OHL suffering from chronic inflammatory conditions related to food allergy, such as asthma and rheumatoid arthritis. To treat these chronic conditions, they were taking large amounts of potent, potentially dangerous anti-inflammatory medications. But as long as they were on such medications, they could not be accurately diagnosed by the cytotoxic test. If they attempted to discontinue the medication abruptly, their symptoms would flare up with a vengeance, forcing them to retreat back to the medication for relief, again postponing the possibility of testing and healing.

Another problem is that, due to the fragility of white blood cells, the test must be done within three hours of the blood draw. Since few facilities still perform cytotoxic testing—few, if any, that I could recommend, at any rate—many people have been forced into expensive and time-consuming travel in order to be tested. Also, with the cytotoxic test, there is potential for many false positives—that is, the test shows allergy but the patient does not react symptomatically when he eats the food. Also, the reproducibility of the cytotoxic test, especially between competing laboratories, is very suspect. (In 1983 an investigative reporter had four cytos done on four consecutive days at four different L.A. labs—and each of the cyto results were different from all the others!) Finally, the cytotoxic test does not pick up the small percentage of food allergies that *are* IgE-mediated.

FICA: THE BREAKTHROUGH

It was in Vancouver, British Columbia, August 1982, at the Second International Symposium on Food Allergy, sponsored by the American College of Allergists, that I had the first hint that a new food-allergy test was being developed.

Research was reported as demonstrating that the fundamental mechanism behind delayed food allergy was the penetration of partially digested and undigested food from the digestive tract through the paper-thin mucosal lining into the bloodstream. According to these authorities, even in so-called healthy systems, this mucosal barrier is not perfect; that is, even in nonsymptomatic people, trace amounts of undigested food are able to get into the bloodstream, where they don't belong. If *large* quantities of these incompletely digested foods get into the bloodstream, you are soon suffering from food allergy. *The big difference between a food allergy sufferer and a nonallergic person is the amount of food that permeates the mucosal barrier and reaches the bloodstream of the allergic person.*

When the undigested food enters the bloodstream, antibodies against that food (*not* primarily the IgE antibodies implicated in airborne allergies but IgG) attach themselves to it, forming an immune complex. Circulating throughout the body in the bloodstream, these immune complexes (CICs), if not cleared and eliminated by the immune system, end up penetrating the walls of the small blood vessels and being deposited at various sites in the body, where they become sources of irritation, inflammation, and ultimately dysfunction of bodily tissue.

Late in 1983, I became acquainted with an exciting series of developments in delayed food-allergy testing using the IgG/immune complex concept. An extraordinarily sensitive assay had just been developed at the University of Kansas Medical School. This new test measures *the actual presence of food-specific immune complexes and food-specific IgG antibodies in the blood.*

It is presently the only automated, commercially available test for delayed food allergy. The FICA process essentially involves taking a nonfasting blood sample and testing it for the presence of IgG antibodies and immune complexes against some 100 different foods. The results are read by computerized laboratory equipment, not technicians. If your blood serum contains a food-specific immune complex or an IgG antibody against a particular food, the anti-IgG antibody (subsequently introduced and radioactively labeled) will attach itself to it; if the measurement as determined by the lab equipment is high enough, you're allergic to that food. If there are no detectable levels of food-specific IgG or immune complex in your blood for that particular food, there's nothing for the antiantibody to attach to, the computerized equipment doesn't detect it, and you're not allergic.

Because the FICA actually measures the presence of IgG- and IgE-mediated reactions *and* immune complexes in the blood, it is a true and more complete test for food allergy. More than that, it has other substantial advantages over existing tests:

- Discontinuation of medication is not necessary. Patients can be tested while they continue to take the medications they need for relief of symptoms.
- It is not necessary to fast or to monitor the diet carefully just before the test. The FICA is much less dependent on the recent ingestion of test foods than the cytotoxic test.
- It is an automated test; therefore, it is more accurate, with significantly fewer false positives and false negatives. It is much more reproducible and simpler to conduct than the skin test or cytotoxic test. The subjectivity of the lab technician is eliminated, along with many of the difficult-to-maintain quality controls. A sample printout of a FICA test result is in Figure 6 on pages 226–27.
- The test can be done with blood samples sent through the mail, as long as the sample reaches the licensed reference labs within seventy-two hours of the blood draw.

The FICA represents a long-awaited breakthrough in the field of delayed food-allergy testing, for it removes the barriers of inaccuracy, poor reproducibility, and difficulty of access that plagued all earlier tests. As of this writing, the FICA is available only at Immuno Nutritional Clinical Laboratory (a division of OHL). It is this simple, fast, accurate test that I highly recommend to anyone starting on the Optimum Health Program.

THE CANDIDIASIS COMPLICATION

One additional factor needs to be taken into consideration in the diagnosis of allergies. Candidiasis, an overgrowth of the common yeast *Candida albicans,* often mimics and exacerbates the symptoms of allergy,

INCL

IMRE A. FISCHER, PH.D.
LABORATORY DIRECTOR

Immuno - Nutritional Clinical Laboratory
6700 Valjean, Van Nuys, California 91406
(818) 780-4720 • 1-800-344-4646 outside California

FEDERAL INTERSTATE LICENSE # 04-1294
FEDERAL MEDICARE PROVIDER # 55-8348
CALIFORNIA LICENSE # 4188

FOOD IMMUNE COMPLEX ASSAY

LABORATORY REPORT STATUS: FINAL

REFERRING PHYSICIAN:

BRALY, JAMES M.D.
5363 BALBOA BLVD. SUITE 536
ENCINO, CA. 91316

LAB NUMBER: 6432

PATIENT DATA

NAME
AGE 22 SEX F ID #:
COLLECTED 6/10/85 9:40
RECEIVED 6/10/85 12:00
TESTED 6/12/85 16:00

IGG RAST

RVS # 84231
FED. TAX ID# 95-3515812

REFERENCE RANGE

NONREACTIVE:0= 0- 3952
BORDERLINE:1+= 3953- 4972
MODERATE: 2+= 4973- 5993;3+= 5994- 7013
SEVERE: 4+= 7014- 8034;5+= 8035 AND ABOVE

FOOD TESTED	CLASSIFICATION 0 NON REACTIVE	1· BORDERLINE	2· MODERATE	3·	4· SEVERE	5·	REACTION SUMMARY BORDERLINE	MODERATE	SEVERE
NUTS									
PEANUT	3918								
PECAN	3096								
CASHEW	2025								
ALMOND	3293								
SUNFLOWER	2003								
COCONUT	3421								
SESAME SEED		4368					SESAME SEED		
VEGETABLES									
AVOCADO	2830								
TOMATO	2478								
BELL PEPPER	1545								
WHITE POTATO	2873								
SWEET POTATO	1670								
ASPARAGUS	1940								
ONION	2455								
CABBAGE	1913								
SQUASH		4398					SQUASH		
BROCCOLI			5001					BROCCOLI	
CARROT	2940								
SPINACH	2885								
LETTUCE	2156								
CUCUMBER	2733								
MUSHROOM	3123								
FRUIT									
STRAWBERRY	3309								
APPLE	2379								
PINEAPPLE	2220								
CANTALOPE	2479								
ORANGE	3099								
BANANA	3115								
GRAPE		4342					GRAPE		
WATERMELON	2138								
SPICES									
BLACK PEPPER			5713					BLACK PEPPER	
GARLIC	3032								
ADDITIONAL FOODS									
BRAZIL NUT									
CAYENNE PEPPER									
ANCHOVY									
CLAM									
HAZELNUT									
HERRING									
PEAR									
MALT									
EGG WHITE	4067								
COW'S MILK			5162					COW'S MILK	
RYE				5563				RYE	
WHEAT	3081								

LAB COPY

INCL

IMRE A. FISCHER, PH.D.
LABORATORY DIRECTOR

Immuno - Nutritional Clinical Laboratory
6700 Valjean, Van Nuys, California 91406
(818) 780-4720 • 1-800-344-4646 outside California

FEDERAL INTERSTATE LICENSE # 04-1294
FEDERAL MEDICARE PROVIDER # 55-8348
CALIFORNIA LICENSE # 4168

FOOD IMMUNE COMPLEX ASSAY

LABORATORY REPORT STATUS: FINAL

REFERRING PHYSICIAN:

BRALY, JAMES M.D.
5363 BALBOA BLVD. SUITE 536
ENCINO, CA. 91316

LAB NUMBER: 6432

PATIENT DATA

NAME
AGE 22 SEX F ID #
COLLECTED: 6/10/85 9:40
RECEIVED: 6/10/85 12:00
TESTED: 6/12/85 16:00

REFERENCE RANGE

NONREACTIVE:0= 0- 3952
BORDERLINE:1+= 3953- 4972
MODERATE: 2+= 4973- 5993;3+= 5994- 7013
SEVERE: 4+= 7014- 8034;5+= 8035 AND ABOVE

IGG RAST

RVS # 84231
FED. TAX ID# 95-3515812

FOOD TESTED	CLASSIFICATION 0 NON REACTIVE	1+ BORDERLINE	2+ MODERATE	3+ MODERATE	4+ SEVERE	5+ SEVERE	REACTION SUMMARY BORDERLINE	MODERATE	SEVERE
GRAIN									
WHEAT	2984								
RYE			5572					RYE	
OATS				6323				OATS	
BARLEY			5707					BARLEY	
GLUTEN	3734								
CORN	3312								
RICE			5039					RICE	
BUCKWHEAT	3800								
MILLET	1895								
MISC.									
BAKER'S YEAST	3122								
BREWER'S YEAST	2601								
DAIRY									
COW'S MILK		4707					COW'S MILK		
CHEDDAR CHEESE	3312								
CAFFEINE									
CHOCOLATE	2546								
COFFEE		4074					COFFEE		
TEA		4761					TEA		
EGGS									
EGG WHITE	3048								
EGG YOLK		4083					EGG YOLK		
MEAT									
BEEF			5573					BEEF	
LAMB	3251								
PORK	3587								
FISH									
SHRIMP			5249					SHRIMP	
LOBSTER	1522								
HADDOCK	2606								
CRAB		4217					CRAB		
TROUT	2162								
FLOUNDER	2715								
CODFISH	1635								
SALMON		4860					SALMON		
TUNA	2923								
POULTRY									
CHICKEN	1625								
TURKEY		4070					TURKEY		
BEANS									
PEA	3140								
KIDNEY BEAN	2007								
GREEN BEANS	1807								
PINTO BEAN	3778								
SOYBEAN		4241					SOYBEAN		
LENTIL			5761					LENTIL	

LAB COPY

complicating diagnosis and treatment. This hard-to-diagnose infestation can show up in many forms throughout the body. When it takes hold in the gastrointestinal tract, it appears to increase the permeability of the mucosal lining of the intestine, thus promoting the passage of allergens through the mucosal barrier into the bloodstream. The presence of candidiasis must either be ruled out or detected and treated before allergy treatment can be successful.

A discussion of candidiasis begins on page 344. A protocol for the treatment of candidiasis is part of the discussion.

METHODS OF SELF-TESTING FOR FOOD ALLERGY

I strongly recommend that you take the FICA to determine your food allergies. But if it is not possible for you to do so, there are several methods that you can use to determine your food allergies yourself. While most methods of self-testing for food allergy can be difficult and time-consuming, they can pinpoint your allergies with a reasonable degree of accuracy if carefully undertaken and monitored. Also, if you suspect that you may have food allergies, you may want to try one of the self-test methods for screening purposes before going ahead with further clinical testing.

Before going into the various means of self-testing, I want to mention some of the drawbacks of these methods:

- If you do not have *obvious* symptoms, it will be difficult to diagnose your food allergies. If you have migraine headaches, rheumatoid arthritis, PMS, irritable bowel syndrome, or such nagging problems as a chronic runny or stuffy nose, fatigue, depression, irritability, or insomnia, you have a barometer by which to measure your responses. If not, it will be hard, using self-testing methods, to determine the exact nature of your allergies with any accuracy.
- False negatives are a problem with self-tests. Allergic reactions are the result not only of eating the allergic food, but of the amount eaten, one's general health at the time the allergic food is eaten, the cumulative stresses in one's life at the time, and possibly other foods or beverages eaten in combination with that food. So it is possible to have negative reaction to a food even if you are allergic to it.
- You cannot test yourself accurately for allergies if you are on medications, especially antihistamines or anti-inflammatory drugs such as Motrin, Indocin, Naprosyn, and corticosteroids, the ones often used by people with allergies and allergy-related inflammatory diseases.

- There may be *many* foods you're allergic to that are involved in your symptoms.
- It is not always possible to be completely objective. In using these self-test methods, you will have to interpret your reactions and monitor your responses to determine whether you are having a reaction, the severity of the reaction, and its source. You must be careful not to be influenced by what you *suspect* you're allergic to or to imagine reactions where none exist.
- Most food-allergy symptoms are delayed. Reactions may occur as long as twenty-four to forty-eight hours after eating the allergic food.

And one caution: Since in rare cases it is possible to trigger an anaphylactic (shock) reaction when testing for allergies, self-tests should not be undertaken (without informed supervision) by those with a history of anaphylaxis, asthma, angioedema, epilepsy, severe emotional disturbances, or previous allergic responses that have required emergency medical attention.

There are three self-testing techniques for you to choose from:

Food Elimination and Challenge. Eliminate from your diet foods you suspect to be allergens for five full days, and then reintroduce each food one at a time to see if it provokes an allergic response.

Fasting and Challenge. Water-fast for five days to clear your system, and then eat the foods you want to test one at a time to see if allergic symptoms appear.

The Least Common Foods Test. Eat a full diet as long as you eat *only* those foods that you rarely eat under normal circumstances. As with the other methods, after five days suspected allergens are then eaten to see if they provoke symptoms.

Determining Which Foods to Test

It would be just about impossible to test every food you eat to see if you're allergic to it, so how do you choose which foods to test? There are three helpful guidelines: the foods that the most people are allergic to (see Table 46, page 230), the foods that you are aware of having some kind of reaction to (that "disagree" with you), and the foods you eat most often (and probably love most).

The questionnaire you filled out in Chapter 13 should give you some of the information you need about the foods you love and eat most often, and perhaps about symptoms that are connected with eating certain foods. Go back through that questionnaire and make a note of

Table 46—The Most Commonly Allergic Foods		
corn	yeast	whole wheat
rye	milk	cheese
eggs	soybeans	coffee
citrus fruit (orange)	chocolate	tomato
white potato	various spices	malt
peanuts	beef	pork

any foods that you can connect to symptoms and the foods that you put down as your favorites. List up to twenty foods, in the order that you want to test them, the ones you like most or that affect you most at the top of the list.

If your questionnaire isn't providing the answers you need, then the best way to ferret out potential allergens is to keep a complete diet diary or record of everything you eat and drink for a week or so, along with notations about any symptoms that you're feeling—from a headache to bloating after eating to congested nose to aches and pains to feeling tired or cranky. It also helps to make note of any "environmental" substances you may have come in contact with, such as cigarette smoke, automobile exhaust, floor polish, dish detergent, perfumes, toothpaste, animal dander, or a mildewed attic. Even though food-allergy tests won't detect an allergy to your deodorant, such an allergy may help to explain otherwise mysterious recurring symptoms.

Taking the Tests

All three self-testing methods require that you abstain from some or all foods for five days, then carefully reintroduce the suspected allergic foods and note what kind of reaction they provoke. The reason for the five-day abstinence is that it takes that long for most allergic symptoms to be "unmasked" to the point that reintroducing the food will usually provoke a marked reaction. With any of these self-tests, you should pay attention to any reactions or symptoms that you notice, including the easing up of symptoms you're used to. Because you are doing without your usual ration of allergic foods, it is possible that you will feel uncomfortable withdrawal or detoxification symptoms for the first few days, but they will disappear thereafter. Treatment for these symptoms is discussed on pages 261–64.

Food Elimination and Challenge

1. Choose five foods that you want to test first—the five that are most suspect.
2. Eliminate those five foods from your diet *entirely* for five days. It is very important to read the labels carefully on any packaged foods during this period—eggs, wheat, sugar, and corn, for example, show up everywhere you look. The easiest way to avoid hidden ingredients is to eat simple, fresh, whole foods. Sometimes it makes sense to avoid the entire food group. Since the glutens and nightshades, for example, often seem to be the bad guys when it comes to rheumatoid arthritis, the problem food might not be just tomatoes or potatoes or wheat and rye, but the whole family of foods. Gluten-free foods are listed on pages 376–77, the nightshades on page 437.

Fasting and Challenge Test

It was Dr. William Rhea, inspired by Dr. Theron Randolph, who developed the idea of testing for allergies in a totally controlled environment. His environmentally controlled hospital in Dallas–Fort Worth provides a sterile setting in which *severely* allergic people can be tested and where they have a chance to recover from the environmental and dietary assaults they are so sensitive to. The idea of fasting to test for food allergies is based on the same principles.

If you suspect that you have quite a few food allergies or if symptoms are severe—and if you have the willpower—water fasting is the most effective way to "clear" symptoms as a preliminary to challenging the system with the suspected allergic foods.

1. You must water-fast for five days, drinking only bottled or distilled water. Don't take vitamins, herbs, or other supplements.
2. Fast at a time when you do not have to maintain a full schedule.
3. Don't smoke, and avoid smoky rooms.
4. Don't use toothpaste (substitute salt or baking soda), mouthwashes, or other personal hygeine products containing chemicals. Avoid smoggy air and environmental pollutants where possible.
5. Don't begin a fast if you're taking an antibiotic; don't continue the fast if you come down with a cold or other infection.
6. Fasting should be closely supervised by a trained physician,

especially if you are an insulin-dependent diabetic, epileptic, pregnant, or disabled by illness.

The Least Common Foods Test

This diet probably involves the least hardship, yet it has the effect of eliminating the foods to which you are likely to be allergic.

1. Make a list of all foods that you eat every three days or more frequently. The list should include coffee, flavorings, and all the ingredients in processed foods that you eat frequently.
2. Devise a diet that *avoids* all those foods—it may include everything else you commonly eat.
3. Eat only the infrequently consumed foods for five days.

Testing Suspected Foods and Evaluating the Results

The way to test your reaction to a suspected allergic food is to eat a *substantial,* unseasoned portion of that food, by itself, as the first food of the day.

To evaluate your reaction:

- *Before eating the food,* take your resting pulse.
- Eat the food.
- While resting and in an unstressful surrounding, take your pulse again fifteen minutes later, and every fifteen minutes for the next hour and a half. If your pulse increases by twelve to sixteen beats, unexplained by stress or activity, you should suspect food allergy. But be aware that this pulse test is not conclusive and, because of physiological idiosyncrasies, does not work for many people. A far more effective evaluation technique is your own monitoring of symptoms, as explained below.
- Pay close attention for other symptoms, especially those you've experienced before. Do you feel warm? Itchy? Have a stuffy nose? Headache? Feel mentally dull or fatigued? Stomach upset? It may help you to refer to the list of potential allergy symptoms in Table 1, pages 44–45. If you experience strong symptoms, you should suspect food allergy.

Let at least six hours lapse before eating your next meal. (The majority of delayed symptoms will appear within one to six hours after eating.) Continue to watch for reactions, and remember that many allergic reactions will not show up immediately. Even if what you eat in the meantime confuses things, remain alert to possible symptoms, and you may still catch reactions that might have slipped by unnoticed.

- Test a new food according to this method each morning. Do not put off the testing, for you must have eaten the food to be tested within the past fourteen days in order for the test to be valid. After about two weeks or so, the body is already beginning to recover, and the allergen may not readily provoke a reaction on just one or two challenges. (If you are tested by the FICA, however, the antibody "fingerprint" will still be identifiable and detectable in your blood.)
- You can repeat the test as often as necessary until you've tested all suspected foods.

Once you know what you are allergic to, you are officially ready to begin the Optimum Health Program.

15

How to Eat: Thirteen Basic Nutrition Guidelines

Because each person is unique, each of us must discover his own path on the Optimum Health Program. But certain basic rules are the same for everyone, the foundation of good eating habits. These are the twelve guidelines on which to custom-tailor your own rotation and health program.

1. Educate yourself about nutrition. If good nutrition and health, so basic to our well-being and understanding of ourselves, were taught in school along with geography and sex education and music appreciation, there would be little need for a book like *Dr. Braly's Optimum Health Program.*

Our program is a simple, commonsense, scientific approach to health that should be part of the education of anyone who has completed high school. Unfortunately many people have their priorities mixed up when it comes to diet. They are more likely to know about gourmet cooking —how to prepare fabulous dishes and present them beautifully—than about the balance and nutrition of these elegant meals. "It struck me when I heard you lecture," a patient told me, "that I can whip up a five-course meal on a couple of hours' notice, but I have no idea of its real nutritional value. Now I feel that if I'm going to eat it, I should know what's in it."

There are those who buy prepared foods described as "enriched" and "good for the whole family," thinking they are dishing up adequate nutrition. Others care only about the number of calories. Still others don't give a second thought to the nutritional value of their junk-food diets and could hardly care less that it represents a long-term danger.

In order to understand how the Optimum Health Program works and to be comfortable with it, you have to learn *how to eat.* This means learning not only how to identify and eliminate allergic foods, but also about food groups and about the nutritional value of individual foods, how to shop for and prepare food, how to read the full story on a label. It means learning about the hidden, often dangerous ingredients in your medications and vitamin tablets, as well as those in prepared foods.

Knowledge makes the Optimum Health Program *make sense* and gives credibility to the changes you must make to carry you through a lifetime of improved well-being.

2. Learn from your ancestors. For better or worse, we've all inherited the digestive systems of our forebears; therefore it is their diet that our systems are designed to eat. Up until the agricultural age—which means very recently in terms of human life on earth—man ate a varied diet of raw or *lightly* cooked food. Rarely was there an abundance of food. He ate dozens of different raw vegetables, nuts, seeds, fruits, and assorted critters, and he was likely to have meat only every few days. All infants were breast-fed, and after that, in most tribes, there was no milk. There was no Hamburger Helper, and you could have raspberries only if you lived in a temperate climate and they happened to be in season. It was on this diet that man's digestive system and nutritional needs evolved—over hundreds of thousands of years. A few hundred years of mass agriculture and a few decades of high-tech foods may have revolutionized the way we eat, but it has made barely a dent in our physiological and biochemical inheritance. Our digestive apparatus and nutritional apparatus haven't caught up. Ten thousand years from now, our bodies may have evolved so that they can process today's diet, but for now we're stuck with the old model. (Besides, by the time —centuries from now—that our systems catch up to today's diet, who knows what people will be eating, or if there will be any such thing as real food left?)

Much of the advice that follows really boils down to taking a leaf from our ancestors' book: Find out how much a varied diet can do for your health.

3. Rotate and vary your diet. One of the best ways to keep from becoming undernourished and allergic and addicted to a particular food is to expand the number of foods you eat and not to eat any one food more than once every four days or so. It is the most important single factor on the Optimum Health Program. To those who are eating the same ten or fifteen foods over and over and whose palate is limited, this seems like a tall order. It is really not so difficult and is in fact one of the most enjoyable aspects of the Optimum Health Program.

Here's where our miraculous modern food chain can help us rather than hurt us. We have so enormous a selection of new and varied things to eat that we need never run out of choices or be bored eating the same foods over and over. Eating is not boring on the Optimum Health Program. Many people who start off at Optimum Health Labs complaining about the foods they are going to have to give up for ninety days come back to report on all the wonderful new foods they've found and enjoy. Learn to try new things; it's part of the adventure.

4. Eat a proper balance of carbohydrates, proteins, and fats. Ideally, your diet should consist of 60–70 percent complex carbohydrates, 10–20 percent protein, and 15–25 percent fats. As with all things, *balance* is important. The right proportions are the key to digestion and to regulation of other body processes and of the 60 trillion cells that make up your body. Even within each food group, balance is important, and nourishment should come from *many* foods in each classification.

Protein. Protein provides all the essential amino acids necessary to life (see page 126) and is the most important factor in tissue building. And it is needed to stimulate the digestive process. As it now stands, however, there is often *too much* protein in the American diet —and whatever protein is not needed to build tissue the body converts to fat and stores. Red meats and dairy products are the villains of the American diet for many reasons. They are the wrong kind of protein —high in saturated fats and highly allergenic. They are not the best source of protein, nor are they the only source. Fish and poultry, beans, peas, vegetables, potatoes, and whole grains are good protein sources. If you are not allergic to milk products and don't suffer from lactose (milk sugar) intolerance, skim milk and yogurt are preferable to cheese and whole milk as dairy sources of protein. Vegetable sources of protein are given on page 445.

Complex carbohydrates. Though all recent research shows that carbohydrates should form the bulk of our diet, the consumption of carbohydrates has actually dropped by about one third in the last fifty years. Worse, more than 50 percent of these remaining carbohydrates are "simple" highly refined carbohydrates—white sugar, candy, refined flour, carbonated beverages—all of which have practically no nutrient value, rely on other foods for their digestion, and are too easily and rapidly absorbed by the system. Whole grains, fruits, and vegetables are the best sources of complex carbohydrates.

Fats. Fats make up 40 percent of the American diet—that's approximately double what it should be. And again they are the wrong kind of fats: cholesterol-laden meats, eggs and dairy products high in arachidonic acid (saturated fats), along with highly processed (heated, pressurized, hydrogenated) oils. Better sources are foods that provide essential fatty acids (Chapter 11): nuts, seeds, raw vegetables, cold-seawater fish, and other marine life. And the oils we use in salads and cooking should be cold-pressed oils from the same sources. Table 47 below shows the staggering amount of calories and saturated fat in nine widely consumed foods.

Because the "good" fats are so hard to come by in our diets, it is best to augment dietary sources of essential fatty acids with supplements—in the form of evening primrose oil and marine lipid (MaxEPA) capsules.

5. When and how much you eat is important, too. Here's one you've heard all your life: "Eat a good breakfast." It's good advice. *Calories consumed in the morning are more apt to be metabolized as heat energy, but calories consumed in the evening are stored as fat.* And it has been confirmed over and over that eating a good breakfast not only provides needed energy with which to face the stresses of the day, but will lead to the consumption of about 600 fewer calories at dinner. Skipping breakfast, or shoring yourself up with the empty calories of coffee with sugar and a Danish, will lead to such a major energy depletion that evening bingeing is almost inevitable.

For energy efficiency and weight control, much of your daily protein should be eaten at breakfast and lunch; dinner should be predominantly complex starchy carbohydrates. Don't eat late at night—calories are stored, not burned, during sleep.

Eat slowly and chew your food thoroughly. These are not idle admonitions. Adequate chewing ensures that the food is properly started on the road to digestion while still in the mouth and provides adequate surface area for the digestive juices to work on. Eating slowly guards against overtaxing your system with too much food too fast. And there's another reason. It takes about twenty minutes, after you begin eating,

Table 47 — Our High-Fat World

Food	Total Calories	Percentage of Saturated Fat
T-bone steak 8 ounces	1,072	80
Big Mac 7 ounces	563	53
Chili (Hormel's) 7 ounces	370	68
Wendy's hamburger 7 ounces	470	50
Stouffer's cheese soufflé 6 ounces	355	66
Fried fish sticks 4 ounces	330	65
Pepperoni pizza ½ frozen	430	46
Ground beef patty 4 ounces	313	65
Spam 3 ounces	260	80

for the intestinal-tract enzyme called cholecystokinin to signal the brain's appetite center that you are full. If all our food is wolfed down, we end up overeating before our system has a chance to tell us that we've had enough.

Take your vitamin, mineral, and essential-fatty-acid supplements with your meals. Dietary supplements are dependent on the enzymatic action of your food for proper absorption. They should be taken in divided doses with or soon after each meal.

Cut down on the amount you eat. More and more attention is being paid to the study of longevity. Anti-aging products and regimens—of varying degrees of effectiveness and safety—are front-page news, and "life extension" has become a household phrase. Among all the claims to the secret of long life, one simple fact keeps turning up over and over: *The simplest and surest thing you can do to add time to your life is to eat less.* A varied rotation diet gets rid of the cravings and usually leads, subtly but surely, to a diet far lower in saturated fats and refined sugars. You'll feel as if you are eating more because you won't feel hungry, but your consumption level may actually have gone down. By lightening the digestive burden on your system, by efficiently burning up rather than storing the calories you consume, you're saving a lot of wear and tear on the system.

With each decade of life, calories should be reduced by about 10 percent. In study after study, laboratory animals that were *slightly* underfed lived significantly (30 percent to 200 percent) longer than those who ate a "normal" unrestricted amount. Those who eat to obesity, of course, shorten their life spans significantly.

Pay attention to the pH factor—the acid/alkaline balance of your diet. The system favors a slightly "alkaline" state, which is often thrown off by the typical diet. Meats, cola drinks, and citrus fruits are highly acidic. Grains, vegetables, and most other fruits are alkaline.

6. Eat as much of your food as possible in a natural uncooked state. The further that food is removed from its raw, natural state, the more it loses its nutrients and natural fiber. This includes not only the effects of heating and cooking and improper storage, but just about everything that the food industry does to it in the way of refining, bleaching, homogenizing, and processing. And of course further damage is done by the many additives that are supposed to improve the product: preservatives, colorings, artificial flavorings, blenders, emulsifiers, bulking agents.

Common additives such as sodium benzoate, sulfites, and monosodium glutamate, colorings such as FD&C Yellow No. 5 (tartrazine), nitrates and salicylates, BHT and BHA are responsible for some of the most common chemical hypersensitivities; several of them are contributing factors to hyperactivity in children (page 302) and migraine headaches (page 378). "Enriching" the food after it's been so badly massacred doesn't begin to make up for the damage. It doesn't restore the natural balance of the raw food, doesn't convert trans fats back to cis fats, and much of the fiber value of the original is lost as well.

Dietary fiber—ideally about 20 grams a day of the stuff—is crucial to proper digestion and elimination. It also helps maintain a healthier level of serum cholesterol and may play an important role in the prevention of diabetes, hemorrhoids, varicose veins, colitis, diverticulosis, and appendicitis. A good working definition of dietary fiber is that it is that portion of food that cannot be easily broken down by our own intestinal digestive juices and therefore passes through the bowel undigested. It speeds up the transit time through the intestines and rectum, and makes the stools larger and softer by virtue of the increased water trapped within the undigested fiber.

In a properly functioning digestive system, most bodily waste products are excreted though the skin, lungs, and kidneys. Feces would ideally be made up only of dead bacteria and sloughed off mucosal cells from the intestines, leftover bile and pancreatic juices and fiber (cellulose, lignin, pectin, semicellulose, for example). There should be no undigested food in the stool. If recurrent and in large amounts, it's a sure sign of digestive problems and a diet too low in fiber. Fiber acts as a cleanser, stimulator, and "detoxifier" of the system.

Unfortunately refining and processing, and even excess cooking, remove most of the valuable fiber from food. There is no fiber in meat and dairy food, in sugar or fat, and little in sweets and processed foods. You can see that the typical American diet is a constipating diet.

Bran is the classic fiber food. Whole grains, fruits, and vegetables all contain fiber, as does guar gum. Fiber supplements are available in most vitamin and health food stores. Beware of the term "nonnutritive fiber" on food labels—this usually means that sawdust or wood by-products have been added to your food. (Also beware that in search of a higher fiber diet, you do not load up on high-fiber foods you are allergic to! Remember that wheat, bran, and other grains are frequently allergenic foods.) A table listing nongrain sources of fiber appears on page 453.

Finally, refined foods are not only guilty of providing "empty" calories and dangerous additives, they often contain dozens of ingredients, which makes it almost impossible to follow a rotation diet without using up all your food choices. Eating packaged foods with their multiple ingredients means eating the same foods over and over, day after day, which leads inexorably to the development of allergies to those foods in allergy-prone individuals.

7. Beware of CATS. CATS is a useful acronym for four of the greatest spoilers of good health: Coffee, Alcohol, Tobacco, and Sugar. All four of these dietary disasters are frequently associated with allergic individuals. Coffee, alcohol, and sugar too easily permeate and adversely affect the digestive tract and seem to enhance one's allergic response to other foods and beverages consumed in conjunction with them, in addition to having their own unique ways of damaging our health.

Coffee. Coffee stimulates the nervous system, but doesn't provide any nutrients to support that nervous energy. Too, it appears to irritate the mucosa of the jejunum and ileum, resulting in abnormal mucus secretion. High coffee consumption also causes a significant increase in serum cholesterol levels (about 14 percent). It depletes B vitamins, and excessive magnesium is lost via the urine in coffee drinkers. Iron deficiency, already a problem for so many, especially women, is made worse by drinking coffee. Coffee (or tea) can reduce the intestinal absorption of iron by as much as 80 percent.

A cup of coffee or tea contains anywhere from 40 to 85 percent of the daily need for fluoride; heavy coffee drinkers often suffer from fluoride overload similar to the industrial disease fluorosis. Many coffee drinkers become dependent on coffee to wake them up and give them energy (not realizing that late afternoon fatigue is the frequent consequence); without coffee they feel listless and nervous. If they drink too much coffee late in the day, they're jittery and can't sleep. Tremors, dizziness, and even hallucinations can occur as a result of drinking coffee, for it can scramble the brain's chemical neurotransmitters. Coffee may also be related to high blood pressure, magnesium deficiency, irregular heartbeat, calcium oxalate kidney stones, low blood sugar, benign enlargement of the prostate, cystic mastitis, headaches, fetal damage, and irritation of the stomach lining. Coffee addicts are damaging their systems in many ways.

Caffeine is present not only in coffee, but in medications for weight control (Appedrine, Dexatrim), stimulants (NoDoZ, Vivarin), painkillers (Anacin, Bromo-Seltzer, Excedrin, Vanquish), cold and allergy drugs (Dristan, Sinarest), menstrual aids (Midol, Femicin, Pre-Mens Forte), soft drinks (Coca-Cola, Tab, RC Cola, Dr Pepper, Mountain Dew, and Pepsi-Cola, though some of these manufacturers are finally offering a caffeine-free variety), teas (both brewed and instant), and even some ice creams.

Coffee should be consumed only on occasion (if at all), and it should be drunk before or between meals and ideally in midafternoon, when it will interfere with neither morning energy nor nighttime sleep. Note: Beware of decaffeinated coffee. Recent studies indicate that the chemical residue found in most decaffeinated coffees, methylene chloride, is associated with cancer in laboratory animals.

Alcohol. The problems of alcohol allergy/addiction and its treatment are discussed on pages 317–23, but I want to mention here just a few of the devastating nutritional dangers of alcohol. Alcohol is a highly addictive drug, which affects the central nervous system, the heart, the brain, the stomach, the pancreas, and the liver, among others, and tragically destroys the lives of both those who become addicted and those around them.

Alcohol is a combination of highly allergic substances in solution. When alcohol is chemically analyzed, the grain, gluten, yeast, protein, and sugars used in its production are still detectable. Therefore, alcohol consumption can lead to allergy/addiction to the grains, sugar, and yeast it contains. (Table 53, page 319, lists the common food substances found in alcoholic beverages.)

Alcohol, like marijuana, causes a reduced secretion of hydrochloric acid into the stomach, with all the predictable consequences: maldigestion, poor absorption of food and nutrients, overgrowth of intestinal flora, and eventually significant malnutrition. Even at moderate consumption levels, alcohol (again, due to delta-6-desaturase inhibition) leads to a "leaky gut"—increased permeability of the mucosal lining of the small intestine—permitting the increased absorption of partially digested food molecules (and perhaps microorganisms, enterotoxins, and drugs) that normally would be screened out.

Tobacco. There is no need to go into detail about the risks of smoking, which are by now well-documented. Cancer, heart disease, strokes, emphysema, chronic bronchitis, and damage to the unborn fetus head the list of dangers. (Parenthetically, tobacco may induce such diseases in much the same way as alcohol—by the inhibition of delta-6-desaturase, leading to PGE1 and PGE3 deficiencies.)

There is one additional smoking danger worth mentioning, however. More and more convincing evidence shows that smoking is also damaging to those around the smoker, who have to breathe secondhand tobacco-filled air. Such victims, when tested, have 80 percent of the blood level of carbon monoxide of smokers.

Sugar. There are more than 100 recognized substances described as sugars. The most common one is white table sugar or sucrose. Other sugars with which we should be familiar are raw sugar, brown sugar, honey, corn syrups, dextrose (corn sugar), fructose or levulose, lactose or milk sugar, total invert sugar, sorbitol, mannitol, and xylitol. (A list describing these sugars appears on pages 454–55.) Fascinatingly, recent studies demonstrate that each individual handles and reacts differently to the various sugars.

In 1979 the average American consumed 125 pounds of processed sugar, as contrasted to only 10 pounds or less 150 years earlier.

Sugar is potentially a highly allergic and addictive substance and as such may be a complicating factor in diabetes and hypoglycemia, as well as obesity, hypertension, hyperactivity, mental and nervous disorders, elevated cholesterol and triglycerides, ulcers, depression, and anxiety.

Refined sugars do not contain the essential nutrients necessary even to metabolize them properly. Thus the body has to cannibalize its own nutrients for their digestion. Sugary processed foods are also unlikely to contain much fiber, so the high consumption of sugar-laden foods contributes to a harmful low-fiber diet.

In a sensitive individual, sugar has been shown to be the direct cause of inhibition of blood cells, and to lower the immunity of certain important "scavenger" white blood cells. Consider the following scenario: After you consume a soda or a couple of cups of coffee with sugar and a Danish, these phagocytic white blood cells will pick up 75 percent fewer bacteria than before, and it will take about six to eight hours to recover their former protective powers. But if, before those six hours are up, you eat a piece of pie a la mode or a couple more cups of sugared coffee, the immune defense system will be further depleted. If before the recovery period is up, you have a typical dinner—perhaps a couple of drinks, a steak, and french fries with wine, followed by dessert with coffee and sugar, 90 percent of the white blood cell's defenses will have been lost.

Refined sugars should be avoided as much as possible, but this is difficult to do since so many processed products contain sugars of various kinds. Read the labels of packaged foods; if sugar (under any of its many aliases) is listed among the first three or four ingredients, it makes up a large percentage of the product. Learn to eat refined sugars sparingly, with a full meal, not as a snack, and to eat fresh fruit to satisfy your sweet tooth.

On the Optimum Health Program, it is recommended that you give up coffee, alcohol, and refined sugars entirely during the three-month allergen removal and general healing period. Help in withdrawing from these substances (and from food allergies) is outlined in the following chapter on pages 261–64. If and when you go back to these substances, consume them only occasionally, on a rotation basis, to assure that you will not become readdicted.

8. Go easy on the salt. Not everyone is sensitive to additional salt in his diet. But some people, especially those with a concomitant deficiency in calcium or magnesium, respond to salt with an elevation in blood pressure. Hypertension is the main reason that excess dietary sodium should be avoided, for hypertension can also lead to problems related to the circulation, heart disease, and the nervous system. Excess salt (second only to food allergy) is a major cause of water retention and may be associated with depletion of the body's store of potassium. The higher the consumption of sodium, the greater the urinary loss of potassium. Low potassium may contribute to life-threatening cardiac arrhythmias.

Most people consume more than ten to fifty times the amount of sodium that is considered necessary—approximately 500–1,000 mg a day. Sodium chloride is found naturally in many foods and *un-naturally* in many more, for it is added to almost all prepared and packaged food products, often in exorbitant amounts. Check food labels if you need evidence: Sodium is often listed among the top ingredients. It may go by any of several names: salt, MSG (monosodium glutamate), sodium saccharin or sodium nitrate, baking soda, sodium benzoate, sodium citrate, or sodium propionate. Even sweet foods like jams and soft drinks contain salt.

Avoid products that are high in salt, including bacon and sausage, pretzels and potato chips. If you are going to salt, use a mixture of potassium chloride and sodium chloride. You will probably find, anyway, that simple, fresh foods that haven't been overrefined and overcooked retain much of the flavor that salt attempts to put back, and that within a week or two, you'll regain your ability to enjoy the taste of your food without adding salt. (If you continue having difficulty tasting and smelling your food at this point, consider a possible deficiency in the mineral zinc.)

9. Watch out for milk. Cow's milk and milk products are one of the two or three most allergic foods, both in children *and* adults. Also, the overwhelming majority of the world's populations are intolerant of lactose, or milk sugar (i.e., unable to digest it well), because of a deficiency of the intestinal enzyme lactase necessary for the digestion of milk lactose. Third, most milk products are high in saturated fats, specifically in the already overconsumed arachidonic acid.

From birth on, humans should consume cow's milk in very limited amounts, and you should keep an eye on your milk consumption to be sure you are not masking an allergy to milk or suffering digestive symptoms (excess gas, bloating, diarrhea, abdominal cramping, for example) as a result of lactose intolerance. Don't worry about calcium deficiency. Most non-Americans consume very little milk after weaning—perhaps one half to one tenth what we consume—and yet they *often* have much stronger and denser bones and teeth far later in life than we. (Incidentally, 50 percent of cow's milk-sensitive people are probably sensitive to goat's milk as well.)

There are many other good absorbable sources of calcium. Yogurt seems to be an easily tolerated form of milk, and the chart on page 441 lists numerous other high-calcium foods. Who needs cow's milk? Only calves!

10. Water is good for you if it's good water. Drinking six to eight glasses of water a day has long been touted, and rightly so, as a vital part of any good health regimen. Water may *assist* digestion when consumed with meals and dilutes toxins in the system and helps flush them out. Water also replaces lost fluids, especially important during vigorous exercise or work, during hot weather, and when feverish. The latest research shows that a glass or two of water should be drunk with meals to stimulate the desired level of gastric secretion in the stomach and to facilitate the secretion of the proper amount of pancreatic enzymes and bicarbonates in the small intestine.

But there may be problems with drinking large amounts of tap water. It is possible to overdose on chlorine and fluoride from drinking tap water, especially if you are a heavy drinker of coffee or tea, or if you use other fluoridated products like toothpaste and mouthwash. Excessive chlorine elevates serum cholesterol and has been reported to damage the walls of arteries. Excess fluoride can discolor one's teeth and cause brittle bones. Too, there is increasing danger that your water supply is contaminated from unregulated toxic wastes and spillage. Contaminated water tables and wells in various parts of the country are turning up in the news with some regularity these days. Drinking carefully selected bottled or distilled water eliminates most of the danger of petrochemical contaminants, as well as an overdose of chlorine and fluoride.

11. Be watchful and prudent about medications. There are two points to be made about prescription and nonprescription medicines. The first is that many people take too much medicine, too easily —everything from over-the-counter drugs to widely used potent prescription drugs in the form of tranquilizers, antidepressants, painkillers, sleeping pills, antacids, and anti-inflammatory drugs. Such foreign chemicals do little or nothing to bring about a cure; if effective, they only relieve symptoms and *mask* causes. Many of them have serious side effects (often requiring additional medication or hospitalization to counteract their undesired effects); others require increased doses to be effective; many are addictive. As we have seen, more than 10 percent of the millions of hospital admissions each year are the consequence of reactions to *prescribed* medications. While in the hospital an additional 5 percent of patients become increasingly ill on *other* prescribed medications.

At OHL, we encourage our patients to cut down on their medications as soon as they start feeling better—but gradually and under close medical supervision. We also encourage people not to take medications unnecessarily. It is not unusual for newcomers to our program to be on half a dozen or more *prescribed* medications, often several to offset the side effects of other medications. But within a few months many are able to reduce their medications to one or two and on occasion to eliminate drugs altogether.

The other point to be made is that there are unseen dangers to many medications. Most medications contain hidden ingredients, such as fillers and binders, colorings and preservatives, that provoke hypersensitive reactions. Sodium benzoate, a preservative, and the food coloring tartrazine (FD&C [Food, Drug, and Colors] Yellow No. 5), two common *chemical* causes of migraines, hyperactivity, and asthmatic attacks, show up in many medicines. A common asthma medication, theophylline, was recently revealed to contain metabisulfites, which *themselves* are potentially powerful asthma provokers. Tagamet, an antacid used to treat duodenal ulcers (having replaced Valium as the most frequently prescribed medication in the world), has recently been demonstrated to be ineffective against ulcers because at least two thirds of ulcer sufferers do *not* oversecrete hydrochloric-acid. The reduction in hydrochloric acid production and pepsin therefore only further decreases digestion and absorption. The thought of it all is enough to give you ulcers!

Then there's aspirin. The problem with aspirin is that many millions of people take this drug liberally without thinking anything about it. Eighty million Americans take aspirin; 25 million take it almost every day for pain. But it's not quite so harmless as it's cracked up to be. The trouble with aspirin (and many other over-the-counter anti-inflammatory drugs, including the new ibuprofen) is that it is indiscriminate in its internal biochemical actions. Aspirin blocks the action of certain of the symptom-producing inflammatory prostanoids, but at the same time it promotes the production of other inflammatory allergy-causing prostanoids.

Even the common practice of taking aspirin or Tylenol for fever may do more harm than good. Fever is an extraordinarily important immune defense that, in most cases, should be allowed to run its course. Fever stimulates the immune system in the presence of certain prostaglandin hormones, as a consequence of which the immune system is better able to fight off the infection. Here again, the prostaglandins are at work to heal you—but aspirin and other widely used and abused anti-inflammatory drugs inhibit or redirect the synthesis of prostaglandins. Fever is a *correct response of the body to disease*—it stimulates certain white blood cells of the immune system to destroy the infection. By eliminating the fever, you remove a most valuable weapon; you prolong the infection and perhaps make it worse.

Aspirin plays a particularly ominous role in the treatment of children's fevers, chiefly flu and chicken pox. Recent reports indicate that children treated for these ailments with aspirin run the risk of developing deadly Reyes syndrome, a set of symptoms that include recurrent fever, irritability, and lethargy, leading to confusion, coma, and sometimes brain damage. Twenty percent of its young victims die. The incidence of Reyes has increased twenty-five times in the last few years, and aspirin has been pinpointed as a leading culprit.

12. A word about water fasting. There are times when a water fast can make sense. It is one useful way to self-test for food allergies (see page 231), and it can be a good way to "clear out" the digestive tract and get a head start on a new diet. Periodic, short-term fasting may be a beneficial adjunct to an anti-aging regimen (page 325), serving to stimulate the immune system. There are people who fast frequently, for religious or spiritual reasons, and many people report that fasting makes them feel extremely good. Fasting often does have the ability to make many of us feel better, but much of the reason is that we're no longer eating allergic foods that make us feel so poorly. Avoiding allergic foods and rotating and varying the nonallergic foods produce the same end result without risk. A fast can be dangerous for certain individuals if it is undertaken without supervision, or if it goes on for too long. It is definitely not a good idea for most athletes in training. Active people who fast for one to three days not only deplete the high-octane energy glycogen stores they need for strenuous exercise, but break down their own skeletal muscle and other essential tissues to provide an alternative fuel source. Eating the right nonallergic foods is better than eating nothing, and you can get the same short-term symptom-relieving, energizing benefit.

13. Nobody's perfect. Remember, you do not have to give up everything you love *forever* to get results on the Optimum Health

Program. Mistakes and backsliding are to be expected at times. You can learn from mistakes—sometimes the hard way, when you prematurely reintroduce an allergic food and provoke a strong allergic reaction. I still manage to do myself in from time to time with milk products. Afterward I often feel rotten and swear I'll never do it again. With the assistance of aerobic exercise and Vitamin-C-to-bowel-tolerance, I quickly control the allergic process(es), and within six to twelve hours I am again symptom-free.

Desperate all-or-nothing cold turkey reforms are often doomed to failure. The best way to change your nutrition and life-style on a permanent basis is to make a list of the things *you* would like to improve or change, in the order *you* want to deal with them. (Just for encouragement, you might make a list of the good diet and exercise habits you already practice.) A sample list might look like this:

1. Drink more water—starting with two glasses of bottled water with each meal. Make ice cubes with bottled water.
2. Take supplements with each meal instead of all at once in the morning on an empty stomach.
3. Make it a point to eat a better breakfast and get some protein in the morning. Possible choices: cottage cheese, bran cereal, cold leftover chicken, lean hamburger.
4. Lay off the saltshaker.
5. Begin reading about exercise. Start an exercise program. Start playing tennis again.
6. Try three new foods every week.
7. Eat a lighter dinner earlier—8:00 P.M. at the latest—and no meat for dinner.
8. Give up coffee. Start by cutting back to one cup in the morning *with a full breakfast* and one with dinner. No coffee after two weeks.
9. Cut way back on drinking. Start by switching from hard liquor to beer or white wine, two glasses maximum. After two weeks, no booze on weekdays.
10. Slow down when I eat and chew my food better.

Your list should be very specific to your diet, life-style, habits, and problem areas. Start with the first couple of items on the list and stick with them until you have them under control before moving on to the next. You may find that the improvement you feel on the rotation diet may spur you on to accelerate the pace of your reforms.

16

The Rotation Diet: Backbone of the Optimum Health Program

Rotation, rotation, rotation! What location is to a real-estate property, rotation of nonallergic foods is to the Optimum Health Program—the single most important factor among the many that determine its value and success.

For the first three months of the Optimum Health Program you will follow a strict regimen in which all allergic foods are eliminated from your diet completely and no one food is eaten more frequently than once every four days. After those three months, you'll be able to reintroduce most of the formerly allergic foods. But the principals of rotation will still guide what you eat, though on a more flexible basis. The principles of rotation are the foundation of a lifetime diet.

WHAT MAKES THE ROTATION DIET SO SENSIBLE AND EFFECTIVE FOR EVERYONE?

1. A rotation diet helps prevent the development of allergies and thus addictions. Allergies develop for a wide variety of reasons, but a major one seems to be too frequent exposure to a potential stressor. It's almost unheard of to become addicted to something that is consumed only once or twice a week, whether that something is food, tobacco, caffeine, or alcohol.

2. Rotation encourages a much more balanced and varied diet and therefore more needed nutrients. In order not to repeat foods more than once every four days, it is necessary to break out of one's rut and go beyond the ten or fifteen foods and beverages that make up most people's diets. This means trying new foods and whole new groups of foods that may have been all but absent from the diet. Those who normally live on fatty red meats and sugar are forced to eat more grains, fruits, and vegetables in order to have enough foods to choose from.

3. Rotation dictates a simple, unrefined, unchemicalized diet. It is almost impossible to continue to eat packaged, processed, or complicated foods on a rotation diet. Many packaged foods contain dozens of ingredients, which pretty quickly "use up" foods that cannot then be eaten for ninety-six hours. The same goes for recipes with multiple ingredients and elaborate sauces. By the fourth day of the diet, if you haven't simplified your meals, you're eating celery sticks with peanut butter or even fasting. Slowly and inexorably the Optimum Health Program leads you away from junk food and toward the foods that are good for you.

4. Rotation unstresses the digestion. A rotation diet is what your digestive system was designed to handle. Because it is relieved of the burden of coping with chemicals and additives, with coffee and alcohol, and with too much of the same foods over and over, the system has a chance to strengthen and repair itself. The increase in dietary fiber is also a boon to digestion: People on the Optimum Health Program don't remain constipated for long.

5. Rotation leads to weight loss. A rotation diet clears up the allergies that lead to food cravings, a slowed metabolism, and water retention. Fats and sugars are of necessity reduced. Even those who continue to eat large meals and whose calorie consumption doesn't change much (though this is unusual once food cravings go away) manage to lose weight naturally on a rotation diet.

CAN ALLERGIES BE ELIMINATED THROUGH ROTATION ONLY?

Patients at Optimum Health Labs have asked if it is possible to become allergy-free just by rotating the diet, without going to the trouble of testing for allergies and without the strict three-month abstinence from allergic foods. It is possible, but it would be difficult and would take a much longer time.

What would happen if you were rotating foods that you were allergic to is that you would be *unmasking* them on a rotational basis. Under normal circumstances, you mask the symptoms of allergy by eating the toxic food to keep from feeling withdrawal symptoms. On the rotation diet, if you did not eliminate allergic foods, you would eat an allergic food, then go through withdrawal during the four-day avoidance period. At the end of the four days, just about the time that the withdrawal symptoms subside, you would eat the food again. And what would happen? You would probably have a stronger-than-usual reaction—you would *unmask* the allergy. And this would occur again and again each time you rotated an allergic food.

However, it is possible that over a period of time, if these allergic foods were rotated and you were taking appropriate supplements and exercising, the system would get stronger, and slowly but surely these allergies would come under control. But it would take a long time and a lot of needless recurring discomfort. Better to go through the tests, bite the bullet, and forgo those favorite foods for a few months.

PLANNING YOUR OWN ROTATION DIET

Careful planning and record keeping will make following your diet easy and effective.

- You need a list of the foods that you are allergic to—determined either by your own self-tests or OHL's automated FICA test (see Chapter 13).
- It is helpful to make several photocopies of Table 48, the food group list, on the following page; the rotation diet planning form, on page 486; and the diet diary form, on page 487 (one copy each day of your diet).

The first step is to plan four days of menus. The meal plans should avoid all the foods to which you are allergic and should not repeat any one food for four days.

- Cross off the foods that you are allergic to on the food group list; those that remain (and any others you can think of) are the foods that are allowed in your diet. Most people are allergic to five to fifteen or more foods; that still leaves plenty to choose from.
- Use this revised list to devise four breakfasts, four lunches, four dinners, and a variety of between-meal snack foods; it is organized by food groups to help you plan your menus. Each meal must use a different meat, a different grain, a different vegetable, and so on. Even spices and sweeteners must be parceled out over the four days.
- Be guided by what you like, the time you have to spend on preparation, and what's available now in local supermarkets and health food stores. Each meal should involve just a few ingredients so that you don't use up all your available nonallergenic foods with complicated multiple-ingredient recipes.
- Be sure that you are compensating for the nutritional value of the foods you are allergic to. This is especially important in the case of foods high in protein or essential nutrients such as calcium and iron. And be sure you're getting enough dietary fiber. If you will be eliminating or cutting way back on meat

Table 48 — Food Group List

Grains
- Wheat
- Rye
- Oats
- Barley
- Buckwheat
- Rice
- Millet
- Corn

Legumes
- Carob
- Lentil
- Split pea
- Peanut
- Kidney bean
- Pinto bean
- String bean
- Mung bean
- Lima bean
- Navy bean
- Soy bean
- Pea
- Chick-pea
- Black-eyed pea

Meat
- Pork
- Beef
- Veal
- Lamb
- Calf's liver

Poultry
- Chicken
- Chicken liver
- Whole egg
- Egg white
- Turkey
- Duck

Melon
- Cantaloupe
- Honeydew
- Watermelon
- Crenshaw

Fruit
- Lemon
- Orange
- Grapefruit
- Lime
- Tangerine
- Nectarine
- Pineapple
- Banana
- Raspberry
- Blackberry
- Strawberry
- Apple
- Pear
- Plum (prune)
- Peach
- Apricot
- Cherry
- Grape
- Papaya
- Cranberry
- Blueberry
- Kiwi
- Fig
- Mango
- Avocado

Nuts
- Almond
- Walnut
- Pecan
- Pistachio
- Cashew
- Filbert
- Brazil nut
- Chestnut
- Coconut

Seeds
- Pumpkin
- Sesame
- Sunflower

Fungus
- Mushroom
- Bakers' yeast
- Brewer's yeast
- Hops

Seafood
- Shrimp
- Lobster
- Crab
- Oyster
- Clam
- Scallop
- Red snapper
- Herring
- Sardine
- Salmon
- Catfish
- Cod
- Bass
- Tuna
- Swordfish
- Halibut
- Sole
- Perch
- Trout
- Abalone

Dairy
- Goat's milk
- Cow's milk
- Butter
- Cottage cheese
- Blue cheese
- Cheddar cheese
- Yogurt

Oils
- Safflower
- Sunflower
- Soy
- Cottonseed
- Walnut
- Olive
- Sesame
- Corn
- Peanut

Vegetables
- Potato
- Eggplant
- Tomato
- Chili pepper
- Paprika
- Garden pepper
- Sweet potato
- Yam
- Asparagus
- Onion
- Head lettuce
- Romaine
- Artichoke
- Kale
- Cabbage
- Brussel sprout
- Broccoli
- Cauliflower
- Radish
- Turnip
- Carrot
- Celery
- Parsnip
- Cucumber
- Winter squash
- Summer squash
- Zucchini
- Pumpkin
- Beet
- Swiss chard
- Spinach
- Olive

Flavoring Agents
- Garlic
- Cinnamon
- Mustard
- Caraway
- Ginger
- Vanilla
- Black pepper
- Cocoa
- Peppermint
- Sage
- Nutmeg
- Clove
- Oregano
- Cumin
- Thyme
- Rosemary
- Psyllium
- Alfalfa
- Basil
- Chive
- Comfrey
- Dill
- Parsley
- Coriander
- Tarragon

Sweeteners
- Maple sugar
- Beet sugar
- Cane sugar
- Corn syrup
- Honey
- Saccharine
- NutraSweet

Miscellany
- Coffee
- Tea

or dairy products, make sure you get your protein from alternate sources. Consult the protein and calcium tables on pages 445 and 441; a fiber chart is on page 453.

- Be an alert shopper. Some commonly allergic foods show up in dozens of popular food items. This is why it is best to eat simple, fresh foods as much as possible. Tables of foods containing yeast, corn, egg, wheat, milk, and soybean appear on pages 432–40. For those with gluten sensitivity, guidelines for a gluten-free diet appear on page 376. Information on the nightshades for those with arthritis can be found on page 330.

To help you plan your diet, two sample menus are shown in Table 49 on pages 253–54, followed by a list of suggested breakfasts, lunches, and dinners.

Sample Meal Suggestions

Breakfast

Poached or scrambled eggs with whole grain bread and tea.
Whole-grain cereal with fresh fruit and nonfat milk.
Buckwheat pancakes with maple syrup, sliced fruit, and herb tea.
Fruit salad sprinkled with sunflower seeds and bran muffin.
Cantaloupe with berries and whole-grain toast.
Hot rice cereal with maple syrup and fruit juice.
Grapefruit with honey and blueberry muffin.
Whole-grain bread with cashew butter and banana.
Baked apple with yogurt and herb tea.

Lunch

Bowl of hearty vegetable soup and whole-grain bread.
Vegetable crudités with dip and iced tea.
Sandwich (see suggestions on page 299) and small green salad.
Hearty salad with greens, mushrooms, cherry tomatoes, and shrimp or tuna or canned salmon.
Artichoke vinaigrette.
Fruit salad with yogurt or low-fat cottage cheese.
Tomato or pepper stuffed with tuna, chopped egg, diced vegetables, sprouts, shrimp, cold rice.
Tabouli salad and iced tea.
Baked potato with yogurt or cheese and chives, and small green salad.
Omelet with sliced tomatoes.

Table 49—Sample Rotation Diet Planning Form

This diet plan was designed for someone whose tests revealed allergies to wheat, oats, malt, gluten, tea, eggs, green beans, cashews, almonds, pineapple, and oranges.

	Day 1	Day 2	Day 3	Day 4
BREAKFAST	Barley flakes with hot milk and blueberries Diluted apple juice with ½ teaspoon crystal Vitamin C added	Corn bread with unsweetened jam Apricot nectar or baked apple Herb tea	Cream of rice with rice milk and strawberries Cranberry juice	Puffed millet cereal with soy milk Peaches Herb tea
SNACK	Pumpkin seeds and raisins	Corn chips with bean dip	Grapes	Sliced apple with peanut butter
LUNCH	Chef's salad with turkey, tomatoes, avocado, lettuce, etc. Cottage cheese	Beef tortilla Salad	Chicken sandwich on rice bread with lettuce and mustard	Tuna salad on rye with lettuce, cucumbers, celery, and curried soy mayonnaise
SNACK	Barley crackers with apple butter	Tapioca pudding	Pear	Toasted sunflower seeds
DINNER	Buckwheat pasta with marinara sauce Spinach salad Baked bananas	Poached salmon or broiled halibut Baked potato Steamed zucchini	Rice and beans Steamed vegetables	Baked yam Vegetable-tofu platter with carrot, cauliflower, broccoli, and mushrooms

Table 49 — Sample Rotation Diet Planning Form

This diet was planned for a person whose tests revealed allergies to barley, wheat, almonds, dates, cabbage, radishes, vanilla, lentils, cocoa, paprika, coffee, maple sugar, clams, sardines, cow's milk, yogurt, and chicken.

	Day 1	Day 2	Day 3	Day 4
BREAKFAST	Oatmeal with applesauce and cinnamon Strawberries Diluted orange juice with ½ teaspoon crystal Vitamin C added	Spinach omelet with onions Rye Essene bread Half a grapefruit	Fruit mix: grapes, cherries, kiwi, or half a papaya ¼ cup cashews or sunflower seeds Herb tea	Corn flakes with soy milk and sliced bananas Herb tea
SNACK	Oat cookies	Peanut butter and celery	Rice cakes with unsweetened jam and sesame butter	Popcorn
LUNCH	Moroccan salad: red leaf lettuce with chickpeas, kale, celery, coriander, oil and vinegar Salmon (on side or in salad)	Cucumber-sprout salad with butter lettuce Cold boiled lobster or crab legs with mayonnaise or oil and vinegar dill sauce	Turkey sandwich with rice bread and soy mayonnaise Lettuce, pickles, sliced tomatoes	Tuna in water with lettuce, alfalfa sprouts, avocado, and soy mayonnaise Corn chips
SNACK	Watermelon	Pear		Orange
DINNER	Sautéed veal medallions with lemon and capers Zucchini julienne Steamed lima beans Baked apple	Broiled filet of sole or red snapper Fresh sautéed mushrooms Steamed broccoli	Rice and beans casserole with carrots and celery	Broiled flounder or scrod Sautéed string beans Steamed beets with dill

Half avocado stuffed with tuna or crab or shrimp.
Asparagus vinaigrette.

Dinner

Broiled fish, steamed broccoli, fruit cup.
Beef or lamb kebab, sautéed cherry tomatoes, fresh fruit sherbet.
Broiled lemon chicken with brown rice and tossed salad.
Shrimp salad with avocado, cup of soup, watermelon.
Eggplant Parmesan, green salad, baked apple.
Sliced London broil, steamed green beans, custard.
Swordfish steak, asparagus, raspberries with yogurt.
Pasta with pesto or tomato sauce and clams, green salad, pineapple sprinkled with brown sugar.

- For shopping purposes, it's a good idea to write down a few alternative meals and a list of possible snacks, using what's left after you've planned the basic menu. This way, you're prepared if you can't find a particular scheduled food, and you have alternatives in case you get bored or aren't in the mood for the meal in your plan. For most people, fresh fruit is the best between-meal snack, but there are many additional suggestions in Chapter 17. This is a working menu to help you shop and plan. You can make any changes you want, as long as you follow the rules.

You'll be following this rotational, diversified plan for three months. You can repeat the same menus every five days, or devise additional four-day rotations, for variety.

TIPS FOR FOLLOWING THE ROTATION DIET

1. Do your best to avoid caffeine, alcohol, tobacco, and sugar. (Tea, cola drinks, and chocolate also contain caffeine.) Be careful about drinking tea in great quantities. Regular teas contain caffeine, and some herbal teas can be toxic at high consumption levels.
2. Try to have a complete protein at two out of three meals, preferably breakfast and lunch.
3. Have a big fresh salad every day. You will need to rotate oils and seasonings. It is important to select only unrefined cold-pressed oils: safflower, sunflower, soy, corn, sesame, chestnut, linseed, walnut. *Note:* For those who are yeast sensitive, distilled white vinegar is the only vinegar that is yeast-free.
4. Drink a couple of glasses of bottled water *with* your meals.

5. Take your vitamins and other supplements with your meals. (Exceptions to this general rule include iron and individual amino acid supplements, which should be taken between meals.)
6. Try not to eat late at night and make the last meal of the day a lighter meal, low in animal protein, high in starchy, complex carbohydrates.
7. There is no limit, except satisfaction of physiological hunger, on the amount that you eat. Do not remain hungry and do not starve yourself. Concentrate on good nutrition and your health, not your weight.

Your success depends on following your diet as closely as possible. If you follow it consistently, you'll only have to do it once, and you'll be set for a lifetime of good health and good eating. At OHL we find that people with painful or distressing symptoms have little trouble sticking to their diets after the first two weeks or so because they begin experiencing relief in a reasonably short time. The most important initial factor during these first three months is the complete elimination of allergic foods. Remember, after it's over you'll be able to eat most of these foods again, but without doing damage. Strict rotation is most important in the case of grains, eggs, meats, and dairy products, since they seem to cause the most common and serious allergy problems. Fruits (with the exception of strawberries and citrus), vegetables, and oils are least allergenic. If it makes things easier, you can use the same oil (cold-pressed unsaturated) all day on any given day—for low-temperature stir-frying, for salad dressing—and you may also repeat the same condiment through the day. *Note:* Consult the following chapter for help with cooking and shopping on the Optimum Health Program.

KEEPING A FOOD AND SYMPTOM JOURNAL

To succeed on the Optimum Health Program, you must pay attention, and you must be patient. During the first month or so, keeping accurate, current records is a must; it is your record of how you are doing, what problems exist, and what needs to be changed. It takes only a few minutes a day, and at most you will have to keep such meticulous notes for three months. It's been our experience at OHL that those patients who become sloppy in their record keeping end up disregarding the diet, overeating nonallergic foods, and eating allergic foods, even if unintentionally. All the hours of history taking, testing, all the time expended in implementing their diet is lost, for want of a few disciplined minutes a day. Persevere, be conscientious, and the diary will be of immense help in improving your health.

The purpose of this careful daily record is to keep close watch over everything you eat and when you eat it, and to discover which, if any, foods, beverages, supplements, medicines, or other substances may be causing or contributing to your allergic symptoms. The relationship between what you eat and your reactions may be very simple or quite complex. Some foods may cause immediate discomfort, while others may provoke a delayed reaction hours or even days after you eat them. Some foods may bring a reaction at some times, but not at others, depending on the amount eaten and what is eaten with it. Of course, if you follow your diet very closely and your allergies have all been picked up by your allergy test, there should be no flare-up of symptoms after the first few days, when any potential withdrawal symptoms will have run their course, and after your digestion, absorption, and elimination have started to improve. Your record keeping should be as detailed and accurate as humanly possible. If you continue having recurrence of allergic symptoms as days and then weeks go by, look for patterns in your reactions, to see if they correlate with a particular food, a particular combination, or time of day.

Have plenty of copies of the rotation diet planning form (page 486) on hand. As you see, it has parallel columns for what you eat, for the supplements or medications taken, and for symptoms and comments, so that you may be able to discern the relationship between cause and effect. Examples of filled-in diet diaries appear in Table 50, pages 258–60.

Directions for Keeping Your Diary

1. Write down everything that enters your stomach, including the water you drink, medications, supplements, digestive aids, snacks, drinks, chewing gum, etc.
2. List the composition of mixed dishes and combinations of foods. For example, it is not enough to write down "a chicken sandwich." Write down the kind of bread, dressing, condiments: "chicken sandwich—whole wheat bread, butter, mustard, salt, lettuce."
3. Note the time that you eat and the time that symptoms appear (the two usually occur an hour or more apart).
4. List all symptoms, even if they're not specific—"feeling dragged out" or "no attention span"—and indicate when the symptoms started, how long they last, and how severe

Table 50 — Sample Diet Diary Form

Date: Oct. 9

Weight: 148
Hours Slept: 5 3/4 hrs.

Time	Food and Drink	Supplements	Time	Symptoms	Severity (1–4+)
T: 6⁴⁵	Early Morning Papaya	4 Primrose 2 MAX EPA	T: 7³⁰	Ran 1 mile stretching Feel good	1+
T: 7³⁰	Breakfast Cream of Rice Rice milk Cherries Cinnamon	multivite-2 multimin-2 B complex C-2000/mg. cal/mag 400 IU vite E	T: 7⁵⁰	Good Refreshed	2+
T: 10⁰⁰	Midmorning Rice cakes w/peanut butter		T: 10¹⁵	Energetic	
T: 12³⁰	Lunch Chicken Breast Avocado Carrots Green salad (olive oil, lemon, pepper)	multivite-2 multimin-2 B complex C-2000 mg cal/mag	T: 1⁰⁰	Good digestion No withdrawals	1+
T:	Midafternoon Plums	4 Eve. Primrose 2 MAX EPA	T: 3⁵⁰	Feeling good	0
T: 6⁰⁰	Dinner Broccoli Potato skins w/sour cream		T:		
T:	Evening Ice cream		T:		

Table 50 — Sample Diet Diary Form

Date: Oct. 10

Weight: 151 1/4
Hours Slept: 6 1/2 hrs.

Time	Food and Drink	Supplements	Time	Symptoms	Severity (1–4+)
T:7⁰⁰	Early Morning 1 cup lemon grass tea Ran 3/4 mile in 10 min.		T:7⁰⁰	Very drowsy	2+
T:7³⁰	Breakfast Oatmeal w/butter Clover honey Cherries	multivite-2 multimin-2 Vit C- 2000/mg. B complex Vit E-400 4 Primrose 2 MAX EPA	T:7³⁰	Hungry Sore muscles	1+
T:10⁰⁰	Midmorning Banana Spring water		T:10⁰⁰	Very drowsy	2+
T:12⁰⁰	Lunch Ground Beef patty Raw carrots/celery Rice cakes w/sesame seeds	multuite-2 multimin-2 B complex Vit C- 2000/mg. Cal/MAG	T:12⁰⁰	Satisfied	1
T:3⁰⁰	Midafternoon Cinnamon tea		T:3⁰⁰	Very drowsy	
T:5⁰⁰	Dinner Steamed Potatoes Green beans Alfafa sprouts Butter	multivite-2 multimin-2 Vit C-2000/mg 4 Primrose 2 MAX EPA	T:5⁰⁰	Digestion good	1++
T:7⁰⁰	Evening Oat muffin		T:7⁰⁰	Restful	1+

Table 50 — Sample Diet Diary Form

Date: Oct. 11

Weight: 150
Hours Slept: 7½ hrs.

Time	Food and Drink	Supplements	Time	Symptoms	Severity (1–4+)
T: 6:45	Early Morning Blueberry leaf tea		T: 7:00	Felt very good after ran 1 mile	1+ 3+ (Sore muscles)
T: 7:30	Breakfast Millet Blueberries	4 Evening P. Oil 2 MAX EPA multivite-2 multimin-2 B complex Vit C-2000/mg. Calcium/mag	T: 8:00	Feeling very energetic Slight headache muscles not as sore	1+
T: 10:00	Midmorning millet muffin		T: 10:00	Slight headache	1+
T: 12:30	Lunch Broiled halibut Tomatoes Lima Beans w/1 pat butter	multimin-2 multivite-2 B complex Vit C-2000/mg.	T: 1:00	Slight headache Slight overall body aches: neck, head, back	1+
T: 3:00	Midafternoon Peaches		T: 3:15	Same	
T: 6:00	Dinner Steamed Cabbage Peas Butter Black Pepper	4 E. Primrose Oil. 2 MAX EPA multimin-2 multivite-2 B complex Vit C-2000/mg. Cal/MAG	T: 6:15	Satisfied with diet Overall-same mild withdrawals	1+
T: 8:30	Evening ½ Cantaloupe	Tryptophane	T: 9:00	Relaxed	1+

they are. The list of common symptoms of food allergy in Table 1, pages 44–45, will help you to pinpoint or articulate what you're feeling. Rate the severity of each symptom on a scale of 1 to 4; 1 to indicate "mildly unpleasant" and 4+ to indicate "painful, obvious, and/or extremely unpleasant." Take special note of symptoms, or their disappearance or absence, before and after each meal or snack.
5. Any additional information is useful. Write down how much you weigh, how long you slept, when and how you exercised.
6. Don't put off filling in your diary until the end of the day. Write things down at the time you eat and at the time you are aware of symptoms. Even the best memory is often unreliable. Carry your diet diary with you.

HOW TO TAKE YOUR SUPPLEMENTS

Everyone on the Optimum Health Program should take a complete, balanced regimen of supplementary vitamins, minerals, and essential fatty acids. (See Table 3 on page 86 for the recommended *routine* adult dosage schedule.)

Taking your supplements in divided daily dosages is extremely important for optimal absorption. *Please refer again to the Guidelines for Supplementation on page 85.* Individual vitamins, minerals, essential fatty acids, and amino acids are treated at length under the appropriate headings in Part III. Therapeutic applications for individual supplements are discussed under individual symptom or illness headings in Part V.

COPING WITH WITHDRAWAL

Physiological addiction to food is no different from addiction to alcohol or tobacco. It is hard to give up an addiction, not only because of one's attachment to the abused substance but also because of the unpleasant withdrawal symptoms. The person who has many allergies of a fairly severe nature can expect to go through a withdrawal period when he abruptly gives up the allergic foods. It's been our experience at OHL that about half of our patients experience discomfort during withdrawal and that for some, the withdrawal involves considerable suffering—especially when the food allergies are accompanied by addiction to highly allergic substances like coffee or sugar.

Now don't worry. With extremely rare exceptions, food-allergy withdrawal involves no tremors or hallucinations. The most common withdrawal symptoms, especially from long-standing addictions, involve an intensification of the symptoms we may already be experiencing: headaches, irritability, increased stuffiness, fatigue, joint aches, anxiety, digestive upset, and of course uncontrollable food cravings. When Merv Griffin started our program, he spent a couple of difficult days with withdrawal headaches and thought he just couldn't go on unless he had a cup of coffee. By the fourth day he was fine.

Moreover, the digestive system needs time to adjust to the new nonallergic diet and to rebalance its output of digestive enzymes to conform with the composition of the new diet. For example, a change from a high-fat, low-fiber diet to one high in carbohydrates can be the cause of gas and bloating or irregularity for a few days.

Treatment Methods

For most food-allergic people, the discomfort of withdrawal lasts only a few days. While the body is readjusting, the unpleasantness can be eliminated—or its severity at least cut down considerably—by large doses of oral (or in more extreme cases, intravenous) Vitamin C. This treatment does not address the psychological origins of addiction; it just makes it possible to go through the withdrawal phase with a minimum of discomfort.

Why does Vitamin C do the trick? One reason may be that food-allergy sufferers have a tendency to be hyperacidic, and acidity deactivates Vitamin C. Very large quantities of C are needed to make up for this tendency to deactivate it. Yet another explanation for Vitamin C's antiwithdrawal effect is its ability to stimulate the production of the anti-inflammatory prostaglandins (e.g., PGE1 and PGE3), thereby suppressing production of proinflammatory PG's. (See Chapter 11.)

Vitamin C is also a powerful detoxifier of the system. Large quantities may produce a mild diarrhea, which leads to the cleansing of the gastrointestinal tract. This therapy—Vitamin C-to-bowel-tolerance—can be practiced only temporarily and doesn't solve the underlying problem of why undigested foods aren't expelled properly in the first place, but it is quite effective. And, in the course of cleaning out the large intestine, the bacterial flora seem to be brought back into balance. This benefit is the same as that often achieved through the use of colonics (enemas)—gentle irrigations of the large intestine, which clean out fecal matter attached to the intestinal walls that may have been there for months, causing a chronic toxic condition.

Yet another explanation for the effectiveness of Vitamin C in alleviating withdrawal symptoms is that Vitamin C is a natural antihistamine and may also stabilize mast cells, the immune cells responsible for releasing the chemical mediators of allergy. Inhibiting the release of these chemical mediators, one of which is histamine, short-circuits the allergic process and thus the eruption of symptoms.

This same aggressive Vitamin C therapy has been used with great success with other disorders. It has proved effective in treating colds, infectious mononucleosis, flu, and just about any type of viral infection.

Vitamin C's effectiveness in alleviating withdrawal was discovered in the 1960s as a result of research into its use with terminal cancer patients who had been heavily dosed with the addictive drug morphine. Use of this powerful painkiller left patients doped up at times when alertness was more desirable, so attempts were made to withdraw them from the drug. It was found that patients who were given Vitamin C not only complained of less pain but experienced fewer or no withdrawal symptoms.

Since that time, megadoses of C have been fairly routine therapy in nutritional medicine for helping people get off addictants, especially alcohol and drugs. The usual treatment we use is intravenous therapy of 20–30 grams of Vitamin C, along with about a gram each of B5, B6, calcium, and magnesium in 500 cc of a normal saline solution dripped in over a period of an hour or so, usually on three consecutive days. The difference is usually noticeable after the first day. After the second day, cravings are often gone, and the third day is merely a cushion to be sure that all withdrawal symptoms are under control.

Withdrawal Therapy

There are four possible levels of Vitamin C treatment for withdrawal from food allergies.

- People whose allergies haven't reached the addiction level. These patients will not experience withdrawal symptoms, but it's a good idea for them to take extra oral Vitamin C, for reassurance.
- People with mild to moderate withdrawal symptoms. These patients can be treated with 2 to 2½ grams of Vitamin C in crystal or powder form, dissolved in water, half an hour before each meal.
- People with severe withdrawal symptoms. Here the recommended treatment is what is called Vitamin C-to-bowel-tolerance, which means taking about half a level teaspoon of Vitamin C in crystal form, dissolved in one cup of water, every half

hour until diarrhea (watery stools) occurs. (This may be anywhere from a few hours to a couple of days.) Then the dose is reduced to about 90 percent of the amount taken and remains at this level until symptoms are gone. *This treatment should not be followed by anyone with a recent or current history of ulcers, diarrhea, or kidney stones.*

- Patients with very severe addictions. For these people, it may be necessary to receive three days of the above dosage intravenously. At OHL, we find that about 1–2 percent of our patients require this intervention.

For more about withdrawal and its treatment, see ADDICTION, page 316.

DIGESTIVE SUPPORT

Dietary Reform: The First Step

In order to heal and get well, it is necessary to clear up digestive problems, so that the body gets the benefits of the nutrients it takes in. The very best therapy, and a remarkably effective one, is to make improvements in your diet.

The rotation diet—involving as it does greater variety of fresh and unprocessed foods, the elimination of allergic foods so taxing on the digestion, plus cutting down on saturated and trans fats, salt, and refined sugars—is already a major step to correcting any pre-existing digestive problems. *This is the diet your body really craves.* Almost all problems of indigestion are cured pretty quickly by a proper nonallergic diet.

Improvement in digestion is often an early sign of success on the Optimum Health Program, for it indicates that more nutrients are being digested and absorbed, and healing has commenced.

Digestive-Support Therapy

Those with severe allergies and long-standing digestive disturbances often need digestive support *temporarily* during the early stages of the Optimum Health Program. There are four steps you can take to help digestion along.

1. Because allergy sufferers are often undersecretors of hydrochloric acid, capsules containing hydrochloric acid with pepsin (not tablets—they may not dissolve fast enough in

the stomach) are often effective. They create the properly acidified environment for initiation of protein digestion and stimulate the release of pancreatic enzymes and bicarbonates into the small intestines. Treatment with hydrochloric-acid capsules should be under the supervision of a physician. Begin at low doses (½ capsule before each meal) and slowly increase to 2 capsules, or less, whatever you find to be the correct level. The capsules should not cause a burning sensation. *This treatment is not recommended for those with ulcers or hiatal hernia problems, or those taking anti-inflammatory drugs of any kind*.

2. Three to four ounces of aloe vera juice (diluted with water, if preferred) fifteen to twenty minutes before meals. This will aid in protein digestion and take some of the burden off the hydrochloric acid- and pepsin-depleted stomach.
3. Pancreatic digestive tablets, preferably a brand high in protein digestive enzymes but containing fat and carbohydrate digestive enzymes as well (such as Pan-Enzyme), can be taken with meals. These tablets replace enzymes, which the malfunctioning pancreas is underproducing. To begin, take one or two tablets after the first mouthful of food, and another one or two at the end of the meal.
4. A tablespoon of potassium and sodium bicarbonate half an hour after meals will neutralize the small intestine hyperacidity that many allergic people suffer as a result of pancreatic dysfunction. Alka-Seltzer Gold, which contains no aspirin, works reasonably well for this purpose.

With proper diet, and occasional support from HCl tablets, aloe vera juice, pancreatic enzyme supplements, and or bicarbonate, digestion clears up pretty quickly in most cases. As a general rule, digestive supplements should not have to be taken for longer than four to eight weeks. Prolonged dependence on digestive support may undermine the ability of the gastrointestinal system to do the job on its own.

Further Tests and Therapy

Occasionally, if the system is at too low an ebb, even the rotation diet and supportive supplements do not bring about the expected improvement. Those with hair-trigger digestive systems may be additionally benefited by taking predigested protein supplements or free-form amino acids.

It is recommended that those who don't show improvement have further diagnostic tests done.

- A stool analysis can determine whether food and other matter is not being digested and absorbed and is as a consequence passing into the large intestine, where it can cause further problems, destroying the balance of bacterial flora and leading to putrefaction and toxicity.
- Another diagnostic tool is the Heidelberg gastrogram, in which a small capsule, emitting an acid-alkaline dependent radio frequency, is tracked through the digestive system while the patient ingests staggered doses of sodium bicarbonate. The Heidelberg gastrogram is used to determine whether the patient is able to secrete proper amounts of gastric hydrochloric acid and to reacidify the stomach as needed.

INDIGESTION, IRRITABLE BOWEL SYNDROME, CONSTIPATION, and DIARRHEA are treated separately under their individual headings in Part V.

REINTRODUCING ALLERGIC FOODS

Only about 5 percent of delayed IgG-mediated food allergies are "fixed" or permanent. After the three-month elimination period is up, you will be able to reintroduce most forbidden foods to your diet without bad effect. But do be careful. Many of these foods have been favorites, and the temptation may be to go back to eating them every day, as before. *Don't do it.* As long as you can eat them on a rotating basis, every four days or so, you won't become readdicted to them and can enjoy them forever.

The same goes for refined and processed foods and the dreaded CATS. I encourage you to try to eliminate these stressors from your diet and life-style as much as possible, for all the reasons that have been mentioned. But once you have your allergies under control and the practice of good nutrition mastered, no irreversible harm will be done by an *occasional* drink or the *occasional* binge on half a dozen brownies. As long as you fall off the wagon on a rotation basis—rotate your vices—you won't do much harm, and you won't become readdicted.

Directions for Reintroducing Allergic Foods

Make a list of the foods you've been avoiding for the past three months. If you've been tested with the FICA, put the ones with the mildest scores at the top of the list. You will be reintroducing one new food every three days, to allow time for any delayed reaction to show itself, so it may take several months to test out all your allergic foods. There's no rush. Don't try to reintroduce a new food on a day when your schedule prevents you from monitoring your reactions carefully.

- First, take your resting pulse. Eat the food, by itself, in a reasonable quantity (a "double" portion is a good rule since too little may give an inaccurate result), as your first food of the day.
- Take your resting pulse again five, fifteen, thirty, and sixty minutes after eating the food. If your pulse has risen 12–16 beats or more and the increase cannot be explained by emotion or activity, you are probably still allergic to that food and should continue to avoid it.

  Now, I have reservations about this pulse test, because other dietary and health factors affect pulse change and because everyone's cardiovascular system is different. Far more important are your own perceptions. See below.
- Monitor yourself. Be alert for allergic symptoms (other than heart-rate change).
- Do not eat any other food for at least six hours, so you can be alert to any other allergic symptoms that may show up later. If you are unsure of your evaluation, test the food again on another day. Once a food passes this reintroduction test, you can put it back into your diet on a rotation basis.

YOU'VE DONE IT

Once those three months are up, you've done the hard part, and you should have a lot to show for it. You will have cleared up your allergies. You will have made many positive changes in your diet habits. Your digestion will be much improved, your immune system strengthened. You will be less vulnerable to disease.

Now you can be somewhat more flexible with your rotation diet and daily supplementation schedule, as long as you don't get carried away. The rule is variety and rotation. By now you're probably eating all sorts of foods you'd never tried before, so your choices are greater. For those on the Optimum Health Program, variety is more than the spice of life —it's a way of life.

17

Cooking, Shopping, and Coping on the Optimum Health Program

Some of life's greatest pleasures are associated with food: a holiday banquet with the family, a romantic candlelit meal with someone one loves, a quiet solo breakfast on the porch as the sun comes up on Sunday morning.

People just starting on the Optimum Health Program often get it into their heads that they'll be giving up the many pleasures of food along with their symptoms and addictions. It's just not true. What is true is that you will have to make some changes in the way you eat and the way you cook and shop. For a short time—a very short time, I assure you—you may find following the diet confusing and tiresome. You're going to have to read labels and try many new foods and pass up prepared "convenience" foods that may have become your standbys. You're going to have to learn some new tricks and unlearn some old ones.

You'll find that once you get into the rhythm of the diet, it will require very little extra effort. For one thing, though you may be giving up some convenience foods, the quick, simple cooking methods used in following the Optimum Health Program add very little to your chores. And you may be pleasantly surprised to find how tasty fresh, simple foods can be and how many exciting new foods there are to enjoy. Once you get the hang of shopping and pick up a few new cooking tactics, following the Optimum Health Program will be smooth and easy.

When you stop to think about it, the things that make eating most enjoyable won't change. You're not giving up Thanksgiving dinner with the family or that romantic restaurant tête-à-tête. You're not giving up pleasurable, presentable, social cuisine on the Optimum Health Program. When it comes right down to it, *what* you eat isn't what makes the difference in your pleasure. It's whom you share the meal with and where, and the ambience and conviviality of the occasion. But what you eat and how it's prepared make an immense difference in your health.

At first your rotary diet will require a good deal of attention and commitment. If you want to break the habit of automatically dipping into the potato chips in the afternoon, you must be sure you have some alternative nonallergic snack food on hand—walnuts, apples, sunflower seeds, bananas, carob-covered raisins, plantain chips, plums, fresh mushrooms. You'll have to be choosy in restaurants and at parties. But it won't take as long as you think to make these new habits stick. The body is a self-monitoring machine, and it will soon prefer the healthful foods on your new diet.

SHOPPING

First, a few simple rules:

1. Whenever possible, buy fresh, unprocessed food. Nowadays, that isn't much of a problem. Fresh fish, poultry, and produce miraculously appear year-round in markets all over the country. And be flexible. If you can't find fresh peaches, try plums or kiwi or mangoes or grapes.

2. Avoid impulse buying. Take your rotation menu list with you and be sure that you have purchased enough variety to rotate your diet. Don't be tempted by foods that don't belong on your new diet.

3. Carefully read the labels on all canned and packaged food. Learning to translate labels is an adventure and an eye-opener. You will find that such common culprits as salt, sugar, partially hydrogenated oils, food colorings, food preservatives, milk, wheat, and yeast turn up in many unexpected places. (Lists of food containing hidden wheat, milk, egg, corn, soybean, and yeast can be found on pages 432–36.) The simplest-looking foods often boast dozens of ingredients—a real no-no on the rotation diet. The colorings, preservatives, and other additives in many products outnumber those ingredients that can be classified as foodstuffs.

Since ingredients in food are listed in order of their importance in the composition of the product, pay particular attention to those that head the list. You'll be surprised at how often sugar, salt, partially hydrogenated oils, and wheat flour are on top. As for other additives, avoid them all whenever possible.

Here are some additional tips concerning label reading:

Sugar. Sugar comes in many forms and may show up in the same product more than once. It can be listed as sucrose, fructose, corn syrup, dextrose, turbinado, corn sweetener, and more. Sugar should be minimized, refined white sugar should be avoided, and the sugars that remain in the diet should be varied. A list and descriptions of the various types of sweeteners appears on pages 454–55.

Salt. The 500 mg or so a day of sodium (the main chemical component of salt) that your body needs to regulate the water content of cells and tissue is amply provided by the grains and fresh vegetables in your diet. A salad provides about 300 mg. But a 2-ounce bag of potato chips may contain 600 mg, and a tablespoon of soy sauce has perhaps twenty times the daily requirement. Sodium, too, goes by many names: sodium bicarbonate, sodium benzoate, sodium potassium, sodium phosphate, monosodium glutamate.

Look at the label on Nabisco saltines: wheat, flour, lard, dehydrated vegetable blend, SALT, sugar, salt seasoning (which consists of SALT, malic acid, SODIUM acetate, fumaric acid), SODIUM bicarbonate, hydrolyzed vegetable protein. Or the label on Kraft Cheese Spread: processed American cheese, water, SODIUM phosphate, SALT, sorbic acid, monoSODIUM glutamate.

Oils and fats. All kinds of processed foods contain hydrogenated trans oils and/or saturated fats: soups, cheese spreads, biscuits, doughnuts, peanut butter, sandwich spreads, dips, crackers. Be on the lookout for listings such as partially hydrogenated vegetable oil, cottonseed oil, palm oil, corn oil, safflower oil, coconut oil, peanut oil, etc. If you shop carefully, especially in your better health food stores, you can find products containing the safer *cold-pressed polyunsaturated oils;* if you do use cold-pressed oils, use them in moderation, being careful not to overheat them when using for cooking.

Colorings, preservatives, and other chemicals. The number and variety of chemical additives to our food is stupefying, and many of the names are mysterious gobbledygook. The ideal way to be sure that you're not poisoning yourself and your family is to avoid these overchemicaled products altogether. As an alternative there are locally and regionally packaged foods, and these often omit the addition of colorings and preservatives. Those that do are certainly to be preferred to the others. If you do buy packaged foods, you should be aware that some additives appear to be far more harmful than others.

One last word about labels. Don't be conned by words or phrases that imply that food is healthy, such as "lite," "natural," "country-style," "healthy," "life," "farm." Packaging can be misleading, too. The earthy colors or the peaceful farm scene, the wheat blowing in the wind, can cover up just as many additives as a plastic cupcake wrapping.

Where to Shop

On your first rotation-diet shopping forays, you may find it frustrating to discover that most of your usual products are loaded with ingredients you now want to avoid. You may find that you've spent an hour roaming the aisles searching for new foods to eat, but an hour later all you've been able to find is literally hundreds of products containing MSG and FD&C Yellow No. 5, and your market cart is still almost empty. Don't despair. The modern supermarket is far more than a toxic-chemical depot. Many supermarkets have extensive fresh poultry, meat, and produce sections, departments for fresh baked goods, fresh fish, pastas, even dried fruits, grains, seeds, and nuts. Get out of those center aisles and cruise the periphery of the market, where all the "real" food is located. Get yourself in the habit of buying new foods each time out, even though you may not know what they are or how they taste. Don't always buy iceberg lettuce; there are a least a dozen other salad greens—chicory, kale, endive, red cabbage, bok choy, spinach, escarole, arugula (rocket or roquette), watercress. Buy casaba or crenshaw or honeydew or Persian melon instead of cantaloupe. Try salmon or tilefish or bass or red snapper or trout or bluefish or mackerel or cod instead of sole and flounder. At your local health food store, buy a small bottle each of several kinds of cold-pressed polyunsaturated oils—walnut, olive, safflower, linseed, sesame, almond (the darker, the less transparent, the better). Buy a new kind of nonallergenic bread, buckwheat pasta, a puffed-rice cereal.

Take advantage of the fresh vegetable and produce stands along the highways and country roads during the warm weather. Not only is much of this food freshly picked and higher in nutritional value, but it will probably have been grown using fewer pesticides than food grown on larger commercial farms. An increasing number of people (my parents have been doing this for almost forty years) grow their own vegetables and fruits in backyards or local community gardens.

A good health food store is a big shopping plus on the Optimum Health Program, because there you are likely to find a greater variety of certain foods such as cereals, breads, and pastas made with various grains, yeast-free breads, foods made with nonsugar sweeteners, pesticide-free fruits and vegetables, and cold-pressed oils. But please be very careful. Don't think you're safe just because you're in a health food store. You can find as many highly allergenic foods, additives, and preservatives in products sold in such stores as at your local supermarket. Certainly many of the sweets and cereals found in health food stores are just as devitalized and fattening as the supermarket varieties. And *many* contain the metabolic poisons partially hydrogenated vegetable and seed oils. Fattening snacks and prepared dishes are getting to be an unwelcome staple of many health food stores—wheat-containing sauces and grains, cream sauces, nut butters, egg dishes, avocado and sesame dressings, candy bars loaded with processed honey and carob and molasses. What is offered—missing from the supermarket—is more choices: a variety of sweeteners, oils, grains, fruits, vegetables, fish, and new and interesting nonallergenic snacks for the rotation dieter.

SUBSTITUTES FOR ALLERGIC FOODS

One of the trickiest things about eliminating allergic foods from the diet is finding replacements for those foods, especially in cooking. You'll be relieved to know that there are many substitutes even for items that are used over and over in food preparation—gluten, wheat, milk, yeast, eggs, sugar. There are breads that use no yeast and salad dressings in which oil is not necessary. There are ways to get calcium without drinking milk, protein without meat, and fiber without highly allergic grains. Not only are many of these foods ideal cooking substitutes for allergic foods, but they are tasty, nutritious additions to your diet.

Alternatives to wheat and other gluten grains, meat and animal protein substitutes, dairy alternatives, wheat-free high-fiber foods, and types of sugars are listed in the Appendices, beginning on page 441. Substitutions for cooking and recipes using alternative ingredients appear in the recipe section, which begins on page 456.

A FEW COOKING TIPS

There are only a few basic guidelines when it comes to cooking. The most basic rule is that foods are at their best—meaning that they retain their maximum in nutrients and fiber content—in their raw, uncooked state. This leads to the second rule, which is that foods should be cooked quickly and lightly, so as to do the least damage.

Though fruits and vegetables should be eaten raw when possible, there are exceptions. "Tightly packed" vegetables such as broccoli, cauliflower, carrots, dried legumes and beans, sweet potatoes, and rhubarb need to be cooked to "loosen" them up a bit, so that their nutrients can be more easily absorbed by the body. Very few people chew a raw carrot sufficiently to break up its tightly packed fibrous composition. Raw milk may transmit listeria bacteria tuberculosis and other diseases and in *some* people may be more allergenic than pasteurized milk.

Meat and fish should be baked or, even better, broiled; broiling is quicker and seals in flavor and nutrients. Fried food is high in oxidized fats and cholesterol, and the overheating can structurally change the protein polypeptides and cook out nutrients.

Frying, boiling, and overheating all destroy nutrients and fiber in your vegetables. The best preparation methods are steaming and stir-frying.

Steaming involves placing the food to be cooked in a strainer that elevates it above a small amount of boiling water in the bottom of the pot. Pots with a special liner are available for this purpose, or you can buy an inexpensive, adjustable steamer rack that can be placed in the bottom of any pot. Cooking time should be as brief as possible—enough to heat the vegetables thoroughly but still allow them to remain crunchy. Steamed vegetables retain their color, taste, and texture; they don't come out looking grayish and soggy.

Stir-frying, or sautéing, involves cooking food quickly in a small amount of cold-pressed oil. The ideal utensil for this is a wok, with its smooth sides, but any frying pan will do. The way to keep oil from overheating during stir-frying (and thus being converted to the dangerous trans configuration) is to add a few tablespoons of water to the oil. Fish, and even meat if cut into small pieces, can be cooked using this technique.

If you do boil vegetables, try to find a use for the water they were boiled in—as a stock base for soups, gravies, or sauces—so that those leached-out vitamins and minerals won't go to waste.

DINING OUT ON YOUR DIET

It's when you're away from home that your resourcefulness—and willpower—will be tested. The most important consideration in these situations, aside from sticking to your diet, is that you not feel deprived or persecuted by your healthy habits. This is the time to reemphasize to yourself that you are glad to be doing something so good for yourself and to gloat a bit about the people around you who are so blithely poisoning themselves. A general rule when dining out or traveling is to remember that you are the one in charge of what you eat. If you take your dieting seriously, you will be careful in choosing which restaurant to patronize, which foods and beverages to select from the array at a cocktail party, and so on. When you are traveling, you can bring along some of your favorite foods, or you can explore the town you're visiting and find out what its restaurants, supermarkets, and health food stores have to offer.

Restaurants

Be finicky about your choice of restaurants. Avoid fast-food restaurants. Hamburgers and french fries are high in fat, the oil is often overheated and far from fresh, and preservatives, colorings, and fillers are liberally added. At some chains, the "milk shake" contains many chemicals but not one ounce of dairy. In others, burgers are seared on grills, a highly carcinogenic cooking process. Even seemingly healthy salad bars are suspect—at many, the greens are kept fresh by coating them with metabisulfites, which are bad for everyone but especially for those with asthma. And many dressings are high in processed oils, allergens, and salt.

Choose restaurants where the food is prepared to order and order what fits your diet. Just because you are eating in a steak house, don't feel pressured to have a steak with onion rings and a buttery baked potato. Have broiled fish, steamed vegetables, a baked potato with yogurt or sour cream, and a salad.

Don't be afraid to ask questions about how the food is prepared and to be specific about what you want. Ask them to broil your fish without butter and to leave the hollandaise off the broccoli, to omit the salt and the MSG. Ask them what dessert they might have that's low in refined sugar or fat. Request a piece of fresh fruit if they haven't something suitable.

In recent years, many restaurants have responded to the increased interest in good nutrition by eliminating salt and cutting down on the high fat content of many dishes, adding new dishes to their regular menus. The "nouvelle cuisine," "spa cuisine," and "art cuisine" offered in many restaurants all reflect the growing interest in pairing good nutrition with beautiful and delicious food. Health food restaurants, which in their early days were more interested in health than in taste, used to serve up variations on a theme of brown rice, soy, and tofu that stopped cold many people who were trying to eat a healthier diet. Today health food restaurants serve fresh, tasty, elegant food in pleasant surroundings, and in most cases you can be assured that you're not getting refined sugars, salt, and saturated fats. But remember, even "health food" can contain many highly allergenic foods—be careful.

Parties and Entertaining

When you are enjoying someone else's hospitality, you neither have to insult them by rejecting their food nor eat foods that you want to avoid.

At large cocktail or buffet parties, especially if they're business affairs, this is seldom a difficult problem. Usually there are enough choices, even if you end up drinking club soda and eating celery sticks—and usually you can find shrimp and cold chicken and strawberries and grapes or a cold pasta salad. You do have the option of eating at home before you go or bringing something you can munch on discreetly. And don't make yourself miserable. Avoid foods you're allergic to, which would really sabotage your diet and bring on symptoms, but a glass of punch and a couple of Swedish meatballs won't kill you if you're really feeling tempted.

Small dinner parties present a different problem. Don't be embarrassed about discussing your dietary restrictions with your host ahead of time. Explain that you don't expect a special meal prepared for you, but that you want to feel comfortable picking and choosing from what's being served without drawing concern and unwanted attention. In the early days of your diet, it is probably better to forgo the temptation and potential embarrassment of such parties altogether. Once your regime is firmly established, you will have more confidence in your ability to fit it into your social life.

When you are the host or hostess, you have to make a decision about whether you're going to serve only food that you consider healthy and that is on your diet, or whether you should make other food available to your guests. By now you should be convinced that there are many wonderful healthy foods and beverages to serve when you entertain, and you can impress your friends and family with a sumptuous spread that is healthy as well. However, I'm well aware that old habits die hard and that many people will feel cheated unless they get their charbroiled steak, scotch and soda, and three-layer cake. You'll have to decide.

RECIPES

When it comes to recipes, the basic rule is the same as that for methods of cooking: *Keep it simple.* A minimum of ingredients, a minimum of preparation and cooking.

See pages 456–85 for some recipes that you may find helpful. This brief section is not meant to be exhaustive but to present a basic selection of tasty and useful dishes. The section opens with substitutions for everyday baking and cooking ingredients and for widely used out-of-the-bottle condiments. Special attention is given to recipes that avoid or substitute for *commonly* allergic ingredients such as wheat, rye, eggs, dairy products, and refined sugar. There are several recipes for sweets and desserts, since many people struggle with their sweet tooth when they first have to abandon refined sugar. Menu and lunch-box suggestions especially suitable for kids can be found on pages 298–99.

As you go along on the Optimum Health Program, you will quickly learn which of your favorite recipes and which of the new ones you come across in cookbooks and magazines will work on your diet and which need to be adapted, and how.

18

Exercise: Nutrition's Partner

I've mentioned several times that our nutritional needs are powerfully influenced by the way the human species has eaten for hundreds of thousands of years, and that as a result our systems are not equipped to handle the huge amounts of refined, chemically enhanced food in the modern diet.

The same correlation can be made to exercise. Our bodies are not designed to handle the sedentary lives most of us lead these days. We are meant to pump more blood, exchange more oxygen, just plain to *move* more, in order for our systems to function at their optimum.

When we don't exercise enough to meet our body's needs, we are at risk, just as we are when we continue to eat an inadequate diet. Eliminating allergens from our diets and eating healthy food on a rotation basis will go a long way toward the attainment of good health. But *optimum health* is not possible unless exercise is given its proper due in our busy lives.

Exercise is medicine. No single drug can boast the impressive list of benefits that exercise provides. More and more doctors now recommend some form of exercise for almost all medical conditions and are becoming aware that exercise, by stimulating the immune system, considerably slows down the aging process. The converse is also true: Inactivity speeds up human decline.

We are in the midst of a fitness craze in this country—which is a very good thing, for it's a welcome antidote to the junk food/obesity plague. Every drop of perspiration is good news for the health of the nation.

I do not intend to make this chapter on exercise a long one, because many good books and articles on the subject have appeared in recent years, and because you no doubt feel inundated by now with information and exhortations about exercise. But I do want to share with you my basic ideas about exercise and tell you about how exercise fits into the Optimum Health Program, and help you begin to plan and implement an exercise program that is well suited to your health and your goals.

There are two points that are central to my thinking about exercise.

1. Concentrate on the health *benefits of exercise and the* beauty *benefits will follow.* The main benefits of exercise have to do with maintaining and improving health, and those benefits are many and far-reaching.

2. You have no excuse not to exercise. No matter how busy you are, no matter how limited your space and your funds, you can devise an exercise program. Neither is your present medical condition an excuse. Those who suffer from obesity or asthma or arthritis, or have damaged hearts, are the ones who can most benefit from medically supervised exercise. With perseverance, and in slow steps, almost anyone can significantly improve his present level of fitness and add immeasurably to his strength and resistance to disease.

THE HEALTH BENEFITS OF EXERCISE

The increase in heart rate, oxygen intake, and muscular activity involved in exercise directly alters the rate of function of your body's furnace—the metabolism.

The metabolic rate—or basal metabolism—is the measure of how quickly and efficiently your body uses calories to fuel the intricate working of the glandular, hormonal, cardiovascular, digestive, musculoskeletal, immunological, and respiratory systems. While each of us has a given metabolic rate, it can be significantly altered by a number of factors: allergy, addiction, diet, hormonal balance, smoking, drugs, and exercise. When the metabolic rate is low, the body cannot manage its intricate biochemical processes optimally, and this can lead to all kinds of secondary physical and mental problems. Increasing the metabolic rate improves the overall functioning of the organism on a biochemical level, and the most effective way to increase the metabolic rate is to exercise and specifically to exercise aerobically. Run, pedal, walk briskly, swim—engage in rhythmic exercises that involve the entire body.

Here are some of the benefits of exercise and increased metabolic rate:

- The increased caloric expenditure inherent in raising the metabolic rate automatically leads to weight loss. Even after exercise the metabolic rate remains elevated for as long as fifteen hours, during which time your body may burn 25 percent more calories than usual, even though you are at rest.

- It increases the output of noradrenaline, a potent brown fat stimulator, and thus leads to the burning of stored calories, which are hard to get rid of under normal circumstances. Regular exercise also seems to have the effect of regulating appetite.
- Brain functions are stimulated. Exercise generates the production of brain neurotransmitters such as noradrenaline, which stimulates the nervous system.
- The functioning of the immune system improves. Exercise increases the release of human growth hormone, which in turn has a powerful stimulatory effect on the master gland of the immune system, the thymus. Exercise improves the ability of the blood to deliver more oxygen to more tissue more efficiently. This increased oxygen controls inflammatory reactions and promotes healing. If oxygen is suboptimal, healing is also suboptimal. Oxygenation is a detoxifier of foreign or toxic chemicals and other elements that don't belong in the blood, including food-laden immune complexes.
- Exercise stimulates the adrenals to increase the production of adrenaline and cortisol, two of the most effective hormones in temporarily arresting or ameliorating an allergic reaction.
- Both systolic and diastolic blood pressure decrease with even moderate regular exercise.
- Exercise dramatically decreases blood fats or triglycerides. Total cholesterol decreases slightly, as does LDL (or low-density lipoprotein), the "bad" cholesterol. It significantly elevates the "good" HDL cholesterol.
- It dramatically decreases blood sugar and blood insulin levels by literally burning up sugars. Since insulin is not needed during exercise, exercise is an important factor in reducing the insulin needs of diabetics.
- It increases cardiac output, meaning essentially that the heart becomes capable of putting out more blood per beat and therefore operates more efficiently. It increases the total volume of blood pumped through your system.
- It will expand the size of the coronary arteries, which supply blood to the working heart, specifically the 12 inches or so of coronary arteries involved in the deaths of over 600,000 Americans each year. The increased size or diameter allows more blood to flow past the clogging atherosclerotic plaque. And it probably also enhances the development of additional new blood vessels to supply the heart.
- It greatly decreases the incidence of repeat heart attacks. Terence Kavanagh, M.D., a cardiac rehabilitation specialist from Toronto, completed a five-year study, showing that those with a history of heart attack who chose not to exercise had twenty-

two times the incidence of repeat heart attacks of those who chose to run eighteen to twenty-one miles a week for five years.

- It decreases abnormal platelet aggregation, another important factor in atherosclerosis, leading to heart disease, possibly as a result of a decrease in blood lipids and increased production of anti-inflammatory prostaglandins.
- The frequency and severity of allergic reactions such as asthma can be reduced with prudent, medically supervised exercise. Increased metabolism and increased circulating noradrenaline and cortisol appear to stabilize the mast cells in the gastrointestinal tract, skin, and airways. The mast cells in most people who are exercising regularly are much less apt to release symptom-producing chemical mediators such as histamines, leukotrienes, and inflammatory prostaglandins.
- Exercise improves the digestion, absorption, and elimination of food. People who exercise regularly are rarely "irregular."
- Exercise increases bone strength. It stimulates bone cells (called osteoblasts) that aid in the formation of new, strong bone tissue, and it improves calcium retention in the bones. Sufficient weight-bearing exercise can go a long way in the prevention of osteoporosis, so prevalent in postmenopausal women.
- It is excellent therapy for (nonpsychotic) depression, probably through the stimulation of mood-elevating endorphins and other natural neurotransmitters in the brain. It is a great stress reducer (my favorite technique) and all-around mental and physical relaxation technique.
- It decreases addictive cravings. Drinkers drink less; smokers smoke less; overeaters eat less.
- Insomniacs sleep better when they exercise. Sleep requirements in general decrease.
- It is a great builder of self-esteem and confidence.

AEROBIC CONDITIONING: THE MOST EFFECTIVE EXERCISE

Exercise can be divided into three basic categories:

1. Aerobic or endurance exercise conditions the whole body. Aerobic exercise is often referred to as endurance exercise. Very generally, it is any activity involving large voluntary muscle groups that are exercised continuously, is rhythmic in nature, and elevates the heart rate. The classic aerobic exercises are jogging, swimming, bicycling, cross-country skiing, and aerobic dancing. Other aerobic exercises (if done with sufficient intensity) would include hiking, competitive singles tennis and racquetball, trampolining, jumping rope, squash, karate/boxing/judo, soccer or basketball, and—very important for the out-of-shape beginner—brisk walking.

2. Anaerobic or strength exercise conditions specific muscle groups. This type of exercise increases muscle contraction and promotes increased muscle bulk and strength through consumption of oxygen from muscle and tissue—a phenomenon known as oxygen deprivation. Anaerobic exercise promotes muscle strength via short bursts of extreme stress on muscle tissue. This leads to a rapid buildup of lactic acid and muscle exhaustion. Anaerobic strength exercise of a specific muscle group cannot be sustained for more than about ninety seconds. The increased muscle strength benefits of anaerobic exercise enable the body not only to perform athletic feats better, but also to endure more aerobic exercise without danger of overstress or overuse injuries. Also, muscle weight is "lean" high metabolic weight; muscle cells burn calories at a much higher rate than fat cells. Increasing one's muscle-to-fat ratio is an excellent way to assure that excess calories are burned rather than stored as fat. Calisthenics and weight training—using free weights or strength-training equipment such as Universal or Nautilus systems—are the classic forms of anaerobic exercise.

3. Flexibility exercises promote deep relaxation and stretching. Muscles, tendons, ligaments, and joints benefit, and in addition the body gains some protection against injury. Yoga, ballet, t'ai chi, aikido, and other forms of stretching exercise are ways of increasing flexibility.

Aerobic Conditioning

The ideal exercise program is basically a regimen of aerobic exercise, complemented by some form of strength training and some stretching warm-up and *warm-down* exercises.

Very simply, the goal of aerobic training is to raise your heart rate to its optimum aerobic rate, or target range, and sustain it there for at least twenty to thirty minutes at least three times a week.

Your optimum heart rate is 65–85 percent of your *maximum heart rate.* Maximum heart rate is very roughly determined by subtracting your age from the number 220. For example, if you are thirty-four, your maximum heart rate would calculate out to about 186. Your optimum target range would thus fall between 110 and 160. If you exercise *more* intensely than 85 percent of your maximum heart rate, you get into an anaerobic, oxygen-deprivation, lactic-acid-buildup stage, and you may

Table 51 — Optimal Target Pulse Rates During Aerobic Exercise*

Age	Aerobic Heart Rate Range	Age	Aerobic Heart Rate Range
18	141–170	50	125–153
20	140–170	52	124–152
22	139–168	54	123–151
24	138–166	56	122–150
26	137–165	58	121–149
28	136–164	60	120–148
30	135–163	62	119–147
32	134–162	64	118–146
34	133–161	66	117–145
36	132–160	68	116–144
38	131–159	70	115–143
40	130–158	72	114–142
42	129–157	74	113–141
44	128–156	76	112–140
46	127–155	78	111–139
48	126–154	80+	110–138

*Guidelines only.

collapse from exhaustion. Exhaustion should be avoided when exercising aerobically. However, if you exercise at *less* than 65 percent of maximum heart rate, you do not reap the usual aerobic benefits.

It is generally felt that it is necessary to exercise at this level at least three times a week for twenty to thirty minutes in your target pulse range—to reap any lasting aerobic benefit. Exercising in the aerobic target range for thirty to sixty minutes five times a week is ideal for noncompetitive, recreational athletes. The weight-loss benefits of aerobic exercise triple at six times a week compared to only three times. But *too much* can be harmful. Overuse injuries and stress-induced infections are known to increase tenfold if aerobic exercise is increased to six or seven times a week. As usual—our old friend, the bell-shaped curve—the optimum benefit falls somewhere in the middle.

Table 51, above, calculates the optimum target pulse rate for aerobic exercise at various ages. This is meant as a rough guideline only. Your present age, sex, health, and condition, along with your medical history, greatly influence your highly individual target pulse range. Before beginning your own exercise program, you should carefully evaluate the cardiovascular risk factors (listed below) and consult with your personal exercise-oriented physician.

In order to determine that you are within your target pulse range during aerobic exercise, you will have to measure your pulse as you go. You can take your radial (wrist) pulse or your carotid artery pulse (place your thumb on your chin and lay the other four fingers along the throat next to the Adam's apple). The radial pulse is generally easier to take and often more reliable than the carotid pulse, for the tendency is to press too hard on the carotid artery, and this slows the pulse rate. And of course, there are several small, relatively inexpensive, portable heart chronometers on the market that do the job quickly and accurately. After you've been exercising for a while, you will become familiar with how your body feels when you are within your target range, and you will need to take your pulse only once a week or so in order to measure improvement.

EVALUATING PERSONAL RISK FACTORS OF EXERCISE

Exercise is highly beneficial stress—what health professionals call *eustress*—unless you overreach your physiological capabilities. Before beginning an exercise program, it is important that you consider any possible risks involved. Many risk factors can be eliminated by simple, immediate changes in your habits or life-style. Others, which may involve serious health problems, may require considerable caution and planning, in consultation with your physician. Once all risks are known and evaluated, you can devise a program that safely limits those risks as much as possible.

At OHL we aggressively encourage regular exercise for patients who are overweight or who suffer from such maladies as migraine, arthritis, diabetes, heart disease, and asthma. Many of these patients have been previously discouraged from exercising or have felt too overweight, too old, or too debilitated to try it. It's been our experience that, however slow and difficult progress is at first, persistence pays off handsomely, often in huge jumps in overall health improvement. And of course, the leap in self-esteem and confidence can be enormous.

The list below enumerates the standard risks to consider when planning an exercise program. Proper evaluation of some factors will require your physician's help. Exercise guidelines for people with asthma, heart disease, migraine, arthritis, and diabetes are mentioned under the appropriate headings in Part V.

Risks

1. Smoking more than five cigarettes per day implies an impaired cardiovascular system. Target rate should be reevaluated.
2. High blood pressure also implies a reduced target range. Any exercise program should start slowly and cautiously.
3. High serum cholesterol levels are often associated with impaired vascular functioning.
4. Low HDL (high-density lipoprotein) cholesterol levels increase risk of coronary artery disease and depress cardiovascular function.
5. A generally sedentary life-style, even if cholesterol levels are acceptable, dictates that exercise should begin slowly and build very slowly in intensity and duration.
6. Anyone with a family history of heart attack, especially death from a heart attack before the age of fifty, should be tested for potential genetic heart weakness.
7. Obesity—more than thirty pounds of excess weight—puts a strain not only on hip, knee, and ankle joints, but also on all biochemical and cardiovascular functions. Again, exercise should begin and build very slowly.
8. Anyone with a high or low blood insulin level should exercise only under a doctor's supervision. Diabetics, both Type I (insulin-dependent) and Type II (adult-onset, often noninsulin-dependent), should be monitored carefully, but should be exercising.
9. Sedentary men over forty and postmenopausal women should also begin their program following evaluation by a physician.
10. A general diagnostic evaluation is advised for all Type A individuals, who are often prone to undetected high blood pressure, coronary atherosclerosis, muscle tension, and general hormonal imbalances.
11. Those with abnormal platelet stickiness are high-risk individuals.
12. Chronic nutritional deficiencies indicate that careful monitoring is needed. Particularly risky are deficiencies of the following: Vitamins C, B3, B6, E; the essential fatty acids of the Omega 3 and Omega 6 groups; the minerals chromium, zinc, magnesium, selenium, and iron.
13. Diets high in red meat, milk products, egg yolk, margarine, and salt are exercise risks, as are highly processed diets low in fiber.
14. The risks of any known illness should be discussed with your doctor.

YOUR PERSONAL EXERCISE PROGRAM

The evaluation of personal risk factors will provide you with the framework for devising your exercise program. The first question is the kind of exercise you want to do. Table 52, on the next page, presents a list of aerobic exercises, showing their comparable benefits.

Table 52—Comparative Benefits of Exercise*
rated on a scale of 0–100

	Running	Bicycling	Swimming	Handball Squash	Tennis	Walking	Golf	Bowling
Cardiorespiratory endurance	100	90	100	90	76	62	38	24
Muscular endurance	95	86	95	86	76	67	38	24
Muscular strength	81	76	67	71	67	52	43	24
Flexibility	43	43	71	76	67	33	38	33
Balance	81	86	57	81	76	38	38	29
Weight control	100	95	71	90	76	62	29	24
Muscle definition	67	71	67	52	62	52	29	24
Digestion	62	57	62	62	57	52	33	33
Sleep	76	71	76	57	52	67	29	29
Average performance	78	75	74	74	68	54	35	27

*Source: President's Council on Physical Fitness.

It is very important that you plan a program that you are likely to *follow through on.* This means that you should choose the type of exercise you enjoy, the time you're really willing to devote to exercise, what you can afford in the way of equipment or health club costs, and the availability of facilities. If you're always squeezed for time, it doesn't make sense to plan to swim three or four days a week at a pool an hour away. Aim for convenience and be realistic; it's all too easy to be self-defeating when starting out.

Consider the fun factor. Enjoying your exercise time is the best way to guarantee you'll keep at it. Aerobic dancing to disco music may be much more bearable to you than trying to tough it out on a stationary bicycle.

Do not allow lack of funds or space to deter you. Aerobic dancing can be done at home in a small space. Jogging and walking can be done just about anywhere outdoors. Take advantage of the many exercise programs on television. The aerobic workouts you can follow on TV are the equivalent of having a free club membership—without the hassle of travel and crowded classes and locker rooms.

It also makes sense to vary or rotate your exercise. In this way, you work out different muscle groups in different ways, reducing the tendency toward overuse injuries and perhaps increasing your overall aerobic fitness. Also, variety forestalls boredom. At Mission Viejo, California's world-famous swimming training club, Olympic hopefuls train in the water five hours per day; in addition, they augment their swimming with land sports, including running and weight training. Switch from jogging to cross-country skiing in the winter or to tennis singles in the summer. Try walking one day, swimming the next, and cycling the third.

Ideally some strength-promoting exercise should be incorporated into your exercise program, even if it's only ten or fifteen minutes per session. Health-club members can take advantage of Nautilus or Universal gym equipment. Small free weights can be purchased at sporting goods stores for those who exercise at home, and even heavy household tools or books will do in a pinch. As you get more involved in your program, you may want to purchase more sophisticated at-home equipment, converting the extra room or unused garage into your own personalized fitness room. These days the array of exercise equipment sold for home use makes it possible to set up an at-home workout facility comparable to what's available at most health clubs.

How much exercise is the optimum amount? The term I like to use is "heightened moderation," by which I mean more than just enough to get by but not too much. There is such a thing as too much exercise; everyone has a threshold, a limit beyond which he or she is prone to injury or illness.

The axiom that *too* much of a good thing is bad is borne out by the experience of those seemingly indestructible instructors who lead aerobics classes. Studies have shown that their heavy work schedule of several classes, six or seven days a week, leads to an abnormally high injury rate. One study showed that over 75 percent of instructors suffered significant overuse injuries (versus 40 percent of their students) and an average of thirteen sick days a year due to injuries; some had been out of commission as long as six months.

To repeat: In order to get real aerobic benefit from your workouts, you should do them at least three times a week, and the target-heart-range pulse should be maintained for at least twenty to thirty minutes. A better regimen would involve maintaining the target-range pulse for thirty minutes to as long as sixty, five times a week. Every third day or so, you should rest one or two days, to give the body time to heal and to guard against overuse injuries.

Another good tactic is to alternate long and short days of exercise. One day, extend yourself a bit with a long run (or walk or swim) plus a short workout; on the next day, a run of perhaps half the distance plus a good concentration on weights and strength building.

Just Get Started

Whatever your eventual goals, start slowly, and do not set impossible schedules. If you have been very sedentary or are overweight, it is important just to get moving, even just to walk once or twice around the block. Do something, and do as much as you can, as often as you can. Frequency and duration of exercise are far more important than speed. Do not be embarrassed by how out of shape you are or by your appearance or by what people may think. You will quickly gain confidence and will be surprised at how quickly your energy level builds up. If you have been very sedentary, you do not need to run or play squash to raise your heart rate; the effort involved in a brisk walk will do the trick. The benefits of walking, incidentally, should not be underestimated—it is an excellent start-up exercise for people with all sorts of health limitations. Swimming is ideal exercise for disorders involving the weight-bearing joints (arthritis, obesity) and for respiratory problems (asthma, hay fever)

TIPS AND CAUTIONS

1. Exercise increases your nutritional requirements. If you've been leading a pretty sedentary life, three aerobic workouts a week can make a significant difference in your body's needs. To be sure that your body is not starving itself to provide energy for exercise and increasing the risk of injury, do not stint on meals and take at least the routine supplementation recommended on the Optimum Health Program.

2. Always warm up before and warm down after ***aerobic exercise.*** Experts differ on the optimum amount of stretching and warm-up time that should precede each aerobic workout session, but consensus seems to be that you should stretch gently, but not to the point of pain and for only a few minutes, so as not to cause microscopic tears in the muscles needed for aerobic endurance. Start your workout at a slow pace and increase it slowly for the first five to ten minutes until you reach your aerobic target rate. Bring your workout to an end in the same manner, slowing your pace over the last five or more minutes. If important at all, stretching exercises are most important *after* the aerobic workout, to ease out tensions and stretch muscles and ligaments that have been tensed and shortened by repetitive motion.

3. Do not institute a crash program that you expect will bring you to optimum fitness in just a couple of months. It is foolish and self-defeating to be in a rush, for it almost inexorably leads to pain, injury, exhaustion, frustration, and loss of self-esteem. It will take a few months of serious persistent application for you to see the first visible benefits of any exercise program, and your long-range fitness goals should encompass a year to eighteen months or more. Instant fitness programs are no different from crash diets. They're doomed to failure because they're too hard to maintain, and they invite fatigue, stiffness, pain, and injury. Stick with your exercise regimen through the thick, and you'll end up thin and fit. And you will have acquired the new, highly beneficial *habit* of exercising. You'll know you've arrived when you feel upset and out of sorts because you're forced to skip exercising on a particular day.

4. Use the "staircase" or "plateau" approach to increasing your training levels. Do not try to exercise farther or longer every day. Plan your progress in stages. When you reach one level of intensity and frequency, continue to exercise at that level for two to three weeks (or three to four weeks if you are over fifty years old) before kicking up your efforts by 5 or 10 percent and moving on to the next stage. This gives your body a chance to catch up and lessens the chance of fatigue and overstress injuries. Take it from me that the straight-line approach—always trying to go faster and farther each time out, day after day—can lead to disaster.

5. Write down your exercise plan and plot specific goals over a period of time. Keep a record of when and how much you exercise and of your progress, heart-rate increases, etc.

6. Proper equipment and attire are vital. You don't need much gear for most exercise endeavors, and don't let a zealous salesman sell you things you don't need—at least to begin with. But running or walking shoes that offer support and cushioning are important, as are clothes that regulate your body temperature and allow for natural evaporation of perspiration. Any exercise suit that is made of rubber, plastic, or heat-retaining material—and these are widely advertised for their weight-loss benefits—are truly life-threatening.

7. Use common sense about exercising in a hot room or outdoors on hot, humid days, when the amount of fluid loss can be deceptive. A large glass of water or two, consumed half an hour before exercising, is a good basic precaution. Drink additional fluids as you feel the need.

8. Beware of the so-called positive addiction of exercise. Now that fitness is becoming such a mania for many people, it was probably inevitable that exercise addiction would turn out to be the aberration of the eighties. Positive addiction is positive only if it is not carried to extremes. But extremism is what happens when people exercise so much that they abuse rather than improve their bodies, and end up destroying tissue in order to keep going. Preanorexic or anorexic people sometimes use exercise as a tool for dangerously strict weight loss and control. Others may develop psychological obsessions that make self-worth contingent on excessive exercise. Instead of running twenty to forty miles per week, they choose seventy-five to 125 miles per week. The result can be exercise-induced malnutrition and overuse injuries. Women who run to the point of amenorrhea (usually in excess of forty miles per week) develop demineralization or calcium loss in the vertebrae of the lower back. Women who run seventy-five to 125 miles per week appear to have an increased incidence of osteoporosis and cancer. The inability to skip exercise even for one day, the urge to run or work out for hours on end, even when exhausted or in pain, the tendency to neglect other important parts of your life or to allow yourself to eat only if you exercise—these are possible signs of excessive addiction to exercise.

9. Do not run or exercise along crowded highways or on city streets. Research done in New York City shows that joggers who run half an hour on polluted city streets get about the same "benefits" as those who smoke a half a pack to a pack of cigarettes a day. Though it is not known whether this short-term exposure is harmful or whether the cardiovascular benefits outweigh the risks, it's better to plan your exercising away from traffic. Carbon monoxide inhalation decreases by 80 percent just 100 yards from the road.

10. Finally, avoid exercise-induced anaphylaxis (exaggerated allergic response). This is a potentially serious side effect of exercise for those with a topic allergies (hives, hay fever, asthma) and possibly for other people with undiagnosed allergic sensitivities. It is common among athletes, and its occurrence is often the cause of the allergy being diagnosed in the first place. Anaphylactic symptoms normally start with itching, followed by breaking out in hives, and in worse cases by dizziness, then a drop in blood pressure, shortness of breath, and loss of consciousness. As traumatic as anaphylactic shock can be, it is entirely preventable if recognized and treated in advance.

Since it is often brought on by food allergy, it can often be avoided by not eating the allergenic food within three or four hours of exercising. There are medications that will prevent anaphylaxis, and taking Vitamin C in crystal or powder form about thirty minutes before beginning aerobic exercise may be very effective: about 500 mg for a child and 1,000–2,000 mg for an adult. Caffeine, probably because it stimulates the production of adrenaline, also seems to forestall anaphylactic reactions in some people.

If, before beginning exercise, there is a warm or flushed feeling or unusual fatigue or light-headedness, do not exercise. Bouts of coughing or sneezing *after* exercise are often signs of undiagnosed asthma and a potential for anaphylaxis. If symptoms appear after beginning exercise, stop immediately. Try again the next day, three to four hours after a meal, thirty minutes after taking Vitamin C. Some people who are prone to exercise-induced anaphylaxis are able to exercise in short spurts without ill effects. More on this subject under the discussion of asthma on pages 333–36.

19

Notes to Parents: Optimum Health for Children

It is our children who pay the severest penalties for consuming our modern diet—overrefined, unbalanced, highly allergenic—and for the constant assault by chemical pollutants in food and in the environment. Today more children than ever before suffer from asthma, hay fever, eczema, inflammatory bowel disease, and migraine headaches. There is a marked statistical increase in hyperactivity, learning disorders, motor skills impairment, childhood depression, and, most alarming, teenage suicide. In the United States, atherosclerosis begins early in childhood; many male teenagers already have advanced coronary artery disease.

A recent fitness survey in Canada showed that males reached peak physical fitness at age thirteen, females at ten. From there on it's all downhill. A survey of 1,500 fourth and fifth graders in Los Angeles, Santa Monica, and Malibu revealed that 24 percent had high blood pressure, 23 percent had high cholesterol counts, 32 percent were obese (not merely overweight), and 27 percent had only a fair or poor recovery pulse rate after exercise. In other words, they were in rotten physical shape. The study, conducted by the Jonsson Center and Joseph Cullen of the National Cancer Institute at UCLA, covered both wealthy and inner-city neighborhoods. The average serum cholesterol level of the group was over 200; the recommended level for this age group is 140. The black children had higher blood pressure, but the white kids were less fit. More boys than girls were found to be obese.

All these problems can be traced, in large part, to overconsumption, dietary deficiencies, sedentary life-styles, and environmental pollution. Many older adults grew up eating a better diet, getting more exercise, and breathing cleaner air than their children and grandchildren. Some were lucky enough to have grown up before the heyday of hydrogenated oils and packaged foods, sugar-coated cereals and Twinkies, fast-food restaurants, convenient TV dinners, colorings, chemicals, and additives, and serious air pollution.

Parents have both the responsibility and the opportunity to provide a strong nutritional foundation for their children's health and to convince the youngsters, through education and example, that eating well is important and enjoyable. This is no simple task, but it is a profoundly important one. *Nutritional abuse is a subtle form of child abuse.*

Teaching a child about good nutrition and convincing him that he's not missing out on those junk foods requires attention and patience. You'll have to campaign and propagandize as hard as they do on television. But it can be done. Children are capable of discrimination about what they eat. They can be taught that the "secret" of being slim and athletic and popular lies in choosing an apple, for example, over potato chips. And if you think it's not worth the effort, remember that you are giving your child the gift of health and a longer, happier life.

GETTING A HEAD START: PREPREGNANCY, PREGNANCY, AND INFANCY

The few years during pregnancy and infancy are the most influential in determining your child's health. Luckily, during these years, you can pretty much control his diet and activity level, in anticipation of that day when he asks for that sugar-frosted cereal he sees on TV.

The best thing you can offer your child is your own healthy diet and life-style. First things first. If you are planning to have children, the time to begin a good nutritional program for those kids is at least six months to a year *before you even get pregnant.* The health of the woman at conception has a direct and profound effect on the health of the fetus in the womb. If you have allergies, clear them up before you get pregnant. If you eat too many fatty foods and sweets, if you smoke or drink too much wine, beer, or coffee, address those problems now, so that you're healthy as can be when you're carrying that baby.

Pregnancy

Because what you eat and drink during pregnancy has a direct effect on your unborn child, you must be sure you're doing all the right things: eating a varied diet, drinking very little coffee and alcohol, avoiding sugar, and not smoking. And cut way down on milk. Despite what you may have been taught, milk is a highly allergic substance (more about this on page 294). Continue to take your supplements (under medical supervision), and specifically increase your intake of Vitamin C, B complex, essential fatty acids, zinc, calcium, and magnesium.

Most of all, be sure that you've eliminated allergic foods from your diet; research has shown that the fetus begins producing antibodies against allergic substances as early as eleven weeks into pregnancy. Finally, unless there are problems that indicate otherwise, keep on exercising throughout your pregnancy. It will help your unborn child, and it will help you through the rigors of childbirth.

Infancy

Here's where I get on my soapbox. I'm a firm believer in breast-feeding for infants as long as is practicable and possible—at least for six months and preferably twelve, without the introduction of *any* regular food or dairy products. During this time, the mother's intake of cow's milk should also be very limited; nonallergic grains, fruits, nuts, seeds, and vegetables, with supplementation, should provide adequate calcium supplies.

There are many nutritional benefits to breast-feeding, in addition to the obvious psychological ones. Mother's milk is the only available source of gamma linolenic acid, the vital precursor to the production of the prostaglandins of the 1 series. (See Chapter 11.) For several months after birth, the infant appears incapable of producing optimal amounts of gamma linolenic acid; the mother's milk is vital. L-carnitine, an important amino acid in short supply early after birth, is amply available through the mother's milk. The infant's absorption of calcium is better from breast milk than from cow's milk, even though the concentration is much higher in cow's milk. Breast milk contains protective immune substances and cells that are transferred to the infant, including secretory IgA and other critical antibodies. Breast-feeding transmits immune capabilities that cannot be obtained from other sources during the first few months of life. Because breast milk is far lower in arachidonic acid than cow's milk, it decreases the potential for childhood obesity and inflammatory disease. Incidentally, breast-feeding also keeps the nursing mother's weight down. Purely breast-fed babies have a far lower incidence of colic, middle-ear infection, asthma, and eczema. The potential for allergy problems may easily be decreased by at least 50 percent through breast-feeding—even more if the mother has no allergies or poor dietary habits herself. This doesn't mean that a child won't develop allergies from foods once off the breast milk, but it is an excellent head start for all-around good health.

If breast-feeding is not possible, the next best alternative is to try to find an alternative to cow's or goat's milk; there are formulas available using soy and other nonmilk protein bases. A couple of capsules of evening primrose oil rubbed into the skin of the baby's chest and abdomen daily may provide the essential fatty acids to infants who are not being breast-fed. The oil is easily absorbed through the skin. After one year of age, the oil can be mixed with other solid foods. Additional supplements I recommend for infants (up to two years) are as follows:

Vitamin A: 1,500–2,000 IU
Vitamin C: 35–250 mg buffered C in divided doses; this buffered form usually contains calcium, magnesium, potassium, and zinc.
Vitamin D: 100 IU (Preferably 20–30 minutes of direct sunlight on exposed skin areas twice weekly, in place of supplementation)
Vitamin E: 5–30 IU

Be sure that you are using FDA-approved infant supplements that are hypoallergenic, containing no chemical binders, colorings, preservatives, and especially no *alcohol* (widely used in the manufacture of supplements).

Finally, please seek professional supervision of supplementation for your baby.

THE PROBLEM WITH COW'S MILK

Why am I so opposed to cow's milk? It is a misunderstood and vastly overrated food, thanks in great part to the National Dairy Council, which spends millions a year touting its products. Federal farm subsidies paid from your hard-earned taxes make these products even more appealing by keeping prices down and supply up, resulting in some 375 pounds of milk products consumed in the United States per person per year. The Dairy Council tells us that milk is a perfect food and convinces us of its high calcium and protein content, while neglecting to mention that it contains 60 percent saturated fat.

1. Cow's milk is one of the two or three most common food allergens in the American diet, both for children and adults. It is the major contributing factor to middle-ear infections (otitis media) in infants. In one recent Scandinavian study, not one purely breast-fed infant came down with middle-ear infections. Gastroenteritis, which affects 5 to 10 percent of all American children under two, is another common side effect of milk allergy. This is an inflammation and irritation of the digestive-tract lining, which often includes a slow, oozing loss of blood, which in turn leads to iron deficiency anemia. Other symptoms associated with allergy to milk include asthma, eczema, migraines, juvenile rheumatoid arthritis, chronic upper respiratory infections and congestion, bronchitis, pneumonia, bed-wetting, so-called growing pains, fatigue, hyperactivity, and even epilepsy in children who have allergy-related migraines.

2. The majority of the world's people are unable to digest milk sugar. While milk allergy is a response to proteins in milk, the inability to digest milk is explained by the fact that most people cannot digest lactose, a sugar found only in milk. They are lactose intolerant, meaning that they are lacking or deficient in the gastrointestinal enzyme lactase necessary for its digestion. The lactase enzyme appears in the intestinal tract of infants during the last trimester before birth and peaks shortly after birth. However, sometime between eighteen months of age and four years, most individuals throughout the world gradually lose the lactase activity in the small intestine, a clue that perhaps human beings aren't meant to drink milk beyond early childhood. But humans, unlike other animals, continue to drink milk, sometimes in great quantities, throughout youth and into adulthood. The result is cramps, gas, bloating, and diarrhea.

3. Milk inhibits the absorption of iron (by far the most common mineral deficiency in this country) and enhances the absorption of the highly toxic mineral lead.

4. Milk is high in arachidonic acid (saturated fats) and has been shown to be a major contributor to the development of atherosclerosis in young children. More, saturated fats are powerful delta-6-desaturase inhibitors and therefore contribute to all the problems that result from a deficiency of prostaglandins of the 1 and 3 series. (See Chapter 11.)

Cow's milk is for calves. Absorbable calcium is available from many other sources. Do your kids a favor and moderate or eliminate their milk consumption. And certainly if your child is showing signs of allergy, hyperactivity, migraine, colic, "growing pains," chronic infections, or behavioral problems, milk should head your list of suspects.

The romance with milk in this country is a long and persistent one. People are skeptical when told that milk isn't what it's cracked up to be—it's so closely associated with the American Way. But it's so often the wrong way.

HOW TO BRING UP HEALTHY CHILDREN

1. Start early. It is far harder to change a child's diet than to start him off eating a good diet in the first place. Children raised on breast milk from a well-nourished mother and then on healthy foods don't suddenly become junk-food junkies when they start going to school and watching television.

2. Set a good example. Children eat what their parents eat. If you're following a healthy diet, the foods on your shopping list and in your refrigerator and on your table will be the right ones. Don't expect your child to eat an apple if you're eating a Ring Ding.

3. Teach your children about good health and good food. As children get older and are tempted by soda pop, french fries, and hotdogs, it is important for them to know that there's a reason for eating well, to know what the difference is between good and bad food. Let your children get involved in shopping and food as soon as they show an interest.

4. Don't be dogmatic. An occasional soda or hotdog or doughnut won't hurt. *Remember, there's nothing more tempting than that which is forbidden.* There will be times—at school, at friends' houses, at birthday parties—when it will be difficult, and perhaps embarrassing, for your child to forgo the food that's offered. Even at home, there's no need to be a purist. The idea is to minimize the junk food and maximize the nourishing foods.

5. Monitor what your youngster eats in school. The problems of trying to be sure that your children consume a healthy diet are compounded when they head off to school. You can guess what I think of the traditional midmorning snack of milk and graham crackers. And most school lunch programs are worse. The greatest sin of most school food used to be that it was unappetizing, overcooked, and too high in fats and dairy products. Today packaged foods, doughnuts, chips, popsicles, soda, artificially flavored juice concoctions, hotdogs, and french fries can be found on school lunch trays, often the largesse of government-funded programs.

If the school lunch program in your area is as bad as most, the only answer is to have your child take lunch to school. Lunch-box suggestions can be found among the menu suggestions below.

6. Offer variety. Be sure to have the pantry stocked with several choices of food. You want your kids to rotate their diets and not get stuck eating the same food all the time (even if it is supposed to be good for them). That means different kinds of fruit, nuts, seeds, cereal, pasta, vegetables, a choice of sweeteners, etc.

7. Offer alternatives to junk foods and highly refined sweet snacks. This does *not* mean celery sticks and tofu. Everyone has a sweet tooth. Kids who aren't stuffing themselves with potato chips and candy bars and soda need attractive substitutes, so they don't feel deprived by their healthy diet or different from their friends. See the section below for suggestions.

8. Offer rewards or trade-offs if necessary. If you are having problems getting your kids to give up their favorite junk foods, don't hesitate to trade off hamburgers on white-bread buns one night for chicken and fresh salad the next. Sign "contracts" with your children, offering whatever they choose on Saturday if they eat the foods you select during the week. Once they have given the new regime a try, they may not need such special inducements.

9. Take supplements every day. Supplementation is often overlooked, yet the majority of children in national epidemiological studies and surveys are deficient in at least one vitamin, and many have three or more vitamin deficiencies. Comprehensive supplementations should be taken every day, mostly in divided doses with meals, for optimal absorption and utilization. Again, your nutritionally oriented physician will help you plan the best supplementation for each of your children. Suggested supplementation ranges by age group are as follows:

Ages 2–7: ⅓ to ¼ adult doses
Ages 8–13: ½ adult doses
Ages 14–18: Adult doses

The routine adult supplement dosage appears in Table 3, page 86. Individual nutrients and their functions are discussed in detail in Part III. Children's supplementation should always be supervised by your nutritionally oriented physician.

10. Make sure your children get enough exercise. Many parents think that kids move around and play spontaneously, that they never sit still for long. But in fact, many kids choose activities that involve very little physical effort. They avoid gym class at school, hang out with friends, watch television, read, snack, and get fat. City kids, confined to apartments and limited to the sidewalks, have an especially hard time burning up energy.

Children who do not have the chance to develop their natural coordination, strength, flexibility, and endurance find it harder to join games and sports later in life without feeling clumsy and out of the running. A physically active family life is the best setting to develop the habit of exercise and learn a love of sports and physical activity.

MENU SUGGESTIONS

The following section offers suggestions for foods to keep in the refrigerator or cupboard for snacks, for foods that are good trade-offs for standard junk food, and for foods to fill kids' lunch boxes. Additional tips can be found in Chapter 17, and a few mail-order food outlets for foods that may be hard to find in your area are included in the Appendices, page 431.

- "Soda" substitute. Mix exotic fruit juices (preferably freshly squeezed *with pulp*)—papaya, mango, apricot or peach or pear nectar, white or purple grape juice, coconut, guava, pineapple—with seltzer or carbonated mineral water. These are sweet and have the same fizzy effect as soda. If it helps, keep them in pop bottles in the refrigerator. And add 100–200 mg of crystal Vitamin C to each 8 ounce glass of juice—I do.
- Instead of 90 percent trans fat potato chips. Health food stores offer alternatives like plantain chips, banana chips, soy and wheat nuts. While some of these are high in processed oil, they are usually salt-free and provide an occasional variety in the diet.
- Instead of candy bars. Again, try your health food store. Most of them offer a tremendous variety of sweet snacks. Fruit leathers are a good bet, as are candy bars that substitute carob —which is lower in sugar and fat—for chocolate and uncooked honey or molasses for sugar. Don't get carried away with these sweets, however. Many are high in trans fats and calories, and although uncooked honey and molasses are better than refined white sugar, for most people there's a limit. But they do provide variety and a way of appeasing the sweet tooth and putting down home rebellions.

Here are some ideas for snacks to have around the house and to include in your youngster's lunch box:

- Fruit salad lightly marinated in lemon or lime, with a little cinnamon and uncooked honey added. This will keep for several days in the refrigerator. Vary the fresh fruit each time you make it.
- A selection of vegetable crudités and a dip. Be imaginative with the vegetables. Besides the usual celery, carrots, scallions, and cherry tomatoes, try fresh mushrooms, broccoli, strips of zucchini or cucumbers, red and white radishes, endive leaves. Add bits of chicken or turkey. Vary the dip each time you make it.

- More snacks: pine seeds, walnuts, chestnuts, almonds, pecans, pumpkin or sunflower seeds, dried fruit, raisins, dates, figs, fresh fruit, unbuttered popcorn, fruit yogurt, natural fruit popsicles, banana or date or pumpkin bread, hardboiled or deviled eggs, oatmeal or almond butter or cashew butter cookies, bran and berry muffins, baked apples or pears drizzled with carob or uncooked honey or molasses, baked-potato skins with cheese or sprouts, rice cakes spread with uncooked honey or nut butter and sprouts.

Sandwich ideas for lunch boxes (all on a variety of nonallergic whole grain breads, of course):

- Cashew butter or almond butter with unsweetened jam or fruit preserves, or with sliced banana, chopped nuts, sunflower or pumpkin seeds, or alfalfa or bean sprouts.
- Tuna fish, chicken salad, or turkey salad with low-fat mayonnaise or yogurt spread, and sprouts or celery or grated carrots or lettuce or endive or sunflower seeds.

IS YOUR CHILD ALLERGIC?

Allergies can undermine a child's pleasure in life and get him off on the wrong foot in school and with friends and can impair his chances for a healthy future. There are some early clues that indicate allergies in children, and parents should be on the lookout for them.

Watch for cravings or demands for a particular food. Overweight, excessive nose picking, dark circles or swelling under the eyes ("allergic shiners"), eye wrinkles (Dennie's sign), or a horizontal crease across the nose from constant nose wiping—all these are indications of allergic irritation. Look for migraine or other "vascular" headaches, excessive coughing—especially right after exercising—sleep disorders, including nightmares, paleness without anemia, bad breath, fatigue, growing pains, abdominal pains, a constant runny nose, nausea, earaches, recurring middle-ear infections, or ringing in the ears. Bed-wetting often begins when a child first goes to school—not, as doctors and teachers often insist, as a result of school phobia, but because of the abrupt change in diet that often accompanies it. A child who is not thriving or growing normally may be allergic. A temperamental, moody, hard-to-manage child who can't seem to sit still or concentrate on lessons—a hyperactive child—is often the victim of food allergies. A child who has trouble coordinating his movements, who suffers from motion sickness in cars, boats, or on Ferris wheels, may be allergic. A child who behaves worse after such candy-coated holidays as Halloween and Christmas probably has food allergies.

Testing Your Child for Food Allergies

If you strongly suspect food allergy with your child, you may want to test out your suspicions. One very effective way to do that is to eliminate the most common allergens (see Table 46, page 230), along with any favorite foods your child craves, for five or six days. Milk should head the list, along with chocolate, eggs, wheat, oats, rye, and any coloring- or preservative-laden foods in his diet.

This is not easy, for your child is likely to rebel and feel deprived. You can make this abstinence period more tolerable in two ways. First, promise your youngster that on the seventh day, he can have as much of the forbidden foods as he would like. Second, make his new diet as enjoyable as possible by substituting foods that are tasty and fun to eat. This is a good chance to introduce the pleasures of healthy food.

If your child has allergies, he will probably feel pretty rotten the first few days as he "withdraws" from those addictive foods, and if his problems are behavioral, he'll be harder than ever to live with. You can help the child ride out this period by being patient and supportive. You can provide relief for the discomforts of withdrawal with an extra 1–2 grams of crystal Vitamin C in freshly squeezed fruit juice diluted by 50 percent distilled water one half hour before each meal. By the third or fourth day, you should notice improvement in symptoms and behavior. Tiredness or headaches or runny nose or stuffiness or temper tantrums should ease up if allergy is to blame for your child's problem. If the child is old enough, point out to him the difference the diet is making.

On the sixth or seventh day, let the child go back to his regular diet—especially the suspect foods, the milk, glutens, chocolate, and sweets. These foods, if allergenic, should produce a noticeable reaction. This won't be any fun for the youngster, and it won't be any fun to see your allergic child feeling sick or to have your hyperactive child behaving worse than ever, but it will give you some very valuable answers about your child's problems. Often a child will feel so bad when he goes back to his old diet that it will convince him of the need to give up those symptom-causing foods.

Once you determine that your child is allergic, you still have the problem of identifying exactly what he is allergic to. You can do this by repeating the same test as above, but with just a few foods at a time.

Diagnosis may be difficult, however. In all probability there will still be allergic foods in his diet during the testing period, and often the symptoms are delayed by eight hours or more. I highly recommend Optimum Health Lab's new FICA test for children of all ages. We also offer a pediatric panel, which tests for thirteen foods (milk, wheat, rye, chocolate, peanuts, orange, corn, eggs, egg yolk, banana, chicken, and turkey) and is designed especially for children under two years of age, for which only 1 cc of blood is needed. (More about the new automated FICA test on page 224.)

ALLERGY-RELATED CHILDHOOD DISEASES

Children suffer from many of the same allergy-related symptoms and diseases as adults, plus a couple of maladies to which they are peculiarly susceptible. Ten-to-fourteen-year-old children are dying from asthma at three times the rate at which they died before 1978, at a time when more children than ever are being diagnosed and treated for this ailment. Asthma, hay fever, and eczema, which affect large numbers of children, are discussed in one of the appropriate sections in Part V. Here I want to make brief mention of juvenile diabetes (which is not directly caused by allergy but can be greatly eased through better diet) and also talk about hyperactivity, which has reached epidemic levels in the present generation of kids.

Juvenile Diabetes

Unlike Type II diabetes (which can be noninsulin-dependent and usually does not affect children), diabetes mellitus, Type I, is insulin-dependent and can appear in childhood. It is an even more serious disease for children than for adults. Once established, the condition cannot be *cured.* Diabetics produce little, if any, of their own insulin, and therefore they remain dependent on daily injections of this hormone. Insulin's function is to prevent formation of extremely high blood-sugar levels and death from diabetic hyperacidity. (Before 1922, when insulin was discovered, 50 percent of diabetic children died within one year of diagnosis.) Unfortunately, as we have begun to learn, insulin's use has many short- and long-term side effects. It appears to accelerate debilitating vessel-disease problems later in life, among them increased risk of premature coronary heart disease, kidney failure, and blindness. However, the recent research of William Philpott, M.D., and others and our clinical experience at OHL demonstrate that the elimination of allergic foods, combined with a highly varied diet of wholesome foods and certain supplements, including essential fatty acids and their cofactors, can reduce the juvenile diabetic's needs for insulin *by up to two thirds.*

Certain supplements are beneficial to the juvenile diabetic. Chromium, Vitamin C, and essential fatty acids are known to enhance regulation of blood sugar. A common problem of juvenile diabetics is hemorrhaging of the capillaries and other small vessels of the eye; diabetes is the leading cause of blindness in the Western world (as Vitamin A deficiency is in the Third World). It is thought that diabetics have problems with hemorrhaging because of a tendency toward abnormal platelet aggregation. Vitamin E promotes the production of an anti-platelet-clumping prostaglandin, called PGI2 or prostacyclin. Research at the Sydney Eye Institute in Australia shows that 400–800 units a day of Vitamin E significantly reduces this hemorrhaging tendency.

For the same reason, and for benefits to heart health and weight control as well, essential-fatty-acid supplements—6–8 capsules of evening primrose oil and 3–6 capsules of eicosapentaenoic acid (MaxEPA) daily in divided doses—are highly recommended.

Finally, juvenile diabetics should be encouraged to exercise, with a doctor's supervision and permission. During exercising, insulin is not needed to regulate blood-sugar levels. *And* it is a boon to overall health and self-esteem. In 1984, a diabetic triathlete, anxious to prove that diabetes limitations can be overcome, finished the grueling 140.6-mile Ironman Triathlon in Kailua, Kona, Hawaii, without complications.

For additional information, see BLOOD SUGAR DISORDERS and DIABETES in Part V.

Hyperactivity (Attention-Deficit Syndrome)

Chances are that, if you think back to your school days, you remember a couple of kids who giggled or acted up a lot in the classroom. Perhaps one year there was "a real terror" in your classes, but he or she was the exception to the rule. But ask any teacher today about classroom behavior, and she almost unanimously reports that she has several difficult kids in her classes, and that there seem to be more and more of these problem kids every year.

I am convinced that our recent increase in hyperactivity and in various learning, emotional, and behavioral disorders is due in large part to the diet of today's young people and to delayed food allergy. In recent studies evidence has emerged that the diet staples of today's growing kids—milk, soy, wheat, eggs, chocolate, oranges, grapes, cheese, additives, preservatives, colorings—are undermining their health. Another contributing factor seems to be nutrient deficiencies, especially of essential fatty acids (EFA metabolic disorders), which result in a lack of the anti-inflammatory, antiallergy prostaglandin El. It is believed that hyperactive children—especially those from families with a history of atopy (hay fever, hives, asthma, eczema, or angiodema)—either are unable to metabolize essential fats properly or are frankly deficient.

When I use the term "hyperactivity," I mean it to include a broad category of emotional, mental, and behavioral disorders. Symptoms may manifest themselves as aggressiveness, temper tantrums, constant movement, destructiveness, abusiveness, inability to concentrate or to sit still, moodiness, nervousness, anxiety, fright, migraines, distractibility, stubbornness. These kids fall behind in class. They irritate teachers and other kids and can drive their parents to distraction. They're reckless about safety and often try dangerous stunts. They can't sleep, often are bed-wetters, or wake up with nightmares.

Mostly hyperactive children are miserable with themselves. As one ten-year-old said to me: "You wouldn't want to be inside my head. You'd be trampled to death." When these problems are caught early, dietary changes can quickly turn symptoms around. If left unattended, problems become compounded, antisocial behavior becomes ingrained, and schoolwork is neglected. Even if the problem is diagnosed at a later age, dietary changes work, but they take longer to become effective and are by that time coupled with social problems. Hyperactive kids often become school dropouts and delinquent teenagers and beyond that hyperactive adults. Hyperactivity in adults comes in many guises; it may turn up in fairly benevolent form in the high-powered workaholic—the temperamental movie producer, the obsessed athletic whiz—or it can invert itself into apathy and disinterest in life, depression, dependency, criminal behavior, and alcoholism and/or drug addiction.

Feeling as I do that many behavioral problems are traceable in large measure to food allergies and the American diet, it seems to me a travesty of responsible parenthood and citizenship that we allow our food supply to be laden with common food allergens and poisoned by chemicals, and then tout this food to our children via children's television programs.

An accepted treatment for hyperactive kids today (by nonnutritionally oriented doctors) is a combination of counseling and Ritalin therapy. Aside from the fact that Ritalin treats only the surface manifestations of hyperactivity and brings only temporary symptomatic relief, it is loaded with side effects. Ritalin is essentially a mild form of amphetamine, a stimulant of the central nervous system. It makes a normal adult behave hyperactively, but it has the paradoxical effect of calming a hyperactive child—so much so that it may turn him into a dull, unresponsive, semiaware robot. It's not much of a trade-off. To me, it represents a failure to understand and treat properly the underlying biochemical and immunological lesion.

What are some of the potential side effects of Ritalin? It can stunt the growth; if abruptly discontinued, it can bring on depression and suicidal feelings; it may lower the attack threshold of young patients with a prior history of seizures and induce more frequent seizures; it can cause adverse reactions in combination with anticoagulant drugs, anticonvulsants, and antidepressants; it commonly causes extreme nervousness and insomnia. Other reactions include skin rashes, high fever, arthralgia (joint pain), dermatitis, internal hemorrhaging, loss of appetite, nausea, dizziness, palpitations, headaches, dyskinesia (impairment of voluntary movement), drowsiness, changes in pulse and blood pressure, angina, chest pain, cardiac arrhythmias, abdominal pain, weight loss, reduction in white blood count, anemia, loss of appetite, and hair loss. Obviously Ritalin dosage must be monitored and adjusted very carefully. As far as I'm concerned, Ritalin therapy should always be the treatment of last resort.

Over the years several nutritional therapies have been advocated for treatment of hyperactivity. The late pediatric allergist Benjamin Feingold, M.D., is considered the pioneer in the field. The Feingold diet calls for the elimination of artificial colorings, additives, preservatives (especially BHA and BHT), and salicylates, which are found not only in aspirin and other over-the-counter medications but also naturally in a small group of foods. This is fine as far as it goes, but the Feingold diet doesn't address the much more important and frequent problems of food allergy, of high consumption of milk, soy, eggs, caffeinated beverages, glutens, and refined sugar, and of the need to redress nutrient deficiencies. Dr. Egger et al., reporting in *The Lancet,* March 9, 1985, showed that of seventy-six selected overactive children on a hypoallergenic diet, sixty-two (82 percent) improved and twenty-one (28 percent) achieved normalcy.

Barbara Reed, a probation officer from Cuyahoga Falls, Ohio, who herself struggled with nutritional problems, has worked extensively with treating juvenile delinquents through dietary management. It turns out that juvenile delinquents drink three times more milk than nondelinquents, consume 30–100 percent more sugar, and live on coffee and packaged sweets. Reed put her charges on a more natural, low-sugar diet, to see if it made any difference in their behavior. After a year to two years on the program, those who were conscientiously following this diet had only one sixth the incidence of repeat criminal offenses. Similar studies have produced like findings—the relationship between childhood hyperactivity and juvenile delinquency confirmed again and again.

Parents' Questionnaire for Hyperactivity

To help ascertain whether your child is hyperactive, fill out the following questionnaire.

Beside each item below, indicate the degree of the problem by a check mark.

If many of the answers regarding your child are in the 2 and 3 categories, hyperactivity may very well be indicated. See your nutritionally oriented pediatrician as soon as possible.

If hyperactivity is indicated by the above test, you should next try the food-elimination test described on page 231.

Treatment of Hyperactivity

The basic treatment for hyperactivity is simply the Optimum Health Program with a few variations:

- Determine allergic foods and eliminate them from the diet.
- Eliminate all refined sugar and, if possible, molasses, corn syrup, fruit juices, dried fruits, and very sweet fruits.
- Remove from the diet foods containing additives, preservatives, and artificial flavorings and colorings.
- The following supplementation is recommended:

Vitamin C: 1,000 mg in crystal or powder form twice a day with meals
B complex: 1 capsule twice a day with meals (children under eight, 1 capsule)
B3 (niacin): 25 mg twice a day with meals
B6: 100 mg twice a day with meals
Zinc: 25 mg once a day with meals
Magnesium: 200 mg once a day with meals
Calcium: 400 mg once a day with meals
GTF chromium: 25–50 mcg twice a day with meals

Hyperactivity Questionnaire				
	0 Not at all	1 Just a little	2 Pretty much	3 Very much
1. Picks at things (nails, fingers, nose, hair, clothing).				
2. Sassy to grown-ups.				
3. Has problems with making or keeping friends.				
4. Is excitable, impulsive.				
5. Wants to run things.				
6. Sucks or chews (thumbs, clothing, blankets).				
7. Cries easily or often.				
8. Carries a chip on his shoulder.				
9. Daydreams.				
10. Has difficulty in learning.				
11. Is restless in the "squirmy" sense.				
12. Is fearful (of new situations, new people or places, going to school).				
13. Is restless, always up and on the go.				
14. Is destructive.				
15. Tells lies or stories that aren't true.				
16. Is shy.				
17. Gets into more trouble than others same age.				
18. Speaks differently from others same age (baby talk, stuttering, hard to understand).				
19. Denies mistakes or blames others.				
20. Is quarrelsome.				
21. Pouts and sulks.				
22. Steals.				
23. Is disobedient or obeys resentfully.				
24. Worries more than others (about being alone, illness, or death).				

Hyperactivity Questionnaire *(Continued)*				
	0 Not at all	**1 Just a little**	**2 Pretty much**	**3 Very much**
25. Fails to finish things.				
26. Feelings easily hurt.				
27. Bullies others.				
28. Is unable to stop a repetitive activity.				
29. Is cruel.				
30. Is childish or immature (wants help he shouldn't need, clings, needs constant reassurance).				
31. Is easily distractible, has short attention span.				
32. Has headaches.				
33. Changes mood quickly and drastically.				
34. Doesn't like or doesn't follow rules or restrictions.				
35. Fights constantly.				
36. Doesn't get along well with brothers or sisters.				
37. Is easily frustrated in efforts.				
38. Disturbs other children.				
39. Is basically an unhappy child.				
40. Has problems with eating (poor appetite, up between bites).				
41. Has stomachaches.				
42. Has problems with sleep (can't fall asleep, up too early, up in the night).				
43. Has other aches and pains.				
44. Vomits or is nauseated frequently.				
45. Feels cheated in family circle.				
46. Boasts and brags.				
47. Lets self be pushed around.				
48. Has bowel problems (frequently loose, irregular habits, constipation).				

Evening primrose oil: 3 capsules twice a day before meals
MaxEPA: 3 capsules twice a day before meals

Having your child stick to the elimination diet will take love and patience. For the first few days, there may be a flare-up of hyperactivity, due to withdrawal, and your youngster may rebel more than usual. But it is very important that the diet, especially the elimination of allergic foods, be followed very closely. Otherwise you'll fall into a vicious circle: Just as the withdrawal symptoms abate, the child eats a forbidden food, which sets off a reaction that starts him feeling bad all over again.

Rewards, comfort, praise, special treats, and support are extremely important during the early stages. Encourage aerobic exercise five to six times a week. When the child starts feeling better as a result of the diet, when friends and family start noticing the results, when he no longer feels so bedeviled and ostracized, he will be more than willing to stick to the regime without too much prodding.

PART V

Therapeutic Applications for the Optimum Health Program

20

Getting Well on the Optimum Health Program

The patient's letter read:

> I am feeling like a new and different person, and I am very pleased with my progress. I have started back to work and school as well as gained stamina and endurance for my physical exercise, which had fallen off to nothing. I am running more, swimming and bicycling. All of these activities have become fun again as I am not tired and fatigued. I can't tell you how grateful I am for the improvement. I feel great every day, not up one day and depressed another. I have lost about sixteen pounds. I have followed the dietary advice and the special supplementation and the prescribed medication. The weight slowly disappears without coming back while all the time I am feeling better and better. I feel certain I will reach my goal and continue with a healthy life as long as I follow your advice.

Two months earlier, when this now vibrant and animated woman of thirty-seven had first come to Optimum Health Labs, she was not so optimistic about leading a healthy life. There wasn't any one outstanding problem—just enough minor complaints that she was feeling overwhelmed and defeated. Most of all, she was physically and mentally exhausted all the time, for no reason that she could put her finger on. It had gotten to the point where every little task—getting dressed, putting away the dishes, going for groceries—would completely wipe her out. And it seemed to be getting worse: nagging muscle and joint aches that jumped from place to place all over her body; a mild, but constant sinus congestion; a mild, but near-constant headache; mild but persistent diarrhea, alternating with constipation; a creeping weight gain; an occasional loud, frightening ringing in the ears; an occasional night of horrible nightmares.

Any prolonged illness—whether it's headaches or stomach pains or insomnia or arthritis or high blood pressure or cancer—can squeeze the joy right out of life. People dogged by ill health and in pain can think of very little else. Even the srongest and bravest can become limited and resigned. "If I just weren't at the mercy of these migraines . . ." a patient will say. "I'd move back to New Hampshire if it weren't for these damned asthma attacks." "If I could just get a good night's sleep . . ." "My life hasn't been the same since these pains took over . . ." "I can't even help my own daughter move into her apartment." "I would have gotten the job if I weren't such a fat blob." "If only I could go back to work . . ."

"If only" is a phrase we hear often from our patients at OHL. I am often struck by how bravely people endure tremendous pain and disability, and how desperately they want to get well and "be the person I used to be."

Patients who come to OHL are given, in addition to the basic program, a program especially tailored to their symptoms and diseases. This might consist of special exercise suggestions, additional supplements, some suggestions about eating habits and specific foods to eat or avoid, help with withdrawal or digestive problems, medications to take or cut down on, a referral to a physical therapist, stress management therapist, or chiropractor. Over the years we've combined our clinical statistics with the latest research and have refined our approach to a number of disorders that we now routinely treat.

Unfortunately, we cannot give you, the reader, the same customized service. But we can give you the benefit of our experience. In this section you will find a brief discussion of each of the major problems we treat at OHL, along with a suggested program—to be added on to the basic Optimum Health Program—that we have found effective in their treatment.

Now, I don't think that any therapy suggested here poses any real danger, and appropriate precautions are given where there is any doubt. I do not consider it within the province of this book—or for that matter my interest—to discuss surgical, psychiatric, or drug-oriented treatment. If you know yourself and your state of health, you should be able to look up your various symptoms and illnesses and use the information here to refine the Optimum Health Program further to your own specifications, without worrying about doing yourself any harm.

However, as I have stated elsewhere in this book, *I strongly recommend that you work personally with a nutritionally oriented physician as you pursue the Optimum Health Program.* A nutritionally oriented doctor is likely to be both knowledgeable about the principles of the Optimum Health Program and supportive of what you are trying to accomplish. Because your individual physiological and biochemical makeup and your personal health history are such important factors in tailoring an optimally successful program, the initial testing and evaluation and the periodic monitoring and adjusting that your own physician can provide will give you an added margin of effectiveness and safety. A physician's guidance is especially important in the case of additionally needed diagnostic tests, exercise programs, and certain supplements.

My suggestion is that you locate in this section your *every* symptom, even the most minor, and see if there's anything extra you might be doing to correct it. Don't just focus on arthritis and skip PMS or insomnia. Our experience at OHL has been that when the Optimum Health Program is tailored to fit individual needs, many if not all symptoms will improve or clear up completely. "Doctor, my blood pressure is back to normal," one patient told me, "and I used to wake up so terribly depressed. I know I didn't mention that to you. I don't even get a headache anymore or a stomachache either, now that I think of it." There are some common symptoms that almost universally disappear on the diet, such as fatigue, elevated cholesterol, constipation, and indigestion. So even if your menstrual symptoms are minor or your sleepless nights occasional, look up these symptoms, too.

Children, incidentally, because they are prey to so many allergies and nutritional imbalances, often get swift across-the-board results on the Optimum Health Program. My heart goes out when I see these children and their worried, frustrated, often exhausted parents. An obviously distraught mother brought in her slim, dark seven-year-old son, who sat through our interview listless, with a palpable melancholy about him. Once very active and cheerful, her son now rarely slept through the night and seemed to daydream constantly. Sometimes after meals he would double over with stomach cramps, though he was eating nothing out of the ordinary. His nose was always stuffed up, and he suffered from frequent stomachaches and earaches. A mild case of eczema was getting out of hand. But most worrisome of all, he would sometimes burst into tears and be wracked with sobs for no reason that he could explain.

The three-month follow-up visit was very different. The boy, as his mother reported, was "his old self" again. And indeed the boy was talkative and happy and, though only seven, chattered to me with great interest about his new diet and his new well-being. His abdominal cramps, stomachaches, and earaches were gone. His eczema had cleared up, as well as his stuffy nose. He was sleeping through the night and only occasionally remembered dreams. I could well see that he was no longer prey to the crying jags, the mood swings, and that sadness that seemed to hang over him, and even his grades in school had gone up.

You and your family can get well on the Optimum Health Program.

Not just one part of you—your head or your heart or your aching bones—but your whole body, from the inside out. Getting well is the first big step on the road to getting optimally healthy.

HOW TO USE PART V

This section is arranged like a mini-encyclopedia, with symptoms and disorders being entered in alphabetical order. Cross-references, from general to specific entries and vice versa, appear in small capitals (INSOMNIA, ASTHMA). There are no entries for disorders for which there is no specific treatment on the Optimum Health Program. Symptoms and illnesses relating to the basic program—allergy, vitamin and mineral deficiencies, water retention, fatigue—are treated elsewhere in the book. Refer to the index.

Entries are not meant to be exhaustive, but rather to touch on basic information about much of the pertinent nutrition-oriented treatment and research. At the end of each main entry is a "protocol"—recommended therapy that augments or emphasizes certain aspects of the basic program. Each protocol is divided into three sections:

1. Dietary Management. In addition to a reminder about the basic Optimum Health diet, this section lists foods to eat or avoid that are specially important in the treatment of this particular disorder, precautions regarding such things as alcohol or caffeine, and advice about eating habits. *All dietary recommendations assume that you are not allergic to the food.* Be especially careful with regard to rotating grains and dairy products; there is a high incidence of allergic reaction and cross-reactions to these foods.

2. Supplementation. Nutrient supplements over and above the suggested routine supplementation are listed in Table 3, page 86. Where pertinent, refer to Digestive Support on page 264.

Refer to page 85 to refresh your memory on the guidelines for taking various nutrients (for example, water-soluble nutrients should be taken in divided doses with or right after meals).

Micellized Vitamins A and E (see page 90) are always preferred, but because only OHL and a few other companies make them, they are sometimes hard to come by. Therefore, we have only specified micellized supplements where they are particularly important for successful treatment—for example, for irritable bowel syndrome, problems with digestion, acne, eczema, and psoriasis. Because of the greatly improved absorption of micellized fat-soluble vitamins, the dosage is much smaller than the usual amount—as a rule, one half to one third as much.

One ml (20 drops) of micellized Vitamin E equals 150 IU; one drop of micellized Vitamin A equals 3,000 IU.

The supplements listed are adult dosages. **The recommended percentages for children of various ages can be found on page 297.**

When you want to know more about a specific supplement, look it up under its individual heading in Part III.

3. Additional Recommendations. **This section lists suggested diagnostic tests, special exercise or stress-management guidelines, and in a few cases helpful medications. Always refer to Chapter 18 for general exercise guidelines.**

If you are not interested in the discussion of your symptoms, you can skip to the end of the entry and just refer to the protocol in planning your own regimen.

Discussion and Protocols

Acne. See ECZEMA
Acid Indigestion. See DIGESTIVE PROBLEMS and Digestive Support (page 264).

ADDICTION

Addictions of all kinds are complex biochemical conditions with both physiological and psychological impact. An addiction can be viewed as the incorporation of a foreign substance into the system, so that that substance becomes a "necessary" ingredient of body chemistry. When the substance is withheld, withdrawal occurs, for to be able to function with the addictant, the body has made an unhealthy adaptation and needs time to make a healthy readjustment to living without it. Until that adjustment is made, nerve impulses are confused and biochemistry scrambled. Withdrawal symptoms may include pain, nausea, vomiting, fatigue, headaches, irritability, insomnia, depression, confusion, flare-ups of known illnesses, even hallucinations.

We usually associate addictions with such substances as heroin, morphine, Demerol, caffeine, nicotine, alcohol, and prescription medications. But it is of course a basic premise of this book that we can become addicted to foods as a way of adapting to allergic reactions to them. The dynamics of food allergy/addiction are discussed at length in Chapter 5, page 55.

But whether we're talking about food or cigarettes or Valium or alcohol, the fact is that biochemically all addictions are very much the same. (This is not to deny the powerful psychological component involved in addiction to a substance such as alcohol.) Significantly, foods to which we are addicted end up having an internally produced narcotic effect. Treatment for narcotic addictions is most effective if psychological counseling of some type is part of the therapy, assuming that the individual has admitted to the addiction and is committed to overcoming it.

What we are concerned with here, though, is a nutritional approach to treating addictions. At our clinics, we have had considerable success not only with food addiction, but with patients wanting to give up cigarettes, alcohol, and even drugs. Often people come to us who have tried several times to give up coffee or cigarettes and want to try again, but dread those first few days when they know they're going to feel just dreadful—obsessed by cravings, nauseated, nervous, listless, in pain. On our withdrawal regimen (page 321), most of them are able to get through this often hellish period with little or no discomfort. For many it's a tremendous relief not to feel—after many years in some cases—slaves to their destructive habit.

A movie director came to us, very discouraged and distraught, at the end of a long, unsuccessful battle with cocaine, alcohol, marijuana, and barbiturates. Though the public and the people he worked with were unaware of his problems, he felt as if he had been walking a tightrope on his last few projects. "I'm barely holding it together," he said. Now a very big and exciting new film had been offered to him, but he was afraid he'd be found out. He was feeling like an imposter: "When I hear the bravos and praise, I don't know whether they're praising my talents or something that has to do with the drugs. I just want to be myself for once. No hiding. Just to be able to act and direct and enjoy the rewards of doing my work well, knowing that I'm doing it under my own power, and deserve those rewards."

On our program this man was able to detoxify cold turkey from the drugs with no withdrawal symptoms, turn himself around, and go on to success with the new project. For him, like many others, it was a great relief to find an effective way to get over a long-ingrained, often self-destructive habit.

Alcohol

Eighty-two percent of American adults drink socially. Over 15 percent of the population of this country—and this includes a growing number of teenagers—live under the influence of alcohol addiction. The loss due to absenteeism in the workplace is over $20 billion annually. It is implicated in more than half of all auto deaths and in over 75 percent of all crime. What is the reason for this epidemic? And why have we been so unsuccessful in treating it?

The answer is that it has only recently been accepted that alcoholism is a disease (often with a genetic predisposition) and must be dealt with as such. Its victims are not to be blamed but treated. Also, much of the treatment available to alcoholics misses the boat in denying the powerful nutritional components of the disease: food allergy, blood chemistry disorders, essential fatty acid and prostaglandin imbalances, malnutrition, and abnormal permeability of the gastrointestinal tract. To understand fully how alcoholism develops and how to treat it, we have to analyze its relationship to these various biochemical functions in the body:

Many of the foods from which alcohol is made—especially grains, corn derivatives, sugars, and yeast—are highly allergic substances. An alcoholic consumes these allergens with every drink. Food allergy response to these substances can deepen an addiction or may even be the reason that the alcohol became addictive in the first place. As early as 1957 Dr. Theron Randolph reported in the *Journal of Laboratory Clinical Medicine* that alcoholics who had given up liquor often started drinking again after being on a diet of the foods from which alcohol is made. This may well account for the sudden reappearance of withdrawal symptoms in some recovering alcoholics: They are inadvertently eating foods found in the liquor they used to drink, reactivating the addiction syndrome in the body.

Ignorance about the role of food allergy in alcohol addiction compounds the problems of staying away from liquor. Many alcoholics switch from alcohol to a diet very high in sugar and grains—pastries, candy, sugary coffee—not realizing that they are just perpetuating their addiction. At any meeting of Alcoholics Anonymous, you'll see how true this is. Nobody's drinking, but nobody's eating tofu or chicken or a green salad, either. It's coffee with two heaping teaspoons of sugar and Danish and ice cream.

There's no law requiring that liquor labels list ingredients. But whether or not you're a heavy drinker, you should know what hidden allergens are in your alcoholic drink. Table 53 on the following page lists the foods from which various alcoholic drinks are made.

Alcohol, even in moderation, seems to cause a substantial increase in the permeability of the gastrointestinal tract. And the more vulnerable the lining of the gastrointestinal tract, the more unwanted toxins and incompletely digested food molecules are able to enter the bloodstream, forming circulating immune complexes (CICs) and causing allergic reactions and inflammations. This leaky-gut phenomenon, which may persist for two weeks after the patient has begun to abstain from daily alcohol consumption, adds to the already increased possibility of delayed food allergy in alcoholics.

A study reported in the *New England Society of Allergy Proceedings* inadvertently demonstrated how the leaky gut of alcoholism exacerbates allergic reactions. Researchers took samples of centrifuged blood serum from a man known to be allergic to peanuts, which therefore

Table 53—Foods Found in Alcoholic Beverages

(*=commonly used)
(•=less frequently used
or used in smaller quantities)

Alcoholic Beverages	Corn (a)	Barley (malt)	Rye (b)	Wheat (c)	Oats	Rice	Potato	Grape	Plum	Citrus	Apple	Pear	Peach	Cherry	Hops	Cactus	Beet sugar	Cane sugar	Yeast
Wines																			
1. Grape	*							*									*	*	*
2. Champagne								*									*	*	*
3. Vermouth	•	•	•	•	•			*									*	*	*
4. Sherry	*							*									*	*	*
5. Cider	*										*						*	*	*
Malt Beverage																			
1. Beer	*	*	•	•	•	*									*				*
2. Ale	*	*	•	•	•	*									*				*
3. Flavored beer	*	*	•	•	•	*		*		*					*				*
Whiskey																			
1. Straight: (corn, bourbon, malt, rye)	*	*	*	•	•	•													*
2. Blended (d): (corn, bourbon, malt, rye)	*	*	*	•	*	*													*
3. Canadian, blended:	*	*	*	*				*	*	*							•	*	*
4. Scotch whiskey, unblended	•	*															•	•	*
5. Scotch whiskey, blended	*	*															•	•	*
6. Irish whiskey, unblended		*	*	*	*													•	*
7. Irish whiskey, blended		*	*	*	*	*		*	*	•							•	•	*
Gin																			
1. Grain spirits	*	*	*	•	•	•				*					*		•	•	*
2. Cane spirits (e)																		*	*
3. Flavored	*	*	*	*	*	*	*	*	*	*	*	*	*	*	*	*	*	*	*
Vodka																			
1. Domestic	*	*	*	*			*										•	•	*
2. Imported, some	•			*													*		*
3. Flavored	*	*	*	*	*	*	*	*	*	*	*	*	*	*	*	*	•	•	*
Rum																			
1. Domestic (includes Puerto Rican rum)								*										*	*
2. Jamaican																		*	*
Tequila																*		*	*
Liqueurs	*	*	•	•	•	•	•	*	*	*	*	*	*	*	*		*	*	*
Brandy																			
1. Grape	•							*									•	•	*
2. Cognac								•									•	•	*
3. Applejack	•										*						•	•	*
4. Blackberry	•						(contains blackberry)										•	•	*

Notes
a. Although the practice of adding corn sugar to wine for fermentation is common, wines produced in California are guaranteed free of added sugars if they carry the "made in California" label.
b. The majority of people who are sensitive to wheat are either sensitive to rye when first seen or readily become so if rye is employed as a wheat substitute.
c. If you are sensitive to wheat, the chances are extremely high that you will also show a sensitivity to malt (sprouted dried barley).
d. Blended whiskeys, the less expensive ones at least, are more apt to contain potato spirits.
e. Cane-spirits gin also contains hops, mint, and/or herbs.

contained antibodies to defend against peanuts. They injected small amounts of his serum into the skin of the forearms of four doctors. None showed any reaction at the time, but after eating peanuts a while later, three of the four soon developed large itchy red welts on their forearms. So they learned, as they expected, that allergies can be passively transferred from one person to another.

But they also learned something else: Two days later, while eating peanuts with an alcoholic drink at a cocktail party, the fourth doctor also broke out in welts—evidence that alcohol can promote the absorption of allergens into the system.

Alcoholism is often associated with malnutrition. There are several factors involved here. Because alcoholics crave the foods in alcohol—the sugars and pastries and corn-sweetened products and grains—they tend to eat these foods when they're not drinking rather than a healthier diet. Too, alcoholics are often profoundly hypochlorhydric. Alcohol inhibits the enzyme delta-6-desaturase, involved in the production of prostaglandins that control secretion of hydrochloric acid in the stomach. This ultimately leads to underproduction of pancreatic digestive enzymes and bicarbonates and thus to digestive disturbances, malabsorption of nutrients, and eventually malnutrition.

Overconsumption of alcohol leads to an excess accumulation of inflammatory prostaglandins in the pancreas, which is vital not only for digestion but also for maintaining proper blood sugar levels. It has been observed that alcoholics may have blood sugar disorders before they become addicted, implying that essential-fatty-acid disorders antedate the alcoholism and that the craving for high-sugar liquors may be an ill-guided attempt to stabilize blood-sugar levels. Whatever the case, alcohol is extremely dangerous for diabetics and hypoglycemics.

Alcoholics are also prime targets for candidiasis (page 344), an overproliferation of a common yeast, **Candida albicans.** This yeast infection can lead to all kinds of problems, among them severe gastrointestinal disorders, which can add to malabsorption/malnutrition problems. Sugar, the primary food of yeast, is a prime ingredient of many alcoholic drinks.

Depression often goes along with alcoholism, and it turns out that there are logical reasons for this. Food allergy itself can lead to symptoms of depression (page 362). Also, alcoholics seem to be deficient in the "happiness hormone," PGE1, and the fatty acid from which PGE1 is derived, dihomo gamma linolenic acid (DHGLA). This defect in essential-fatty-acid metabolism is a problem that leads not only to depression but to other problems associated with prostaglandin imbalances (Chapter 11). Alcohol is a potent inhibitor of delta-6-desaturase, the enzyme necessary for the conversion of essential fatty acids to prostaglandin E1 and E3. Alcohol, in small doses—and only initially—actually increases the production of the mood-elevating PGE1. But while this may at first make the drinker feel jolly or euphoric, extended drinking eventually depletes the brain's ability to produce more of it and leads to alcoholic depression and hangover. It has been conjectured that alcoholics may drink in an attempt to balance the brain's prostaglandins.

High systolic blood pressure in alcoholics is also associated with delta-6-desaturase inhibition. Systolic blood pressure increases consistently as alcohol intake increases; in moderate and heavy drinkers, the incidence of systolic hypertension was four times that of teetotalers. Studies show, however, that this effect is reversible when drinking is discontinued.

Poor nutrition, often associated with alcohol abuse, further compromises essential-fatty-acid metabolism.

Addiction Therapy the Optimum Health Way

Regardless of the psychological complications involved in addiction, the cause in most cases is at least partially (and in some cases entirely) traceable to nutritional problems. Thus a great deal can be done to break addictions using a nutritional approach.

Withdrawal from narcotic addictions can be especially difficult and potentially traumatic. Such a program should be undertaken only under a physician's guidance and should include psychological help and stress-management guidance.

However, self-management and self-education about your particular addiction problem is crucial if you are to break your habit. You must be responsible for your own nutritional and life-style changes, and these must be made if you are to succeed.

Protocol for Addiction

Dietary Management

1. Basic Optimum Health Program: elimination of allergic foods, rotation diet. See Part IV.
2. Increase quality protein (page 444) and nonallergic complex carbohydrates.
3. Avoid all sugars.
4. Avoid caffeine.

Supplementation

Routine supplementation (page 86) *plus*

Vitamin C: Increase to 90 percent bowel tolerance for withdrawal period (see page 262) or see below for intravenous withdrawal therapy
Evening primrose oil: Increase to 6–8 capsules daily
MaxEPA: Increase to 6 capsules daily
B complex: 1 capsule with breakfast and lunch
Folic acid: 1,000–2,000 mcg (1–2 mg) daily
Pantothenic acid: 1 250 mg capsule with each meal
Zinc chelate: 25–50 mg daily
Calcium: 600 mg daily
Magnesium: 400 mg daily
GTF chromium: 100 mcg daily
Glutamine: 200–500 mg four times a day, between meals and at bedtime
L-tryptophan: 2,000–3,000 mg forty-five minutes before bedtime (for sleep and depression)
DL-phenylalanine: 2,375 mg capsules three times daily, between meals
Stereotrophic adrenal tissue supplement: 2 tablets after each meal for three weeks (if adrenal support is indicated)

See Digestive Support, page 264.

Additional Recommendations

1. Intravenous withdrawal support. Those with severe withdrawal problems can benefit from three or four consecutive days of intravenous therapy consisting of 25–35 grams of Vitamin C, 1,000 mg calcium gluconate, 1,000 mg magnesium sulfate, 500 mg pantothenic acid, and 500 mg B6 in a 500 cc solution of normal saline. It's been our experience that withdrawal symptoms are often completely eliminated after one or two days. (More about this on page 264.)
2. Stress reduction and exercise. A regular exercise program naturally increases mood-elevating endorphins in the brain, improves digestion, absorption, and elimination, improves blood-sugar control and decreases blood insulin, improves oxygenation of body tissues, lowers blood pressure, improves sleep and the ability to handle stress, enhances self-esteem with improved appearance and weight loss, and reduces the craving to smoke, drink, or use drugs. The goal should be a slow buildup to thirty minutes of aerobic exercise five days a week. See Chapter 18, page 277.

See also DEPRESSION, STRESS MANAGEMENT, BLOOD SUGAR DISORDERS, CANDIDIASIS, Essential Fatty Acids (page 137), Withdrawal (page 261), and Digestive Support (page 264).

Adult-onset diabetes. See BLOOD SUGAR DISORDERS and DIABETES.
Airborne allergies. See ATOPIC ALLERGIES.
Alcoholism. See ADDICTION.
Anemia. See IRON DEFICIENCY.
Angioedema. See HIVES, ASTHMA.
Angina. See CARDIOVASCULAR DISEASE.

ANTI-AGING

Life extension has been a hot topic in recent years. Lately the search for the fountain of youth has taken some bizarre turns down exotic and dangerous byways. The latest elixirs of eternal life include large doses of chemical food preservatives (e.g., BHT and BHA) and potentially dangerous prescription drugs meant for treatment of other disorders.

Medical and magical miracles notwithstanding, there is no way to stop the aging process. However, there are many sane and sensible ways to prevent premature aging. And premature aging is precisely the diagnosis for those in whom heart disease, high blood pressure, elevated cholesterol, arthritis, diabetes, and chronic digestive problems show up long before gray hair and Social Security.

What are the major factors involved in the aging process? They include the faltering of many functions: the breakdown of immune functions; the related problem of free-radical proliferation and the breakdown of body tissues, especially the peroxidization (excessive oxidization) of fatty acids in cellular membranes; coronary heart disease, hardening of the arteries and the breakdown of circulation; slow healing of wounds, injuries, and lesions; digestive disorders and the breakdown of nutrient absorption and metabolism; elimination disorders and the breakdown of the body's main detoxifying system; skin wrinkling; autoimmune disease; decrease in size and function of the thymus gland; demineralization of bones and the resulting loss in height and strength. All of the above can be slowed down by lightening the burden on one's overworked system.

Optimal nutrition, in combination with stress management, exercise, and a positive attitude can tremendously reduce premature wear and tear on the system. The Optimum Health Program is by nature an anti-aging regimen, addressing the above degenerative processes in the following ways:

Immune function. The Optimum Health Program preserves immune-system function in several ways. First of all, the elimination of allergies lifts a tremendous burden from the immune system, and the rotation diet helps to prevent the development of new allergies. Many nutrient supplements, all included in the program's routine supplementation, are targeted at immune-system function and the control of free-radical proliferation. Stress management and a positive attitude enhance immunity. Exercise also enhances immune function; growth hormone levels increase, and the two- to three-degree increase in body temperature during aerobic exercise acts like a mini-fever to stimulate immune-system activity, especially white-blood-cell vigilance. These cells are part of the immune system that, among other things, monitors and destroys cancer cells. Restful sleep also improves immune function.

Coronary heart disease. The Optimum Health Program naturally lowers cholesterol, for most people find that they eat less meat, fewer eggs, and little or no margarines, shortenings, and dairy products on the program. Certain supplements (especially essential fatty acids, B3, B6, C, and zinc) lower blood fats, as does exercise, which is well known to enhance heart function and improve circulation. The increased tendency of the blood to become "sticky" and clot more easily that goes along with aging can be slowed tremendously through proper nutrition and the addition of such nutrients as Vitamins E and C, zinc, magnesium, B3, B6, and essential fatty acids.

Digestion and elimination. Efficient digestion and elimination are primary underpinnings of good health. One major cause of these problems is allergies; another is a diet too high in fat and sugar, too low in fiber. Efficient digestion and elimination allows for optimal absorption and metabolism of nutrients, and ensures that the body will have adequate fuel for all its functions. The Optimum Health Program also encourages good eating habits—from preparing food properly to eating well. And of course exercise helps here, too.

There are a couple of other approaches that I would add to round out an anti-aging program. One very important approach—an approach that has turned out to be a longevity factor in study after study—is calorie restriction or systematic undereating. This makes eminent sense, for relieving the body of the task of constantly processing huge amounts of heavy food greatly cuts down on the wear and tear to the system. In his book, *Maximum Life Span,* physician Roy Walford recommends an intake of under 2,000 calories a day (with supplementation) for moderately active individuals. Another determination would be 10 percent less than recommended calorie intake for your age group. A more aggressive longevity program might include periodic water fasts—one or two days a week or a monthly four-day fast.

Finally, amino acids may be added to an aggressive life-extension regimen. Arginine/ornithine and tryptophan supplementation, in particular, are used to stimulate the production of human growth hormone, a powerful immune-system stimulant that decreases drastically with age.

The proper objective of an anti-aging program is not to preserve youth, but to preserve and optimize health, and to prevent unnecessarily premature aging. Here is a suggested anti-aging protocol:

Anti-Aging Protocol

Dietary Management

1. The basic Optimum Health Program: elimination of allergic foods, rotation diet. See Part IV.
2. Eat a diet low in saturated and trans fats, low in sugar, and high in fiber.
3. Reduce caloric intake to 90 percent of recommended levels.
4. Limit alcohol, tobacco, and caffeine.
5. Drink plenty of bottled and distilled water.
6. Consider periodic, short-term water fasts.

Supplementation

Routine supplementation (page 86) *plus*

Vitamin C: Increase to 8–10 grams daily
Evening primrose oil: Increase to 6–8 capsules daily
MaxEPA: Increase to 6 capsules daily
Vitamin A: Increase to 10,000–50,000 IU daily
Vitamin E: Increase to 400–800 IU daily
B complex: 1 capsule twice daily with breakfast and lunch
Calcium 800–1,000 mg daily
Magnesium 600–800 mg daily

See also Digestive Support, page 264.

Note: More aggressive anti-aging supplementation might include periodic Vitamin C-to-bowel-tolerance or intravenous Vitamin C therapy and amino acids such as arginine/ornithine and tryptophan.

Additional Recommendations

1. A program of regular aerobic conditioning. See Chapter 18, page 277.
2. Stress-reduction techniques, if indicated, such as meditation or yoga.
3. Plenty of rest and *restful* sleep.

See also OSTEOPOROSIS.

Anxiety. See STRESS MANAGEMENT.
Arterial Disease. See CARDIOVASCULAR DISEASE.

ARTHRITIS

Arthritis is a very general term for a long list of disorders involving inflammation of the joints and surrounding tendons, ligaments, and cartilage, including some twenty-two distinct conditions with literally dozens of variations. Crippling, painful, and life-limiting, arthritis in one form or another, to one degree or another, affects just about everyone at some point in life. The most common varieties of arthritis (encompassing over 90 percent of arthritis sufferers) are these:

Osteoarthritis, a chronic degenerative disease of the large weight-bearing joints, which comes on with age, overweight, general wear and tear, and a lifetime of inadequate diet and exercise. The basic Optimum Health Program has proved very helpful in the treatment of this form of arthritis.

Gouty arthritis, an inflammation of the joints caused by deposition of uric acid crystals into joints, due to inadequate elimination or overproduction of uric acid. The basic Optimum Health Program is also effective in treating this form of arthritis; a protocol for the treatment of elevated uric-acid levels can be found on page 415.

Rheumatoid arthritis, a serious joint disease associated with crippling disabilities, and painful, tender, stiff swollen, often deformed joints, with fatigue, appetite and weight loss, aching muscles, and even anemia. Of all forms of arthritis, rheumatoid is the most dreaded and serious. The good news is that it has proved to be especially responsive to treatment on the Optimum Health Program.

Rheumatoid arthritis is classified as an autoimmune disease, in which, it is speculated, the body mistakenly attacks its own tissues. A more contemporary view is that the pain of rheumatoid arthritis may well be the result of the local inflammatory response from the depositing of food-containing immune complexes in and around the joints and other affected tissues, provoking the release of painful chemical mediators. Rheumatoid arthritis can attack infants and children as well as adults; the condition may be chronic or may show up in sporadic flare-ups. It is known to affect about 6.5 million Americans, though countless millions of others have mild, undiagnosed, or latent joint diseases. It usually makes its first appearance between the ages of twenty and thirty-five, and affects three times as many women as men.

Rheumatoid arthritis affects the synovial tissue, the membrane that lines the joints, which, when healthy, secretes a lubricant that allows bone to move against bone without abrasion or pain. Early symptoms of the disease are red swollen joints, which are hot to the touch, perhaps accompanied by fever and general malaise. Prolonged bouts with rheumatoid arthritis can cause permanent bone and cartilage deformation, loss of mobility, and severe, constant pain. And the damage has a domino effect. Inflammation of this synovial membrane causes a rapid growth of the membrane cells, which crowd the joint, getting wedged between bones and eventually eating away at the cartilage connecting the bones of the joint. Sooner or later this problem leads to damage of tendons, ligaments, and muscles in adjoining areas, which can in turn lead to misshapen bones.

What Causes Rheumatoid Arthritis?

A primary cause of most rheumatoid arthritis appears to be delayed food allergy and the often related problem of abnormal permeability of the intestinal mucosa. With the Food Immune Complex Assay (FICA), this is simple enough to demonstrate, and there is a sizable body of scientific literature to strongly suggest this belief. Yet the Arthritis Foundation continued for years to deny that food allergy is a factor in arthritis at all and once declared flatly, "If there were a relationship between diet and arthritis, it would have been discovered long ago." As Gardiner B. Moment, professor emeritus at Goucher College and guest scientist at the National Institute of Aging, remarked in 1980: "The National Arthritis Foundation must have set some kind of record for scientific naiveté." Fortunately the foundation is beginning to acknowledge that there might be connections between arthritis and diet after all.

This fact was discovered as long ago as 1914. *The American Journal of Medical Science* published the first study of allergy-arthritis connections by Solis-Cohen over seventy years ago. Since then a steady body of research and reports has supported this view. In 1948 Michael Zeller published his paper, "Rheumatoid Arthritis—Food Allergy as a Factor," in which he pointed out that "rheumatoid arthritis symptoms can be produced repeatedly at will by the ingestion of specific food allergens." He went on to identify likely arthritis sufferers according to their history of allergies and joint disease. The publication in 1980 of *Dr. Mandell's 5-Day Allergy Relief System* further cited the food allergy/arthritis connection. *Medical World News* subsequently stated the benefits of a dietary rather than a drug approach to arthritis.

As we know, food allergy leads to inflammation by allowing incompletely digested food particles to pass through the walls of the digestive tract and into the bloodstream where, if not cleared, they are eventually deposited in tissue, causing the release of such inflammatory chemical mediators as histamines, prostaglandins, bradykinin, and leukotrienes. These inflammatory reactions cause arthritis associated with an autoimmune disturbance in which the body's immune system also begins to attack the joints.

The chemical mediators that are, in part, the source of the pain—the various prostaglandins of the 2 series (PGE2)—may be the by-product of too much dietary arachidonic acid (saturated fats) and inadequate levels of the anti-inflammatory prostaglandins PGE1 and PGE3. Aspirin is the conventional prescription for relief of arthritis pain because it blocks the production of certain inflammatory prostaglandins. Unfortunately, aspirin also encourages the production of the other inflammatory chemical mediators, which explains why it doesn't actually change the course of the disease.

Nutritional Help

Essential-fatty-acid supplements, however, not only increase the production of the anti-inflammatory prostaglandins; they also work to block the release of arachidonic acid from storage and thus block the production of PGE2 and other inflammatory prostanoids. In addition, they may enhance the integrity of the intestinal mucosa.

Because the unchecked proliferation of free radicals is often implicated in mucosal permeability and immune system breakdowns, rheumatoid arthritis sufferers often show marked improvement when aggressive antioxidant nutrients such as Vitamins A, B5, C, E, and selenium are included in a treatment program. The combination of food-allergy elimination, antioxidants, and essential-fatty-acid supplements makes for a powerful antiarthritis therapy.

By now, we have seen countless arthritis patients who experienced significant relief from long-standing, drug-resistant symptoms. They got well on a program that includes the elimination of allergic foods, the avoidance of other specific arthritis-inducing foods, supplementation with essential fatty acids and certain other nutrients, plus exercise to prevent muscle and bone atrophy and to maintain joint mobility.

The recovery of one of our patients, a woman delighted to be playing the piano again after ten crippled years, is quite typical. Years of treatment by a series of doctors had consisted of aspirin, followed by any number of pain-dulling medications, and finally heavy doses of steroid drugs, which were causing debilitating side effects. Nothing seemed to arrest the progressive degeneration of her condition, though, and when she came to see us, she could not walk without a cane and was facing the possibility of having to give up working.

Her tests revealed numerous severe allergies and nutritional deficiencies, for her years of illness had caught her in a downward spiral of increasing vulnerability to an increasing number of allergens. We eliminated the food allergens, placed her on a rotation diet and an aggressive supplement regimen. "The results," she reported, "were rather dramatic. In less than two days, my hands were improved. I almost cried when I realized that I might be able to play the piano again—all I had hoped for was relief from the horrors of the constant pain." Little by little, she regained mobility in her joints and was able to speed up her recovery through exercise. Little by little, she was able to give up the dangerous, expensive drugs. Of course, though her insurance company had been shelling out money for all sorts of drugs and treatments for years, she was unable at that time to get reimbursement for our "non-standard" tests and supplements. As usual, the medical community, and their insurance company cohorts, were locked into a dangerous, costly, and ignorant posture of patient neglect and abuse.

Arthritis Therapy

Arthritis therapy involves a long-term program, which includes dietary management, supplementation, exercise, and stress reduction. The first step, which often results in a rapid reduction in pain, is the elimination of allergic foods. But once you've stopped adding fuel to the inflammatory fire, you must give your body time and help in healing the irritated or destroyed tissues. Recovery can be slow and exacting, but the rewards are great: the gradual abating of swelling, stiffness, and pain, the slow but steady withdrawal from drug dependency, the slow recovery of mobility, and the reopening of horizons that once seemed closed. "My husband can't believe how much I've improved," one patient reported. "This program saved not only my life but my marriage."

Dietary management for arthritis can be quite restrictive. Of course the usual allergic foods must be eliminated. But arthritis patients also seem to do best on a diet that limits fatty meats, margarines and dairy products, as well as caffeine, alcohol, and refined sugar. The rue family, or Rutaceae, which includes such citrus fruits as oranges, lemons, limes, grapefruit, and tangerines, often causes problems for arthritis sufferers. See also GLUTEN SENSITIVITY, page 374.

And while these reactions are highly individual, many people with arthritis are sensitive to members of the nightshade family, or *Solanaceae.* This plant family contains over 1,700 species, all of which contain potentially poisonous alkaloids such as solanin, capsaicin, nicotine, and atropine. The most common foods in this family are the potato, tomato, eggplant, and pepper. Other family members include tobacco, belladonna, which produces the medically important drug atropine, and henbane, used to make the asthma drug hyoscyamine and the sedative scopolamine. These drugs do have medical uses—e.g., to stop bronchial spasms or to cause dilation of the pupil of the eye—but in concentrated form they can cause paralysis and death. Livestock deaths have been reported in North Africa and Europe, where animals have eaten potato vines and peelings that have turned green from overexposure to sunlight.

This is not meant to scare you. It's just a rather fascinating phenomenon and shows how powerful seemingly harmless foods can be when eaten in excess. If it turns out that you are one of those arthritis sufferers who is sensitive to the nightshades, you will have to avoid this whole group of foods. This is not easy, since there are hidden nightshades in many processed and packaged foods. The list on pages 437–439 names the nightshade foods and many of the packaged foods in which nightshades may be squirreled away.

Patients are sometimes understandably skeptical about the idea that the nightshades might be the bad guy behind their aching joints. I had recommended to one such patient, who had chronic bursitislike pains in his shoulders, stiffness in his fingers, and elbow pain, that he try discontinuing potatoes and tomatoes, because although his allergy testing had diagnosed very few allergic foods, it was likely that something in his diet was causing his problems. He resisted my suggestion, pleading his fondness for these foods.

After three weeks on the program, he saw improvement in his mood swings and energy level, and his poor digestion had cleared up significantly, but much of the soreness and stiffness persisted. This time I made a deal with him. If he would strictly avoid the nightshades for three more weeks and still saw no noticeable improvement, I wouldn't mention it to him again.

So? After two weeks, he was *pain-free.* No soreness and not even a trace of stiffness in the morning—usually the worst time. Just for the sake of "science," we reintroduced potato and tomato to his diet a month later; the very next morning he felt twinges of joint pain. Needless to say, he's off the nightshades for good.

As mentioned, the key ingredients of arthritis supplementation are antioxidants, essential fatty acids, and the natural pain-relief amino acid DL-phenylalanine. And one more component: exercise.

Now, people with sore, achy joints have little interest in exercise, since few people care to indulge in self-torture. Left to their own devices, arthritics often curtail their movements and exercise, and slowly become increasingly wasted and rigid as the disease progresses.

This is a terrible mistake, for inactivity hastens the course of disease; exercise can slow or arrest it and can help to relieve pain. Exercise is of crucial importance in arthritis therapy. It is needed to maintain optimal joint and connective tissue flexibility. Inactivity hastens loss of muscle tone and bone calcium and further inhibits the immune system.

Exercise must be done carefully, slowly, and preferably under a doctor's supervision. It should never be done to the point of pain, nor to a level of extreme fatigue or exhaustion. In the early stages, this may mean extremely brief and limited movement, but as pain and swelling abate, increased activity will be possible. And the more you are able to do, the faster you will make progress. The objective is to put the joints through their full range of motion, so that flexibility is maintained. Any form of aerobic exercise will bring added benefit. For example, if your arthritis is confined to your arms, it may be possible to get aerobic benefit from riding a stationary bicycle without straining inflamed joints.

A commitment to a full range of arthritis therapy can help you, no matter how long you have had arthritis, no matter how severe your symptoms. After *thirty-two years* of steadily worsening arthritis, one patient wrote us to report on her first two weeks on the program: "For the first time in memory, I have hope and encouragement. After just two weeks, I feel a change in my condition. Thank you for giving me a new outlook and hope for the future."

Protocol for Arthritis

Dietary Management

1. Basic Optimum Health Program: elimination of allergic foods, rotation diet. See Part IV.
2. Cut down on fatty meats, eggs, margarines, shortening, and dairy products.
3. Cut down or eliminate CATS: caffeine, alcohol, tobacco, and sugars.
4. If indicated, eliminate the nightshade family of foods. (See pages 437–439.)

Supplementation

Routine supplementation (page 86) *plus*

Vitamin C: ½–1 teaspoon buffered powder (or 2,000 mg in buffered capsule form) twenty minutes after each meal If discomfort persists, try the Vitamin C-to-90-percent-bowel-tolerance therapy described on page 262.
Evening primrose oil: Increase to 6–8 capsules daily
MaxEPA: Increase to 9 capsules daily
Micellized Vitamin A: 3–8 drops daily (10,000–25,000 IU)
Micellized Vitamin E: 2 ml daily (300 IU)
Niacinamide: 250 mg after breakfast and lunch
Calcium/magnesium: 2 capsules (200 mg calcium/150 mg magnesium) twice a day after meals
Chelated zinc: 37–50 mg daily
DL-phenylalinine: 2 capsules (375 mg each) three times a day between meals. (If no pain relief is experienced after three weeks, take one aspirin tablet with each 2 capsules of DLP.)

Additional Recommendations

1. Get ample rest throughout the day, especially before and after exercise.
2. On warm, sunny days, expose face and arms to direct sunlight for twenty minutes (two to three times a week minimum) to aid Vitamin D production and soothe sore joints.
3. Working with a physical therapist or physician, maintain an exercise program to the best of your ability, focusing on exercises that encourage the full range of motion in all joints, plus some mild aerobic conditioning. Swimming may prove excellent for some arthritics. Those with severe arthritis can benefit from exercise in a heated whirlpool, to soothe the inflamed tissues and relieve pressure on the weight-bearing joints.
4. With reduction of pain, swelling, and stiffness, slow and gradual reduction in medication.

See also PAIN, GLUTEN SENSITIVITY.

ASTHMA
(Including Hay Fever)

There are more than 9 million asthma sufferers in this country, and the incidence of this chronic respiratory disease is on the rise. Paradoxically, even with earlier diagnosis and more hospitalization, deaths from asthma have almost doubled since 1977; the fatality rate is highest in children between ten and fourteen. Asthma accounts for one out of four school absences.

Why is this debilitating disorder becoming more widespread and dangerous? My guess is that the declining quality of the diet, stressful and inactive life-styles, the increasing toxins in our air and food, and the increased utilizations of potentially harmful drugs for the treatment of asthma all combine to augment the asthma statistics.

Asthma is, in part, an allergic response, in which allergens, coming in contact with IgE antibodies in the mast cells lining the air passages, stimulate the release of prostaglandin D2 and other chemical mediators, such as histamine and potent leukotrienes. This causes the bronchial tubes to constrict, surrounding tissue to become edematous, and thick, tenacious mucus to accumulate in the air passages. The result? Wheezing, coughing, shortness of breath, pressure in the chest, and difficult breathing. Attacks may last for just a few hours or may go on for weeks. The attack may never get past the wheezing stage, or the victim may need all of his energy to keep breathing, so that even simple tasks like talking or eating may be difficult. Fatigue, fear, and loss of confidence are predictable side effects of chronic asthma. For a child, the limitations of asthma, the missed school days, the inability to take part in activities can be a particular burden. Asthmatic children sometimes develop behavior and personality problems; they become introverted and dependent, or unmanageable and bullying.

The allergic responses associated with asthma are similar to those involved in other respiratory diseases that affect an additional 14 million Americans, such as hay fever, perennial allergic rhinitis (runny, congested nose), and anaphylaxis (hypersensitivity shock). All of these disorders may eventually be associated with bronchial spasms and may lead to additional complications such as eczema, hives, migraine headaches, growing pains, even epilepsy, depression, and anorexia.

The allergen involved in allergic asthma may be any number of substances, and varies from one person to the next. There are airborne allergens such as pollen, dust, mold, feathers, animal dander, petrochemicals, perfume, and cigarette smoke. The provocateur may be a food: Wheat, milk, and eggs are common culprits. In many cases colorings (FD&C Yellow No. 5), preservatives (metasulfites, sodium benzoate), and other chemical additives to food are at fault. Aspirin and certain other anti-inflammatory and immunosuppressant drugs, by increasing leukotriene release, can provoke asthmatic attacks. Many asthma sufferers are allergic to numerous things and add more to the list as their condition deteriorates; they spend their limited energy trying to avoid substances that will provoke an attack.

Mainstream medicine is disappointing when it comes to treating asthma. A traditional allergist may hand you a morose little booklet telling you that you have a chronic disorder for which there is no cure. He may state that asthma will give you plenty of trouble. So you should be very careful not to exert yourself and provoke an attack. He may want you to get rid of your dog or your cat or all your feather pillows and be careful to take your medicine—even though it has many potential side effects. If you don't take your medicine, he may warn you, you'll have a bad attack, and then in an emergency they may just have to give you stronger medicine.

Well, I think nutritional medicine can offer many asthmatics a more effective therapy than that and a more optimistic future.

Our approach to the treatment of asthma is to strengthen the immune system. This is accomplished by eliminating those allergens that can be avoided (foods and chemicals in the foods), correcting digestive problems, correcting (with essential fatty acids and their cofactors) the prostaglandin imbalance common to asthmatics, and exercising. A deficiency of essential fatty acids (and other nutrients important to the immune system) may weaken the cell membranes and increase their permeability, so that substances in the environment can permeate the mucosal lining of the airways, skin, and gastrointestinal tract easily and indiscriminately. Once the cell membrane barrier is strengthened, the system is able to screen out unwanted substances, and attacks are averted.

Traditional wisdom states that asthmatics should not exercise because of the risk of provoking an attack. This advice is both unwarranted and detrimental for asthmatics, for exercise improves general fitness, stimulates the immune system, and enhances defenses against attacks, in addition to its benefits in the area of confidence and self-esteem. Any program of exercise may be undertaken, as long as the precautions and guidelines listed below are followed. Swimming especially has been found to be an ideal form of exercise for most asthma sufferers.

Asthma sufferers usually see great improvement on the Optimum Health Program. The number and severity of attacks decrease sharply, the amount of medication needed is reduced, and general health improves. It *is* possible to come to livable terms with asthma. Asthmatic children, especially once their asthma is being successfully managed, should be encouraged to live as normal a life as possible. Diagnosis should be made early, so that treatment can begin, strength and confidence built up.

The following protocol can be followed by both children and adults. A separate supplementation regimen is given for children under sixteen.

Protocol for Asthma

Dietary Management

1. Basic Optimum Health Program: elimination of allergic foods, rotation diet. See Part IV.
2. Avoid all artificial colorings (especially FD&C Yellow No. 5—tartrazine) and flavorings.
3. Avoid all preservatives, especially metasulfites, which are often used to keep food fresh in restaurants.
4. Avoid caffeine, alcohol, tobacco, and sugars.

Supplementation for Adults

Routine supplementation (page 86) *plus*

Vitamin C: Increase to 8–10 grams (during periods of exacerbation, an increase to 90 percent of bowel tolerance, page 114).
Evening primrose oil: Increase to 6–8 capsules daily
MaxEPA: Increase to 6 capsules daily
Micellized Vitamin E: 1 ml (20 drops) daily (150 IU)
Micellized Vitamin A: 3 drops daily (10,000 IU)
Pantothenic acid (B5): 250 mg three times daily after meals
B6: 250 mg twice daily, after breakfast and lunch

Supplementation for Children

Multivitamin: 1 capsule with each meal
Multimineral: 1 tablet with each meal
Vitamin C: 1,000 mg twice daily with meals
Evening primrose oil: 3 capsules twice daily with meals
MaxEPA: 2 capsules twice daily with meals
Micellized Vitamin E: ½ ml (10 drops) daily (75 IU)

Micellized Vitamin A: 1 drop every other day (3,000 IU)
B complex 1 capsule with lunch
Pantothenic acid: 100 mg with dinner

Additional Recommendations

A program of regular aerobic exercise supervised by an exercise-oriented physician is a vital part of asthmatic therapy. Here are some guidelines to ensure that exercise is safe and effective:

- Do not eat a known allergic food before exercising.
- Do not exercise for at least three hours after eating.
- Thirty minutes to an hour before exercising, take 500–1,000 mg of crystal Vitamin C (children under sixteen: 500 mg) to help prevent exercise-induced asthma.
- Exercise level should begin at low intensity and increase slowly over time as fitness increases.
- Warm up *and* warm down. Exercise periods should begin and end at a leisurely pace.
- Do not exercise to exhaustion. Each exercise period should be limited to thirty to forty minutes. Or work out for short periods interspersed with rest.

See also ATOPIC ALLERGIES.

Atherosclerosis. See CARDIOVASCULAR DISEASE.

ATOPIC ALLERGIES

Atopic allergies (asthma, angioedema, eczema, hives, hay fever, conjunctivitis) are often associated with classic, IgE-mediated, Type I allergic reactions. Atopic allergies are frequently associated with an immediate outbreak of symptoms, triggered by the sudden release of chemical mediators from mast cells lining the oral cavity, skin, and air passages. Such allergies are the bailiwick of the traditional allergist. Identification of the offending allergen is often made with the scratch test, prick test, or IgE RAST blood test; the traditional treatment is medication, allergy shots, and, when possible, avoidance of the offending allergen.

For several good reasons, we do not approach the diagnosis and treatment of atopic allergies in a traditional fashion at OHL. Conventional test methods used in identifying food allergens, by anyone's estimation, are unreliable. Existing medications—antihistamines, decongestants, theophylline, corticosteroids, Alupent, adrenaline, etc.—offer partial relief but no treatment of the underlying cause of allergy. And just how do you go about avoiding pollen or dust or mold or petrochemicals, without moving to another planet? Too, it has been our experience that many of those with atopic allergies have abnormal mucosal permeability and/or a weakened immune system and easily pick up new allergies; most suffer from multiple allergies. Thus, a hay-fever victim who manages to move away from a pollen-infested area will often develop allergies to mold or another pollen irritant. Someone who gets rid of his beloved pet will transfer the allergy to pollen, food, or cigarette smoke. An infant who gets over his eczema may later develop childhood asthma and still later in life may break out in hives from a chemical in his office.

A better, more rational way to treat atopic allergies is to address the underlying problems of abnormal permeability and a weakened immune function. For this reason, the Optimum Health Program is often very effective in treating atopic allergies. As might be expected, the great majority of people with airborne or contact allergies also have food allergies. The restoration of good digestion, good nutritional status, normal permeability, and the reclaiming of immune system strength, along with attention to stress reduction and supplementation, make it possible to withstand the onslaught of environmental allergens.

Life can be a nightmare for those who are susceptible to just about everything they come in contact with—mildew in the summer, pollen in the spring, animal dander at home, formaldehyde at work. One patient came to us feeling as though he were under attack from all sides. He was sniffling, which he described as a permanent condition, what with the pollen and the dust and his allergy to cigarette smoke and the sulfites in so many foods. His hands were covered with a fiery rash, and now he was having terrible bouts of light-headedness in the office. Was it all in his head, he wondered, because his company had just moved to new quarters, and maybe he had hidden apprehensions he wasn't aware of? He had been to several doctors and was afraid of adding yet more medications to the several he was already taking. He came to us after he heard Phyllis Diller mention us on television.

The light-headedness we traced pretty quickly to the petrochemicals in the drapes and rug in his new office; they were soon replaced by tile and slatted blinds. But the most effective treatment was the elimination of food allergies—he had eleven—and aggressive supplementation to build up his immunity. Eight months later his symptoms were so much improved that for the first time in his life that he could remember, he didn't have to carry around a packet of Kleenex "like a security blanket."

Table 54, showing the most common environmental toxins and allergens, appears on page 339.

A list of environmental toxins and allergens would not be complete without a brief mention of some of the common chemical culprits found in food:

- MSG (monosodium glutamate) is common in Chinese food and much restaurant fast food and many canned and packaged foods.
- Metasulfites/metabisulfites are common in factory-prepared foods, wines, and beers, and are often added to potatoes, avocados (guacamole dip), shellfish, greens, and vegetables in restaurants to keep the food looking fresh. Asthmatics often have severe reactions to these preservatives.
- Tartrazine, used widely as a food coloring (FD&C Yellow No. 5), is a known provocateur of hyperactivity, migraines, and asthmatic attacks.
- Sodium benzoate, a commonly used preservative (e.g., in carbonated soft drinks), is associated with migraines and related symptoms.

As yet, no reliable test exists to diagnose sensitivity or allergic reactions to most chemical toxins. In the first place, there are thousands of such toxins, so the testing process would be exhausting and expensive. Besides, like dust or pollen, there's not much you can do in most cases about completely removing them from your environment—they're in the air, in your food and water, in the furniture, in the very fabric of your life. All you can do is to try to avoid them as much as possible. As problems of chemical hypersensitivity become more common (as they will continue to do until we stop poisoning our air, our water, and our food), solutions and antidotes will probably be found for the most troublesome. For example, it's known that 50–200 mg of Vitamin B6 an hour before consuming MSG will prevent or minimize a reaction. A dose of 1,000–4,000 mcg of oral B12 is often effective in arresting a reaction to metabisulfites. Tartrazine sensitivity can be reduced by increasing the essential fatty acids in the diet.

Discussion and therapy protocols for the major atopic disorders—ASTHMA, HIVES, and ECZEMA—can be found under individual headings in this section. Hay fever is discussed under ASTHMA.

Atopic Dermatitis. See ECZEMA.

Bad Breath. See DIGESTIVE DISORDERS and Digestive Support (page 264).

Bloating. See DIGESTIVE DISORDERS and Digestive Support (page 264).

Table 54	
Pollutant	**Major Emission Sources**
Predominantly Outdoors	
Sulfur oxides	Fuel combustion, smelters
Ozone	Photochemical (sun) reactions
Pollens	Trees, grass, weeds, flowers
Lead, manganese	Automobiles
Calcium, chlorine, silicon, cadmium	Drinking water, industrial emissions
Organic substances	Oil-derived solvents, vaporization of unburned fuels from natural sources
Predominantly Indoors	
Spores	Fungi, molds
Radon	Building construction materials such as concrete and stone—radon, a gas, is held in high concentration in these substances
Formaldehyde	Insulation, furnishings, cosmetics, plastics, particleboard
Asbestos and synthetic fibers	Fire-retardant materials, insulation
Other airborne particles	House dust, dust mites, animal dander
Microorganisms	Bacteria and viruses from people, animals, and plants
Aerosols	Consumer and industrial aerosol products
Mercury	Paints, fungicides, thermometer breakage
Ammonia	Cleaning products
Organic substances	Cosmetics, cleaning solvents, adhesives
Polycyclic hydrocarbons, arsenic, carbon monoxide, sulfur dioxide, nicotine, acrolein, etc.	Tobacco smoke

BLOOD-SUGAR DISORDERS: ADULT ONSET DIABETES AND HYPOGLYCEMIA

The regulation of the body's blood-sugar level is a delicate process involving the digestive tract, the liver, the pituitary, the pancreas and adrenal glands, plus a full roster of enzymes, hormones, chemical mediators, and secretions.

When the whole system is functioning smoothly, the pancreas, adrenals, and pituitary gland release hormones that maintain a steady blood-sugar level. For example, the adrenal medulla releases adrenaline, which stimulates the release of sugar stored as glycogen in the liver and muscles. The pancreas has multiple functions: It produces and secretes the eleven enzymes that metabolize all foods, including the conversion of complex carbohydrates to simple sugars; it releases a bicarbonate fluid that maintains proper acid/alkaline balance in the digestive tract; and it produces insulin to carry blood sugar into cells; finally, the pancreas produces yet another hormone, glucagon, that serves to raise blood sugar and suppress appetite.

This complex process of checks and balances should ensure a healthy blood-sugar level, since the liver, the pancreas, and the adrenals serve as double-checks against the presence of too much or too little sugar in the blood. What goes wrong?

For something is surely wrong. Diabetes mellitus is rampant. It's predicted that by the year 2000, one in three adults will have diabetes. This is neither natural nor inevitable. It just means that once again our chronically high level of food consumption and low level of nutrition, our dependence on processed foods, our laid-back sedentary life-style, and our national sweet tooth have gotten us into serious trouble. It just means that once again we've failed to recognize the incredible influence of allergy and nutrition.

"I knew something was getting dangerously out of whack," a patient recalled to me. A toll collector (now *there's* a "desk job"), forty pounds overweight, he had a lifelong history of allergies and always kept a stack of candy bars and a bag of doughnuts in his tollbooth. Suddenly his lethargy and his mood swings began to get out of hand, and he was having headaches. "Some days I'd feel OK, but then suddenly I'd get all shaky. Other times I'd just want to cry. Or I'd just feel like falling asleep forever."

A great many people like this man come to our clinic—people who for years and years have abused their bodies with inactivity and inattention to what they were eating. One day they realize that lots of little things are wrong and further along they discover that one of those nagging little things is now a big, serious thing. Often that big thing is diabetes mellitus or hypoglycemia. Both of them can become serious, debilitating diseases. Both of them are related to allergy and nutrition. Both can be tremendously improved or controlled on the Optimum Health Program.

See also DIABETES MELLITUS, HYPOGLYCEMIA.

BRAIN ALLERGIES

The brain is no more immune to the effects of allergy or poor nutrition than any other part of the body. The brain's chemistry can be thrown off by allergic reactions to foods, inhalants, or any number of brain-scrambling chemicals in the environment. When the brain is the target organ of allergy, the repercussions mirror those that are diagnosed in the traditional psychiatric lexicon as depression, anxiety, irritability, phobia, hyperactivity, insomnia, mental fatigue, even perhaps stuttering or severe psychosis.

There is no mystery about this. The brain, like any other organ in the body, is an interconnected web of biochemical actions and reactions. We know, for example, serotin, which is vital for the transmission of electrical impulses in the brain, is manufactured from tryptophan only in the presence of B6. If B6 is in short supply, because of allergy-induced digestive problems or generally poor nutrition, this brain process breaks down. If the brain is *your* Achilles' heel, circulating immune complexes will settle in your brain, causing cognitive or emotional upset; in another person they might do their inflammatory damage in the joints or the liver or the sinuses.

Mental disturbances can result from an inadequate concentration of many nutrients in the brain. Many enzymes, hormones, and neurotransmitters that are essential for clear thought and mental health are contingent on good nutrition. Mental patients in numerous hospital studies have gotten better with improved nutrition and an allergy-free diet. It was Linus Pauling who led the way in identifying the nutrition/mental health connection. Coining the term "orthomolecular" (meaning "correct molecules") medicine, he demonstrated that both physical and mental health can be optimized by giving the body the right amounts of the right nutrients.

Dr. Ben Feingold's controversial diet for hyperactive children (page 304) is another example of the emerging awareness that "mental" disease can be helped best by improved nutrition.

In *The American Journal of Psychiatry,* Dohan and Grasberg reported in an article entitled "Relapsed Schizophrenics: Earlier Discharged from the Hospital After Cereal-Free Milk-Free Diet" that schizophrenics seem to have a high intolerance to gluten and milk. On a controlled diet, their symptoms abated, and they were able to be discharged well ahead of "schedule." Other studies have shown that a five-day water fast will often bring dramatic relief from the diagnosed problems of mental patients. Symptoms reappear when they go back to their regular diet—and thus to their allergies.

The Scope of Brain Allergies

Considering the fact that there are over 1,000 known separate chemicals involved in brain function and that at any given moment more than 20,000 biochemical reactions are occurring simultaneously, the potential effects of food allergies on our mental and emotional well-being is enormous.

At our clinic, we see emotional and mental problems clear up all the time. Many people who come to us for headaches or arthritis or obesity report back to us at a later visit that they are now feeling more alert or that their depression or irritability is gone, that they are sleeping through the night or they no longer feel "fuzzyheaded."

One patient came to us after years of seeking a psychiatric solution to his bouts of deep depression. During these periods, he was unable to work and had lost five jobs in as many years. He'd tried many medications; most had affected him adversely. Now he was on a mood-elevating drug that left him feeling listless and nauseated and seemed to interfere with his concentration. Needless to say, he'd had lots of "talk" therapy.

The FICA test revealed that he was highly allergic to both milk and grains. Furthermore, he was very sensitive to the petrochemicals he encountered in his work as a mechanic. In addition to the elimination of allergies and a strict rotation diet, we had him take several supplements targeted at boosting his immune system and suggested that it would be well worth it to seek training in a field that would not expose him to the chemical irritants that plagued him. After four months he had managed a career switch. "The cloud has lifted," he said, and his energy level was better than it had been since he was a teenager. Pretty good, as he put it, for a guy who was dragging himself through life. A year and a half later he called in to say that he had been free of depression and that his family enjoyed "having me back."

Here are some additional instances of the alliance between food allergy and emotional problems.

Clinical tests show that even mild allergies can cause mood swings. *The Journal of Psychology* reported a 1979 double-blind study by Singh and Kay, showing that cognitive/emotional symptoms can be produced by exposure to allergens. In other studies, common irritants such as tobacco smoke have been found to impair the thinking ability of 48 percent of the smokers surveyed.

It is accepted that blood sugar and insulin imbalances affect psychological states. Hypoglycemia, in large part an essential-fatty-acid and/or food-allergy disorder, can cause crying jags, despondency, and even suicidal feelings. When blood-sugar and insulin levels stabilize, these feelings disappear.

There are yet other manifestations of brain allergies. Hyperactivity and other learning disabilities (page 302) often associated with such conditions as dyslexia, stuttering, the inability to concentrate or to retain information, are well-established consequences of brain allergies. A 1983 article in *The Lancet,* "Are Migraines Food Allergy?" reported that, in a double-blind, placebo-controlled study, thirty-five of forty-one behaviorally disturbed children improved with elimination of allergic foods.

Across the country, general IQ levels, as well as reading and math scores, have declined dramatically in the last three decades. Everyone is blaming someone: parents, teachers, the federal government. But few have thought to look at the changing diet of American schoolchildren. The average school lunch is a nutritional nightmare. Cake and coke and candy are not just for after school; you can get them in the lunchroom and probably at home as well. This chemical-, fat, and sugar-laden diet, not to mention the daily milk intake, could fry anyone's brain.

Even crime may well be connected to allergy and diet. Seventy to 75 percent of incarcerated criminals were hyperactive children —that's ten times the incidence of hyperactivity in the general population. Childhood nutrition problems don't go away; they become antisocial, alcoholic, and/or violent behavior in adults.

Mental impairment in the elderly is directly tied to nutrition. That catchall term for everything from memory loss to mental confusion, "senility," may be the work of poor nutrition combined with allergies and the reduced ability to digest and absorb nutrients.

Now the finger is being pointed at food allergy as an explanation for phobias—irrational, inappropriate, immobilizing fears. This is good news for those who are frightened not only by heights or cats or crowds, but by their inexplicably intense reaction to them.

Such was the case with a young New York woman who started college in New Mexico. She was not aware of more than average homesickness and nervousness, but one night about three weeks into the term she returned from dinner in the dorm shaky and dizzy, with chills and a headache. The same thing happened the next day. Every time she went to the dining room for a meal, the symptoms would reappear. Her immediate thought was that she was nuts. Slowly she developed a fear of open spaces, anywhere, at any time; she was agoraphobic. She went home, but it was several years before she sought help from us for her closed-in life. It turned out that she had many food allergies, probably brought to a head by the repetitiveness of the highly allergic foods they served in the dorm, combined with the stress of her new life. Once relieved of the dizziness and anxiety, she was able to dismantle the fears that they produced as well. She returned to college, aware that she'll be fine as long as she avoids caffeine, rye, wheat, and other allergenic foods.

Any mental or emotional problem requires prompt medical attention. Just be sure that your doctor is open to the possible relationship of allergy and nutrition to human psychology and behavior.

Discussions of individual "brain" allergies can be found under DEPRESSION (CHRONIC), INSOMNIA, PMS, and HYPERACTIVITY (page 302).

Bursitis. See ARTHRITIS.

CANDIDIASIS

Candida albicans is a normally harmless yeast, which we all harbor from birth in the intestinal tract. Normally candida, along with bacterial flora with which we coexist, remains under control. But during periods of prolonged stress or lowered immunity it can proliferate to the point of infestation, changing from its benign yeast form to an invasive fungal form.

Candidiasis is the name given to the condition resulting from the overproliferation of *Candida albicans.* A common, though often undiagnosed disorder, it is of particular importance because its symptoms often mimic those of food allergy and because the two are sometimes interrelated and must be treated together.

The invasive, fungal form of candida appears to permeate the gastrointestinal mucosal lining, breaking down the barrier to the bloodstream, permitting allergic substances to penetrate easily, form immense complexes, and perhaps promote food-allergy reactions. Food allergies, on the other hand, are often associated with hypochlorhydria (deficiency of hydrochloric acid), but since HCl kills yeast, it is needed to keep the candida under control. Thus it is often necessary to correct food-allergy and related nutritional problems (increase production of HCl) in order to get rid of candidiasis. And vice versa.

The symptoms of candidiasis range from the bland to the bizarre; you will quickly see why it might be confused with allergy.

- Digestive problems such as gas, bloating, indigestion, elimination problems, heartburn, colitis, and diarrhea.
- Respiratory problems such as lung congestion, hay-feverlike sneezing and watery eyes, earaches, hives.
- Genitourinary disorders: vaginitis, menstrual irregularities, premenstrual syndrome, endometritis, cystitis, kidney and bladder infections, localized itching and pain.
- Central nervous system imbalances: depression, false reading of autism, memory loss, and headaches (all have been reported).
- Generalized symptoms such as fatigue, lack of energy, loss of libido (particularly with rampant vaginal infections).

As you can see, candidiasis can wreak all sorts of hard-to-pinpoint havoc. One bizarre case of candidiasis occurred in a young boy, who seemed to have severe emotional problems and had been diagnosed as autistic. After years of ineffective treatments, his parents began to suspect that his food allergies were connected to these conditions. Eventually they were able to trace a complex network of hypersensitivities back to a childhood ear infection, which had been treated with a prolonged exposure to antibiotics. It was then that many of his food allergies had first showed up, perhaps the result of the invasive *Candida albicans* infestation permeating the digestive tract, a situation created by the antibiotic therapy. When the fungal infection was brought under control, allergies abated, and symptoms of "autism" disappeared.

Yet another documented case of candidiasis involved a child who demonstrated all the symptoms of alcoholism. It turned out that his system was apparently producing so much yeast that his gastrointestinal tract was manufacturing ethanol (alcohol) from the sugars in his diet.

Fortunately for most candidiasis sufferers, the symptoms are limited to fatigue, indigestion, anxiety, worsening allergies, or repeated vaginal infections. Even so, it is a tenacious, debilitating, health-sabotaging disorder, often requiring prolonged treatment.

Several factors contribute to the overgrowth of candida:

- Antibiotics. These seem to be the number-one offender, for they kill off the friendly but competitive bacteria in the intestines that keep this yeast under control. Our widespread, chronic exposure to antibiotics in our meat (via its presence in animal feed) and the common and often unnecessary use of antibiotic medications have made us increasingly vulnerable to candida overgrowth.
- Lack of adequate hydrochloric acid in the stomach. This deficiency, often associated with essential-fatty-acid deficiency, alcohol abuse, and food allergies, permits *Candida albicans* to flourish.
- The use of birth control pills. This is sometimes a factor in candidiasis, since the fungal organisms seem to thrive in the presence of estrogens.
- A diet high in alcohol or sugar. This encourages the growth of candida, as does a diet low in fiber.

Given this set of causes, it's no wonder that candidiasis problems are becoming so common. However, it can be tricky to diagnose. The symptoms can indicate many other conditions. Moreover, the traditional stool culture for candidiasis is not accurate, since just about everyone will show the presence of some candida, and the exact level is hard to measure with precision. At this time, there is no generally accepted and scientifically verifiable test for gastrointesinal candidiasis.

Treatment for candidiasis involves getting rid of food allergies, clearing up digestive problems, and bringing the rampant candida growth under control. Sugars and alcohol must be avoided, because yeasts are sugar metabolizers and simple sugars are just what candida thrives on. HCl capsules with meals along with lactobacillus acidophilus supplements seem to help restore the proper balance of intestinal flora. Biotin supplements may be important, because candida is partially dependent on biotin deficiency for the conversion to the destructive fungal form. (*Note:* Some researchers disagree with this treatment and feel that biotin may enhance candida growth.) Essential fatty acids, which are thought by some researchers to be deficient in cases of candidiasis are added to the diet to provide a source of oleic acid. And a high-fiber diet hastens the elimination of nonabsorbed metabolic toxins. Treatment for candidiasis must be continued for six to twelve months in most cases. The reward is disappearance of long-standing symptoms and improved general health—well worth the prolonged effort.

Protocol for Candidiasis

Dietary Management

1. Basic Optimum Health Program: elimination of allergic foods, rotation diet. See Part IV.
2. Increase dietary fiber. See page 453 for a list of high-fiber foods.
3. Avoid all sugars, including white sugar, honey, molasses, and most fruits. Small amounts of aspartame (NutraSweet) can usually be tolerated. Limit complex carbohydrates to two servings a day. Rice, millet, and oats are good choices; limit starchy vegetables like yams and sweet potatoes.
4. Avoid all alcoholic beverages.
5. Hydrochloric acid (HCl) and pepsin capsules with meals as needed. Begin with 1 capsule at the start of the meal and increase cautiously to 2 capsules with each meal if needed.

Supplementation

Routine supplementation (page 86) *plus*

Vitamin C: Increase to 8–10 grams daily
Vitamin E 1 400 IU capsule daily
Evening primrose oil: Increase to 6–8 capsules daily
MaxEPA: Increase to 6 capsules daily
Pantothenic acid: 250 mg daily
Zinc chelate: 25–50 mg daily
Lactobacillus acidophilus: 1 dry teaspoon three times daily (if allergic to milk, use nonlactose acidophilus)

See also Digestive Support (especially HCl supplements), page 264.

Additional Recommendations

The elimination of *Candida albicans* often requires some form of medication. In all cases, treatment of candidiasis, because of the prolonged therapy, should be undertaken with the supervision of a healthcare professional familiar with this condition. The first medication tried is usually a preparation of caprylic acid; if progress is not made, antifungal drugs such as Nystatin or Nizoral are added.

See also Chapter 14: Testing for Food Allergies, page 221.

Cardiac Arrythmias. See CARDIOVASCULAR DISEASE.

CARDIOVASCULAR DISEASE (INCLUDING HYPERTENSION)

Heart disease will kill hundreds of Americans while you read this chapter. There were 1 million heart attacks in this country in 1984, over half of them fatal. A surprising number struck down relatively young people who had no idea they were at risk. Perhaps the worst irony of these awful statistics is that many of these heart attacks could easily have been avoided.

What is behind this modern epidemic? Why do we continue to spend over $6 billion a year on more than 170,000 questionable coronary bypass operations? Why are countless millions more spent on drugs that treat only symptoms and in some cases have side effects as perilous as the problems they are designed to treat?

Once again, the answer is "Because we do not yet take seriously—deadly seriously—the power of nutrition and life-style to cause, and by the same token prevent and reverse, heart disease." That's why I've chosen to write at some length about this subject, even though, on the surface, it is not as closely related to allergies as most health disorders we focus on at our clinic. I hope that, after reading this discussion, you too will take the heart disease/nutrition connection seriously.

Before going any further, let me re-emphasize the importance of working with your physician when it comes to treating something as complicated as heart disease. At our clinic, we work with patients whose strong family history of heart disease makes them prime targets for future problems and with patients recovering from heart attacks. These latter patients we monitor very carefully, especially with regard to certain supplements, such as niacin, essential fatty acids, Vitamin E, and amino acids, and with regard to exercise levels.

Happily, there are clear signs that heart-related deaths are down some 35 percent since 1968, after years of skyrocketing statistics. The explanation seems to be that people are smoking less, exercising more, and cutting down on fatty foods. Gains have also been made in the regulation and control of hypertension and in emergency treatment for heart attacks. Even so, the statistics remain alarming. We still consume more artery-clogging foods than we did sixty years ago. The overprocessed, high-sugar, high-fat, nutrient-depleted diet we feed our kids casts a shadow over their future health. *Time* magazine reported that autopsies of soldiers killed in the Korean and Vietnamese conflicts showed that 77 percent had signs of arterial disease. Their average age: twenty-two. Autopsies of their Korean and Vietnamese counterparts, raised on diets high in unrefined rice and vegetables, revealed no such damage.

The Risk Factors in Cardiovascular Disease

Cardiovascular disease is a catchall term for a number of disorders related to the circulatory system and the heart. All these problems—from high cholesterol to high blood pressure, to blood-clotting abnormalities, to atherosclerosis—are steps on the road to the ultimate crisis: heart attack and stroke. There are predictable risk factors connected to the development of cardiovascular disease. Most, as you'll see, are amenable to changes in diet or life-style. Even those that involve hereditary disposition can be minimized by the way we live and eat.

Smoking. Smoking not only cuts down on the amount of oxygen the blood transports to the cells, it also damages the lining of arteries, promotes abnormal blood clotting, interferes with prostaglandin production, and pollutes the body with gases and chemicals. Smokers are especially at risk for the coronary artery vasospasm type of heart attack.

High blood pressure. No matter what its origin, high blood pressure is an often silent but deadly contributor to cardiovascular disease. It puts a strain on the heart muscle and the arterial walls and damages the kidneys.

Elevated serum cholesterol. Most of our diets are dangerously high in the type of cholesterol that causes the arteries to become clogged with fatty deposits. This atherosclerotic plaque cuts off the blood supply to the heart and brain, causing oxygen deprivation, heart damage, and strokes.

Sedentary life-style. Exercise increases oxygenation, stimulates the immune system, increases muscle and heart strength, controls harmful cholesterol and triglyceride levels, reduces the percentage of body fat, reduces excess stress, prevents abnormal platelet stickiness, and stabilizes enzyme and cellular activity. A slow-moving, chair-centered life-style cancels out those benefits and causes a general lack of metabolic vigor in all bodily systems.

Heredity. A tendency to heart disease is often inherited. This should not condemn family members to the same fate, but should be taken as a signal to take active control of other risk factors.

Blood insulin and blood glucose levels. Diabetics, hypoglycemics, and others with blood-sugar disorders have greater susceptibility to heart disease, probably because of the associated abnormal platelet aggregability, increased blood fats, and abnormal prostaglandin metabolism, all of which affect the strength and integrity of veins and arteries.

Elevated uric-acid levels. Problems with overproduction or improper elimination of uric acid tend to indicate systemic imbalances in the renal and cardiovascular systems.

Body fat level. Although weight is not always a true measure of general health, percentage of body fat often is. The average American male carries 20–30 percent of his body weight in fat, his female counterpart 30–45 percent. Anything above 19 percent for men and 22 percent for women constitutes an added risk, for it implies the consumption of too many metabolism-inhibiting foods and not enough exercise, which can lead to clogged arteries and poor circulation.

Alcohol abuse. The abuse of alcohol and all drugs cripples the body's self-regulating systems, altering prostaglandin and enzyme production, and increasing blood pressure. Alcohol also interferes with nutrient absorption and use.

Nutritional deficiencies. Poor diet, food allergies, digestive disturbances, and malabsorption problems can all lead to lack of nutrients especially needed to maintain cardiovascular health, from Vitamins E and C to essential fatty acids and certain trace minerals.

Atherosclerosis

Atherosclerosis is "clogging of the arteries" due to proliferation of smooth muscle cells and the buildup of lipids (cholesterol/fat deposits) and fibrin in the linings of the artery walls. These protruding deposits, known as plaque, may lead to heart attacks, strokes, and kidney failure —the causes of over 50 percent of all deaths in the United States.

Atherosclerosis appears to begin when the lining of an artery, called the endothelium, is roughed up, torn, irritated, or otherwise damaged. Theoretically, this damage may be accomplished by abnormal platelet aggregation, excess cholesterol, high blood pressure, food immune complexes, infection, or even smoking.

When the lining of the vessel is damaged, the collagen layer underneath is exposed. A healthy blood vessel can repair any damage easily and quickly, without aftereffects. But an unhealthy artery—one constantly imperiled and eroded by high blood pressure, aggregated platelets, poor nutrition, too much cholesterol, or smoking—eventually becomes too weak to perform its usual self-healing tasks. Instead, the damage escalates.

Unhealed injuries to the blood vessels lead to three interrelated reactions and subsequent problems. First, the tear itself signals the blood to send Band-Aids, in the form of more *platelets,* to the site of the injury. The function of platelets is to assist in blood clotting, and hence they thicken the blood in the injured vessel and stop the bleeding.

Second, once the lining is damaged, the smooth muscle cells located toward the outside of the blood vessel walls are activated by the chemicals (released earlier by the aggregated platelets), which begin to multiply wildly and to migrate to the site of the damage. Once these cells are present at the damage site in large numbers, they attract more and more platelets. They also attract another another type of white blood cell, known as a *macrophage.* While the platelets are stimulating more runaway growth of the smooth muscle cells, the macrophages are gorging themselves on fats (cholesterol) contained in the blood. They become bloated and turn into *foam cells.* When they have stuffed themselves to the breaking point, they explode, spewing their fatty contents into the blood vessel wall at the site of the initial tear. The presence of this added cholesterol signals the blood to call in more macrophages to clean up the mess. They gorge themselves, explode, and the cycle repeats itself.

It may be an excess in the blood of this particularly dangerous form of cholesterol (LDL, or low-density lipoprotein), along with the abnormally sticky platelets, that turns a limited arterial injury into the beginnings of atherosclerosis. LDL cholesterol stimulates smooth muscle-cell growth and contributes to this vicious cycle; smooth muscle cells in turn stimulate the collagen layer within the blood vessel. The more smooth muscle cells there are, the more collagen is manufactured. It is this collagen that accounts for the tangled, scarlike fibrous tissue that ends up deposited at the site of the tear. And it is this collagen tangle that attracts and holds cholesterol deposits.

The result of all this is the formation of excess plaque—the overaccumulation of smooth muscle cells, cholesterol, fibrin, and some calcium. Dense and lumpy, it narrows the opening of the blood vessels, constricting blood flow and causing pressure to spread to adjacent tissue lining.

Coping with Cholesterol. The way to avoid this cycle of degeneration and damage is to limit those factors that can cause the cycle of destruction. One very important factor is the level of total serum (LDL) cholesterol and how your body processes it.

Cholesterol and other blood lipids (fats), such as triglycerides, are necessary for health. Cholesterol and fatty acids contribute to the synthesis of hormones, cell membrane integrity, prostaglandin production, formation of bile salts, cellular metabolism, and the health of skin and nails. Without adequate lipids, liver function is impaired and our digestion compromised. So what's wrong? Why is excess serum cholesterol seen as one of the three or four major health threats to Americans of all ages?

Cholesterol and other body fats are produced in part in the liver. Our liver was designed not only to synthesize cholesterol, but to reprocess and filter it. Even if we didn't eat much cholesterol, our body could produce enough to maintain health. However, many of the foods we eat are high in cholesterol and saturated fats. There are complex liver, blood, and endocrine systems designed to manage added fats, but they can become overloaded, particularly when our diet consists of too many foods high in saturated fats and LDL cholesterol. What are those foods? Red meats, milk, cheese, butter, egg yolks, warm-seawater shellfish, and other crustaceans—the staples of many a diet.

Despite a decline in the consumption of saturated fats in red meat, butter, and eggs, the average American man eats a stunning 500 mg of cholesterol a day, the average American woman, 350 mg. That's 60 percent more than the American Heart Association's already liberal recommendation of 300 mg a day for men, 225 for women.

There are 56 mg of cholesterol in three ounces of lean beef, 372 in three ounces of beef liver. One egg contains 274 mg of cholesterol, a cup of milk 33 mg, a tablespoon of butter 31 mg. If you have two eggs in the morning (548 mg), fried in oil or butter (31 mg), and three slices of bacon (30 mg), you've had a heart-stopping 600 mg of cholesterol before you've gotten out of the house. On the other hand, a breakfast of high-fiber cereal, low-fat yogurt, and a sliced peach gives you about 11 mg of cholesterol.

Good and Bad Cholesterol. But too much saturated fat and cholesterol in the diet is only one aspect of the cholesterol problem. As Figure 7 on page 353 shows, there are several kinds of cholesterol in association with lipoproteins, the substances that transport cholesterol in the bloodstream: high-density lipoprotein (HDL), low-density lipoprotein (LDL), and very-low-density lipoprotein (VLDL). Recent study shows that HDL cholesterol is the "good" form of cholesterol; LDL and VLDL cholesterol are the "bad." If there is too low a level of HDL lipoproteins, cholesterol remains in circulation and in the tissues and cannot be reprocessed through the liver. If the level of LDL cholesterol and saturated fats in circulation rises, the cycle of trauma to the arteries begins the process of atherosclerosis.

Improving serum cholesterol levels is not only a matter of lowering LDL and VLDL cholesterol. It also involves increasing HDL cholesterol and improving the *ratio* of HDL:LDL cholesterol.

Conventional medical wisdom states that overall cholesterol levels should be at the national average, or about 220 mg, of which at least 45

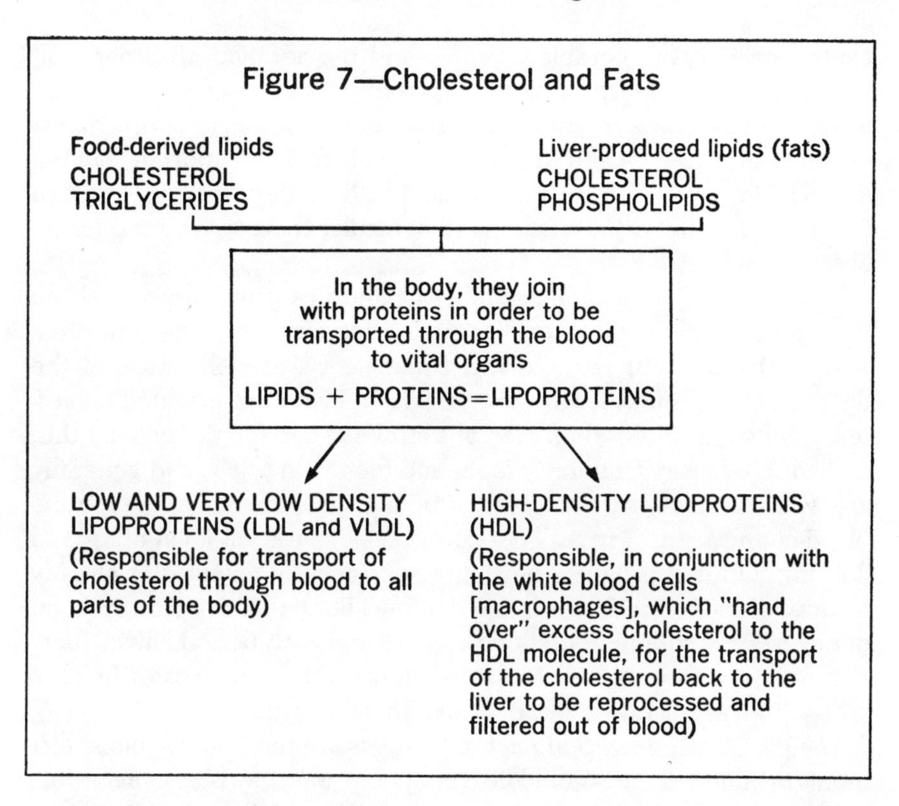

mg should be HDL cholesterol: that is, a ratio of five to one. Statistically a five to one ratio means a 25 percent chance of having a heart attack by the age of sixty-five; a ten to one ratio doubles that risk.

Figure 7—Cholesterol and Fats
Food-derived lipids
CHOLESTEROL
TRIGLYCERIDES
Liver-produced lipids (fats)
CHOLESTEROL
PHOSPHOLIPIDS
In the body, they join with proteins in order to be transported through the blood to vital organs
LIPIDS + PROTEINS=LIPOPROTEINS
LOW AND VERY LOW DENSITY LIPOPROTEINS (LDL and VLDL)
(Responsible for transport of cholesterol through blood to all parts of the body)
HIGH-DENSITY LIPOPROTEINS (HDL)
(Responsible, in conjunction with the white blood cells [macrophages], which "hand over" excess cholesterol to the HDL molecule, for the transport of the cholesterol back to the liver to be reprocessed and filtered out of blood)

Both are unacceptable and unnecessary. At OHL, we aim for an *optimal* total serum cholesterol level of 160–180 mg, with a minimum HDL level of 65 mg. The optimum ratio is probably two to one; a three to one ratio reduces by 50 percent the risk factor of having a heart attack by age sixty-five.

The bell-shaped-curve distribution appears to apply to cholesterol (Figure 2, page 32). Cholesterol over 180 is increasingly risky, as is cholesterol under 160 mg; less than 160 mg is statistically associated with an increased risk of cancer, stroke, and sudden death.

Correcting Cholesterol Imbalances. Lowering the overall cholesterol level is a matter of cutting way down on margarines, shortenings, and other saturated fats (particularly animal fats), increasing fiber and carbohydrates in the diet (a cup of oat bran a day can lower cholesterol by about 20 percent), cutting out smoking and caffeine, and increasing Vitamins B6, C, and niacin, and essential-fatty-acid intake. The most effective ways of *raising* HDL cholesterol are weight loss, nonsmoking, control of diabetes, aerobic exercise, and the addition of either food sources of essential fatty acids (such as unprocessed vegetable and seed oils and cold-seawater fatty fish), or essential-fatty-acid supplements (evening primrose oil and MaxEPA), to the diet. The importance of the essential fatty acids in cardiovascular health is discussed at length in Chapter 11. A full discussion of cardiovascular therapy begins on page 358.

While a diet low in nonessential fats and oils is important, it is no guarantee of low cholesterol, for such a tendency may be inherited. Mark, a twenty-four-year-old retail manager, was well aware of the danger of a high-fat diet; his father, with a history of elevated cholesterol and triglycerides, had died of a stroke at age forty. Knowing this, he had shied away from fatty foods and too much sugar, and generally ate well and made sure to exercise on a regular basis. Yet his routine blood-chemistry test revealed a consistent cholesterol level of around 280 mg. On our program he didn't substantially change his already healthy diet (though he eliminated a few allergic foods). However, on our aggressive supplementation program and with periodic liver function tests, he brought his cholesterol down to the much safer level of 189, with a HDL rating of 50, in just three months.

The Platelet Aggregation Factor. Platelets are the smallest blood elements (a billion of them could fill a teaspoon), but they play a major role in cardiovascular health. Their primary role in the body is to keep the blood inside the blood vessels by rushing to close up any tears, wounds, or punctures in the vessel wall—whether these injuries are caused by a knife stab or the trauma of high blood pressure.

As long as the walls of the blood vessels are smooth, platelets slip easily over their surface. But as we've noted, when a blood vessel is damaged and the underlying collagen is exposed, the platelets rush in to cover the gap. And once the platelets are activated, they do more than form a plug. They also release potent chemical vasoconstrictors such as serotonin and the powerful platelet aggregator, thromboxane A2. Though this reaction is desirable when the body has sustained a wound, this healing tactic is inappropriate here; abnormal platelet stickiness may increase atherosclerosis and further narrow the artery walls, the preliminary to most strokes and heart attack.

Platelet clumping can be triggered by traumas other than an actual wound. A tendency toward abnormal blood clotting is also brought on by smoking, psychological stress, excessive fat intake, diabetes and other blood sugar disorders, high LDL cholesterol, suboptimal levels of certain vitamins (C, A, E, beta carotene, B3 and B6), minerals (calcium, magnesium, zinc, and manganese), and essential-fatty-acid imbalances, leading to excess thromboxane A2. Someone who's had a heart attack might have a platelet adhesion index as high as 90, compared to an index around 20 for someone in good health. And the dangers of excess platelet aggregation are not confined to atherosclerosis; it is also implicated in migraine, arthritis, lupus erythematosus, diabetes, cancer, and stroke.

Hypertension

Now let's look at atherosclerosis' frequent partner in cardiovascular disease: high blood pressure. This silent, sneaky killer affects, conservatively, about 35 million people in the United States—or about 15 percent of the adult population. (If you want to include all the Americans with average—i.e., unhealthy—blood pressures over 120/80, the numbers are much higher.)

The occasional symptoms of high blood pressure—dizziness, headaches, fatigue, flushed face, nosebleeds—are often ambiguous and seem innocuous—if they are present at all. Often it is not until damage has been done that the condition is finally diagnosed. And that damage may take the form of a heart attack, a stroke, retinal hemmorhaging or swelling of the optic nerve, congestive heart failure, or renal (kidney) failure.

Blood pressure is the measure of the force with which the blood presses against the walls of the arteries. It is a two-part measurement: Systolic (contraction) pressure indicates the force *during* a heartbeat; diastolic (expansion) pressure is the force *between* beats. The "average" person has a blood pressure reading between 100/70 and 140/90. Medical standards say that a reading higher than 140/90 may indicate hypertension. Once again that norm is dangerously unhealthy. Scientific studies now indicate that adult blood pressures above 120/80 are risky and should be lowered, regardless of whether they are "average" or "normal."

Reasons and Risk Factors in Hypertension. Because it is hard to separate cause and effect in hypertension and because the pumping of the blood affects all the bodily systems, its origins are not fully understood. But some of the underlying causes have been identified:

Essential-fatty-acid deficiencies and prostaglandin imbalances. Certain essential fatty acids and their resultant prostaglandins (including PGE1 and PGE3) act to lower blood pressure; their potent vasodilator effects prevent and counter the constriction of blood vessels, due to malnutrition and stress. They are also important in regulating sodium, potassium, and water excretion, and renal blood flow through the kidneys.

Mineral balance. There are several minerals that must be in proper balance to regulate blood pressure.

Magnesium is needed at proper levels to ensure vasomotor tone. A deficiency leads to an increase in sodium uptake, and a consequent increase in fluid retention. Additionally, magnesium deficiency can cause constriction of the arterial walls, lack of vascular response to prostaglandins, and increased blood pressure.

Sodium. Any disturbance of fluid levels in the body, combined with mineral deficiencies, excesses, or imbalances, can lead to high blood pressure, particularly when combined with other risk factors such as obesity, excess stress, or alcohol consumption. The level of sodium in the body, in conjunction with other minerals, is crucial to the regulation of fluid balance and affects everything from blood pressure to the closely related problem of kidney function.

Potassium is as important as sodium in maintaining internal fluid balance in cells. It also affects the electrically active tissue of the heart pacemaker cells, which react quickly to changes in the concentration in potassium outside the cells. Low potassium levels can cause cardiac arrhythmias and blood-pressure fluctuations. High levels can lead to premature ventricular beats, ventricular fibrillation, and sudden death.

Calcium. Recent studies have shown that calcium supplementation can also lower blood pressure in certain hypertensive patients.

Risk factors for hypertension overlap somewhat with those of atherosclerosis and include the following:

Heredity. A family history of hypertension usually encompasses both genetic predisposition and learned habits and behavior. Such a history indicates that you should be aware of your susceptibility and extra careful about how you eat and live.

Obesity. Hypertension affects the fat and the skinny. But obesity is an increased risk factor, and it increases the strain on cholesterol-clogged heart vessels.

Smoking. Smoking increases LDL cholesterol, hardens the walls of the arteries, and increases abnormal platelet aggregation, which together can clog blood vessels and increase blood pressure. It also deprives the heart of oxygen and affects heartbeat and respiration.

Excessive salt intake. As was mentioned, the sodium/fluid balance within the body's cells is monitored by the kidneys. When there is too much sodium in the system and not enough potassium, magnesium, and/or calcium, the kidneys retain fluid and minerals to keep the ratio in balance. When there is so much sodium that the kidneys can't excrete it, they are forced to maintain permanently high fluid levels, which increases the volume of the blood. You end up with more water running through your pipes than you have space for. Pressure against the blood-vessel walls increases as the greater volume is pumped through the circulatory system.

This is why salt should be consumed in moderation. But many people are not aware of the enormous amounts of salt in processed and prepared foods; they often top them off with more from the ubiquitous salt-shaker. The quantity of sodium chloride we need (about 500 mg daily) can be found in a big salad or a small fillet of fish.

Stress. Chronic, nagging, unreleased, destructive stress contributes to hypertension in several ways. It throws the adrenal system out of whack, affecting the hormone and mineral levels in the blood. It causes increased vessel-wall tension. It compromises the heart, for repeated adrenal surges pump up the heart rate on a permanent basis, and the "fight or flight" response gets reinterpreted as "stand and quake."

Atherosclerosis. As noted, arteriosclerosis (the hardening of the arteries often found in association with atherosclerosis) creates high blood pressure, as the blood is forced to pass through too inflexible and narrow an opening.

Hypersensitivity of the sympathetic nervous system. Some individuals, for reasons that are not quite understood, seem to have very strong, almost hair-trigger, nervous system reactions; these responses control the dilation and contraction of the blood vessels. There may be a genetic component to this, or it may be the product of hormonal imbalances brought on by stress, nutritional deficiencies, adrenal insufficiency, allergy, or some unknown brain chemical response in an area of emotional/biological interplay.

Sedentary life-style. Prudent, regular exercise lowers both systolic and diastolic blood pressure. A sedentary life-style raises both.

The Dangers of Drug Therapy in Hypertension. The nutritional and life-style basis of high blood pressure seems clear. Mineral imbalances, problems of essential-fatty-acid metabolism and prostaglandin production, excessive stress, too much alcohol, not enough exercise, too much salt, and high-fat foods are all clearly implicated. It stands to reason then that a preventive or remedial program for high blood pressure would be one of nutritional and life-style change.

However, the usual approach to treatment is powerful drugs. Some are chemical diuretics used to decrease fluid volume, such as chlorothiazide, the potential side effects of which include potassium and magnesium deficiency, weakness, muscle cramps, cardiac arrythmias, gastrointestinal irritation, skin rashes, pancreatitis, and impotence. Then there are the sympathetic nervous system suppressors, used to control vascular constriction and dilation, such as Serpasil, Minipress, and Ismelin, with such side effects as headache, nausea, gastrointestinal irritation, fatigue, liver malfunction, and impotence or lack of ejaculation. The beta blockers, such as Inderal, are used to control vascular response; although less toxic, they are known to cause fatigue, gastrointestinal disturbances, impotence, depression, and bizarre mental aberrations. There's more: The vascular smooth muscle relaxers such as Hydralazine may cause the same problems, plus palpitations, fluid retention, angina, hirsutism (unwanted hair growth), psychosis, and a lupuslike syndrome.

Now, no one should suddenly discontinue hypertensive medication; the body's snapback response could be damaging or deadly. But it is possible, working with your doctor, to combine drug therapy with a nutritional approach. Slowly, the amount of medication taken can often be decreased and in some cases stopped altogether.

Therapy for Cardiovascular Disease

The therapeutic program for heart disease, preventive or remedial, is pretty much the same whether the problem is atherosclerosis or hypertension. The only variations are in the supplementation guidelines; in several cases particular supplements are indicated for hypertension, the control of platelet aggregation, and cardiac arrythmia disorders.

First of all, any treatment for heart disease should be conducted under the care and supervision of your physician. Do not attempt self-diagnosis and treatment in this area. Supplementation and exercise especially must be monitored by a qualified professional.

Protocol for Heart Disease

Dietary Management

1. Basic Optimum Health Program: elimination of allergic foods, rotation diet. See Part IV.
2. Severely restrict consumption of saturated and trans fats: red meat, eggs, whole milk and dairy products, warm-seawater

shellfish, chicken skin, margarines, shortenings, processed foods containing partially hydrogenated oils.

3. Restrict consumption of sugars, including fruit juices high in sugar (and low in pulp), dried fruit, honey, dates.
4. Severely restrict salt (sodium chloride) intake; this is especially important for some people with hypertension, though just about anyone can benefit from this advice. If you do use salt, make sure it contains equal amounts of *potassium* and *sodium* chloride. Also, supplement with calcium and magnesium.
5. Increase consumption of high-fiber foods: whole grains, fresh fruits, and vegetables. (See the table on page 453.)
6. Increase consumption of garlic and onions, on a rotation basis.
7. Increase consumption of cold-seawater fish such as cod, mackerel, salmon, sardines, herring.
8. Increase consumption of foods rich in magnesium and potassium (See Tables 29 and 32, on pages 179 and 182.)
9. Here is a good way to reduce serum cholesterol and triglycerides further. Add 3–5 teaspoons of alfalfa seed to your diet every other day. Alfalfa seed, which is available in health food stores, contains a class of chemicals called saponins, which have the ability to reduce serum cholesterol, because they bind certain blood fats and facilitate their removal from the system via the liver.

   Toast the seeds in the oven (to dry them out) at 250 F for about fifteen minutes; grind them fine in a blender. In this form they can be blended into juice or mixed into cereal and salads. Store in refrigerator. (Alfalfa tablets, 8 per meal, can be substituted.)

   Do not continue this therapy for more than three weeks; it is possible to remove *too much* cholesterol from the system.
10. Severely restrict alcohol, caffeine, and tobacco.

Supplementation

Routine supplementation (page 86) *plus*

Vitamin C: 8–10 grams daily
Evening primrose oil: Increase to 6–8 capsules daily
MaxEPA: Increase to 6–9 capsules daily
Vitamin E: (may increase blood pressure at first; must be supervised by physician) 400–800 IU daily
Niacin: (only under supervision of health-care professional) 2,000–3,000 mg daily (begin with 50 mg daily and increase slowly)
Vitamin B6: 250 mg daily
Beta carotene: 25,000 IU daily
DL-carnitine: 600 mg three times daily between meals
Magnesium/calcium orotate: (for hypertension and cardiac arrythmias) 400–800 mg magnesium/800–1,200 mg calcium
Lipotropic formula: (Phosphatidyl choline, inositol, lecithin) 1 capsule three times daily

Additional Recommendations

1. Exercise is immensely beneficial in treating and preventing heart disease. Cardiologists now agree (after years of discouraging exertion by heart patients) that it is essential for both physical and psychological health, especially *after* a heart attack. A Harvard study of 16,000 graduates over a twenty-year period shows that those who exercised regularly had *half* as many heart attacks as those who were sedentary. Even more impressive, Terence Kavanagh, M.D., reports that heart attack victims who do not follow a medically supervised aerobic exercise routine have a *twenty-two times greater risk of a second attack over a five-year period.* An exercise program must begin gradually and be tailored to your needs. See Chapter 18 *and your physician* for help in planning an exercise routine suitable to your condition, even if it is nothing more than a regular, brisk walk.
2. Relaxation and stress-management techniques.
3. Weight loss, if indicated.
4. Diagnostic tests: coronary lipid panel (total cholesterol, LDL-, VLDL-, HDL-cholesterol, triglyceride), periodic liver-function tests, blood glucose, blood insulin, platelet aggregation determination, treadmill stress test, periodic blood pressure checks, blood vitamin and mineral tests, Food Immune Complex Assay (FICA).

See also STRESS MANAGEMENT

Celiac Disease. See GLUTEN SENSITIVITY.
Childhood Asthma. See ASTHMA.
Cholesterol (Elevated). See CARDIOVASCULAR DISEASE.
Chronic Allergic Rhinitis. See ASTHMA.
Cluster Headache. See HEADACHE.
Cold Sores. See HERPES.
Colitis. See IRRITABLE BOWEL SYNDROME.
Congestive Heart Failure. See CARDIOVASCULAR DISEASE.

CONSTIPATION

Constipation, like so many gastrointestinal disturbances, can undermine the whole system, affecting digestion, the clearing of toxins from the system, energy level, and the absorption of nutrients. Food allergy, poor dietary habits (especially lack of fiber in the diet), low fluid intake, stress, and lack of exercise all contribute to this common, distressing, often painful condition. In many people it alternates with diarrhea and abdominal cramps in a common condition known as IRRITABLE BOWEL SYNDROME.

Attempts to treat anything other than occasional constipation with laxatives is bound to fail and, if laxative use becomes chronic, will end up making things worse. One patient at our clinic, a banker in his midforties, came to us complaining of fatigue, lower back pain, dizziness, nausea, overweight, high blood pressure, headaches, and severe constipation. Dependent on laxatives, he was also taking two prescription medications and six to eight aspirins daily. Within ten days on the program, his chronic constipation disappeared, along with all his other problems, except for the low back pain. He was able to give up his medication, and he had lost 8 pounds. Now, this man had not been eating such a terrible diet, but he was severely allergic to several of his favorite foods. No amount of bran or other fiber would have done the trick alone; the elimination of allergies was the crucial factor.

The fact is, the problem of constipation simply and predictably goes away on the Optimum Health Program.

Protocol for Constipation

Dietary Management

1. Optimum Health Program: elimination of allergic foods, rotation diet. See Part IV.
2. Increase dietary fiber. A list of nongrain high-fiber foods appears on page 453. (Be careful using wheat and oat bran—both are common allergens.)
3. If constipation persists, take 2 teaspoons, twice daily, of rice bran and soy bran on a rotation basis.
4. If constipation persists, add 1–2 teaspoons of ground flaxseed or psyllium to breakfast cereal, or mix into beverage every day. (Be careful—recent reports suggest that it is possible to develop a severe allergic reaction to psyllium.)
5. If constipation persists, drink 3–4 ounces of aloe vera juice, diluted by half with water or juice, before each meal and at bedtime.
6. Drink six to eight large glasses of bottled or distilled water daily.

Supplementation

Routine supplementation (page 86) *plus*

Vitamin C: To 90 percent bowel tolerance (see page 114)
Evening primrose oil: Increase to 6–8 capsules daily
MaxEPA: Increase to 3–6 capsules daily

Additional Recommendations

Regular exercise is extremely effective in stimulating the bowels. The best program is a brisk walk of at least thirty minutes after one meal daily, combined with aerobic exercises four to five times weekly. See Chapter 18, page 277.

See also DIGESTIVE PROBLEMS, CANDIDIASIS, Digestive Support (page 264), and Chapter 6.

Contact Dermatitis. See ECZEMA.
Coronary Heart Disease. See CARDIOVASCULAR DISEASE.
Crohn's Disease. See IRRITABLE BOWEL SYNDROME.

DEPRESSION
(Chronic, Nonpsychotic)

Occasional episodes of depression affect most of us at one time or another, often for a very good reason, though sometimes it seems to spring out of nowhere, with no easily identifiable cause. Then the crisis, or the feeling, passes, and the sun comes out again. But sometimes depression comes and stays. When it lingers on with no apparent explanation, the suffering is particularly befuddling and unbearable.

Classically, depression can be viewed as an inability to enjoy life, combined with feelings of sadness, impotence, and the inability to think and act with purpose. As one patient said: "It got to the point where I considered it a good day if I got out of bed, a great day if I got dressed. It seemed like I tried for so long to make sense of it, tried for so long to lift my spirits out of the mud. I hated myself and my life, hated the crying and the weight on my heart. Sleeping was the only thing that gave me any comfort."

Chronic depression is a serious life-limiting, immune-system-suppressing state that disrupts the lives of more than 30 million Americans. Eighty percent of terminal cancer patients have a history of chronic depression with resignation *prior* to the initial diagnosis of cancer. When it is persistent, when it becomes woven into the fabric of one's life, medical assistance is needed, for both body and soul. So-called neurotic or psychotic depressions require psychiatric help. But a great deal of depression has no apparent neurotic or psychotic basis. In such cases, nutritional therapy can be far more beneficial than years of psychiatric intervention.

In most cases depression can be viewed in terms of biochemical disturbances: dopamine/noradrenaline deficiency, serotonin depletion, or low levels of PGE1 often accompany depression. This explains why our drug-happy culture has produced such a panorama of biochemically active drugs to treat it. But these drugs do nothing to treat the underlying cause of depression, and they have myriad, serious, long-term side effects.

There are often better ways to treat depression. Chronic food allergies and chemicals in our food are often responsible, especially in cases where there is no discernible reason for the depression. And there are natural substances that can correct biochemical imbalances and elevate mood without side effects. The amino acid DL-phenylalanine, for example, increases the presence of neurotransmitters such as phenethylamine, dopamine, noradrenaline, and endorphins—all potent mood elevators produced naturally in the brain. Another amino acid, tryptophan, increases the levels of the natural antidepressant serotonin. *The Archives of Psychiatric Nerve Disease* reported a study done in 1979 confirming that DL-phenylalanine was as effective as standard antidepressant drugs in elevating mood but without side effects. Finally, there have been reports that evening primrose oil and MaxEPA have demonstrated potent antidepression effects in the depressions of childhood, alcoholism, and PMS.

(Nonpsychotic) Depression Therapy the Optimum Health Way

Severe, chronic depression should not be self-treated. However, in conjunction with medical and psychiatric guidance, the following program of dietary, supplemental, and stress-reduction guidelines can provide the wide-spectrum approach needed to pull out of long-standing depression.

Protocol for Depression

Dietary Management

1. Basic Optimum Health Program: elimination of allergic foods, rotation diet. See Part IV.
2. Eliminate sugars and refined foods. Use only fructose and that sparingly. Dilute all fruit juices by half with water.
3. Avoid all chemical additives such as food colorings, preservatives, and artificial flavorings.
4. Avoid alcohol, caffeine, and tobacco.

Supplementation

Routine supplementation (page 86) *plus*

Vitamin C: Increase by 4–6 grams daily
Evening primrose oil: Increase to 6–8 capsules daily
MaxEPA: Increase to 6 capsules daily
B6: 250 mg with breakfast and lunch
Niacin: Start at 25 mg daily, increase to 50–100 mg daily as flushing subsides (see page 102)
DL-phenylalanine: 2 275-mg capsules three times daily between meals, especially if depression is associated with chronic pain
L-tryptophan: 2–3 grams daily between breakfast and lunch

Additional Recommendations

Though it's the last thing on your mind when you're depressed, and though it seems beyond your capabilities, exercise is excellent therapy for nonpsychotic depression. In fact, the Menninger Hospital reported a study in which patients in psychotherapy to treat depression fared no better than a group following a routine of stretching, swimming, and physical games. Other studies have produced similar findings. Exercise stimulates the production of brain neurotransmitters like norepinephrine and endorphin, both powerful mood elevators, and it forcibly takes you away from the cycle of negative thinking. The goal: thirty minutes of aerobic exercise five to six days a week. See Chapter 18.

See also BRAIN ALLERGIES.

Dermatitis. See ECZEMA.

DIABETES MELLITUS (Adult-Onset Diabetes, Diabetes Type II)

Diabetes is a serious, life-limiting disease. Type I, or juvenile diabetes, involves dangerously high blood sugar as the result of the inability of the pancreas to produce ample insulin. Those with Type I diabetes, many of them children, are dependent on regular injections of insulin and contend with many side effects both of the disease and of the insulin, both associated with severely damaged blood vessels. Such children are discouraged from exercising, and later in life develop heart, eye, and kidney problems.

While the adult Type II diabetic usually produces sufficient insulin, this hormone doesn't function properly in the transport of glucose and other nutrients into the cells. Though adult-onset diabetics may have all the problems of Type I diabetes, and though some may become insulin dependent, their disease is frequently and easily controllable, via changes in diet and life-style.

Both types of diabetes appear to be directly linked to a wide variety of degenerative, life-threatening diseases. Some degree of cardiovascular impairment (atherosclerosis, microscopic damage to small blood vessels, e.g.), abnormal platelet aggregation, elevated cholesterol and triglycerides, digestive disorders, and liver malfunction—all are common to both types of diabetes. Insulin-dependent diabetes can lead to blindness, coronary artery disease, and perhaps kidney failure. Gangrene of the limbs, stroke, and heart attack are further hazards. Diabetes is not to be trifled with.

We have been very successful in treating adult-onset diabetes at OHL. I think one reason is that the increase in Type II diabetes over the last thirty years or so is directly related to the deterioration of our diets and to the increasing number of desk jobs and decreasing activity. It is foolish to rely on insulin or other diabetic medicines when dietary and life-style changes can do the job better—without insulin's long-term complications.

Research appears to have confirmed that good nutrition can reduce the amount of insulin needed to manage juvenile diabetes as well. Given the prognosis of future problems for insulin-dependent juvenile diabetics, I feel it is extremely important that the parents of such children get them on a closely supervised allergy-free diet and make sure that they follow a prudent supplementation and exercise program. Overprotective parents who keep diabetic children out of games and play are doing them no favor.

What Causes Adult-Onset Diabetes?

Once again, think of the body as a complex network of interconnected systems that must all be in balance if the whole is to function well. Now add these "disturbances" to the system: a repetitive diet, deficient in nutrients and high in fat; overweight; long-standing undiagnosed food allergies; lack of exercise; and stress.

From all this you get a system that goes into a tailspin from continually trying to right the balance. Hormones no longer function properly. This in turn impairs the ability of the cells to absorb nutrients such as glucose and amino acids. Food allergies associated with digestive disturbances may lead to the release and accumulation of excess inflammatory prostaglandins that further inhibit an already malfunctioning pancreas in its production and use of insulin. When challenged by an increase in blood sugar, the pancreas responds inadequately and blood sugar rises dangerously.

Correcting the diet and eliminating allergic foods gives the body a chance to break the debilitating cycle of damage and restore immune-system and pancreatic functions, while healing an irritated gut.

Symptoms

Adult-onset diabetes usually creeps up slowly, with subtle indications that are easily overlooked until there is a serious problem. But the following symptoms should alert you to the possibility of adult-onset diabetes mellitus: overweight; a history of allergies; extreme tiredness two to four hours after meals; blurred vision; drowsiness; tingling or numbness in hands and feet; skin infections or slow healing of cuts (especially on the feet); *Candida albicans* infestation of the vagina and/or intestines; excess hunger; excess urination; excess thirst.

Adult-Onset Diabetes Therapy

Dietary changes are the first order of business for diabetics. This entails not only the elimination of allergic foods, but a diet that controls blood-sugar levels. Such a diet is high in vegetables, protein, essential fatty acids, and complex carbohydrates, low in sugar and saturated fat.

Complex carbohydrates are found in all beans, nuts, whole grains and rice, seeds, vegetables, and fruits. Composed of long molecules of carbon and hydrogen that digest very slowly, they may take hours to convert to glucose, rather than minutes as refined carbohydrates do. (Simple carbohydrates, or sugars, turn up in ice cream, white bread, candy, and other sweets.) Consequently, if a person is not allergic and digesting properly, these complex sugars provide a steady flow of glucose into the bloodstream. However, recent studies show that blood sugar and insulin response is much more complicated than just simple sugars versus complex carbohydrates. Certain individuals respond in the opposite way: with slow, gradual increases in blood sugar and insulin to simple sugars and with fast elevations to complex carbohydrates. Based on my clinical experience I believe the individual differences will prove to be attributable to food allergies.

In addition, most complex carbohydrates are high in fiber. Its spongelike effect is a major factor in proper digestion. Once the diabetes (and the underlying problems of allergy, digestion, and weakened pancreas) are under control, it is possible to be more flexible. But strict adherence to the diet is important for the first few months.

The pancreas and digestive tract, and the entire blood-sugar mechanism, are compromised by stress, overweight, and lack of exercise. When there are no other medical conditions limiting physical ability, a diabetic should undertake a medically supervised routine of regular aerobic exercise. High blood-sugar levels can be controlled in part by the metabolism of glucose through exercise. While exercising, blood-sugar regulation does not appear to need insulin.

Protocol for Adult-Onset Diabetes

Dietary Management

1. Basic Optimum Health Program: elimination of allergies, rotation diet. See Part IV.
2. Diet should consist of
   50–60 percent nonallergic complex carbohydrates
   20–30 percent fats
   15–20 percent nonallergic protein
3. Avoid simple sugars, trans-fat foods, refined and processed foods, food colorings, and additives. Reduced saturated fats. NutraSweet may be used sparingly.
4. Restrict fresh fruit to one serving daily.
5. Avoid alcohol, caffeine, and tobacco.

Supplementation

Routine supplementation (page 86) *plus*

Vitamin C: Increase to 8–10 grams daily
Evening primrose oil: Increase to 6–8 capsules daily
Max EPA: Increase to 6 capsules daily
GTF chromium: 50 mcg with each meal
Zinc chelate: 50 mg daily
Calcium: 600–900 mg daily
Magnesium: 400–600 mg daily

Additional Recommendations

1. Recommended diagnostic blood tests: glycohemoglobin, fasting blood insulin, fasting blood glucose, platelet aggregation, FICA,

serum cholesterol, HDL cholesterol, triglycerides. If allergic symptoms persist, consider gastrointestinal candidiasis (see page 344).
2. Exercise, under a doctor's supervision, with a goal of thirty minutes of exercise five times weekly.
3. Weight loss, if indicated. See Chapter 12.

See also BLOOD SUGAR DISORDERS, Juvenile Diabetes (page 301).

DIARRHEA

Chronic or recurrent diarrhea is commonly caused by a disruption in the digestive tract due to food allergies, viral or bacterial infection, parasitic infestation, stress, or medications. It is often a factor in more complicated digestive disorders such as candidiasis, irritable bowel syndrome, Crohn's disease, and ulcerative colitis. Diarrhea causes or contributes to all manner of nutritional deficiencies and metabolic imbalances and must be treated promptly to avoid complications such as dehydration and vitamin, mineral, fat, and calorie loss.

Over-the-counter remedies are not long-term answers to diarrhea treatment. They, as well as stronger prescription drugs, often have harmful side effects, and their chronic use undermines the system's ability to regulate itself. Because they coat the lining of the intestines, they may further hamper absorption. Moreover, if bacterial or viral infection are causing the diarrhea, such treatment holds in the infection instead of expelling it.

Because food allergy is a *major* cause of diarrhea, the basic Optimum Health Program is often enough to clear it up. For acute or chronic cases, the protocol below is prudent therapy. Persistent diarrhea, however, warrants further testing to rule out parasites, infection, or more serious organic disease.

Protocol for Diarrhea

Dietary Management

1. Basic Optimum Health Program: elimination of allergic foods, rotation diet. See Part IV.
2. Decrease consumption of saturated and trans fats.
3. Eliminate *raw* vegetables and fruit (except for bananas every four days).
4. Eliminate fried foods.
5. Eat well-cooked nonallergenic grains such as millet and amaranth.
6. Avoid alcohol.

7. If diarrhea persists, drink 3–4 ounces of aloe vera juice before each meal.

Supplementation

Routine supplementation (page 86) *plus*

Evening primrose oil: Increase to 6–8 capsules daily
Max EPA: Increase to 6–9 capsules daily
Micellized Vitamin A: 2 drops (10,000 IU) daily
Calcium: Additional 600 mg daily
Magnesium: Additional 400 mg daily
Zinc: Additional 25 mg daily
Iron: 50 mg if indicated by serum ferritin test.

See Digestive Support, page 264.

Additional Recommendations

1. In case of chronic diarrhea, gastrointestinal X ray, sigmoidoscopy, stool analysis, and general physical checkup to rule out parasite, infection, or other disease.
2. Delay exercise until three hours after eating. See Chapter 18.
3. If indicated, use stress-reduction techniques such as deep relaxation, biofeedback, meditation, or yoga.

See also DIGESTIVE DISORDERS, CANDIDIASIS, Digestive Support, page 264, and Chapter 6.

DIGESTIVE DISORDERS

The intimate connection between good digestion and good health has been emphasized many times in this book. You cannot get well until you clear up digestive disorders, and you cannot clear up digestive disorders until you get rid of your allergies.

Digestive disorders may be experienced in any combination of the following: belching, flatulence, constipation, diarrhea, mucus or undigested food in the stools, bloating after meals, drowsiness, fatigue or depression after meals, heartburn, bad breath, acid stomach, nausea, vomiting, coated tongue, stomach pains or discomfort. Though just about everyone has complaints of this nature, in a healthy system digestion should take place without calling attention to itself.

It has been our experience that people on the Optimum Health Program clear up their digestive problems rather quickly with the elimination of allergies, a rotation diet high in fiber, and digestive support during the early stages of the diet.

It is vital that digestive problems be attended to, for not only do they undermine basic health, but they may lead to more serious gastrointestinal disorders, such as irritable bowel syndrome, duodenal ulcers, diverticulitis, Crohn's disease, or perhaps even ulcerative colitis. Tums or Alka-Seltzer are not the long-term answer to digestive problems.

The protocol for a comprehensive program of digestive support is given on page 264. Specific protocols for IRRITABLE BOWEL SYNDROME, DIARRHEA, and CONSTIPATION can be found in this section under the appropriate headings.

See also Chapter 6.

Digestive Support. See page 264.
Diverticulitis. See IRRITABLE BOWEL SYNDROME.
Drug dependency or addiction. See ADDICTION.

ECZEMA

Both immediate (IgE-mediated Type I) and delayed (IgG-immune complex mediated Type II and III) allergic reactions are implicated in eczema, a chronic, itching inflammation of the skin. People with eczema usually develop other allergic conditions, e.g., childhood asthma and/or hay fever.

Many in the orthodox medical community still seem to be unaware that both adult and childhood eczema is often related to food allergy and malnutrition. This in spite of the fact that study after study has confirmed that food allergy is responsible in perhaps the *majority* of cases. Glutens, eggs, and milk and other dairy products are common offenders. Perhaps this explains in part why so many babies who are not breast-fed end up with "cradle cap," a form of this condition that affects an infant's scalp. At OHL we've seen the disappearance of enough unsightly eczema problems to be totally convinced of the food allergy/malnutrition connection.

As with asthma and other atopic allergic disorders, a problem with fat metabolism—essential-fatty-acid metabolism in particular—is often an underlying condition with eczema. Over two thirds of eczema sufferers improve dramatically with supplementation and topical application of evening primrose oil alone. Also, Vitamins A and E, which are especially important in the maintenance of skin health, are often poorly absorbed.

Another common factor in people with chronic dermatological disorders appears to be digestive disturbances, particularly hypochlorhydria. Seventy-two percent of eczema sufferers, 75 percent of contact dermatitis sufferers, and 52 percent of those with psoriasis have inadequate HCl levels.

In our experience, the best approach to treating eczema and other chronic skin problems consists of getting rid of food allergies, correcting digestive problems and thus improving fat-soluble-vitamin absorption, correcting prostaglandin imbalances, and taking care to avoid unnecessary irritation of the affected skin areas. See the guidelines below.

Eczema Management Guidelines

- Use lukewarm (not hot) water for showers and baths. Add bath oil to soften dry, scaly skin. Never use soap. Use soap substitutes that do not dry the skin.
- Avoid extremes of temperature and exhausting exercise that induces excessive sweating.
- Avoid long-haired cats and dogs, fuzzy or furry toys and pillows.
- Wear soft, absorbent cotton next to skin, never wool or fabric with pile.
- Avoid chemicals, dust, aerosols, solvents.
- Avoid lanolin in cosmetics, lotions, cleansers, and oils.
- Do not use petroleum jelly or greasy ointments that can block evaporation of sweat and aggravate itching.
- Avoid over-the-counter salves, particularly those with benzocaine or antibiotics in them.
- Do not wear rubber gloves for household chores, unless you wear cotton liners inside them.
- Avoid nutritional, psychological, and environmental stresses that lower immune-system resistance. Physical and emotional upset can trigger inflammation.
- Try not to scratch inflamed areas; it makes the inflammation much worse.

Protocol for Eczema

Dietary Management

1. Basic Optimum Health Program: elimination of allergic foods, rotation diet. See Part IV.
2. Increase consumption of cold-seawater fish: sardines, herring, mackerel, cod, salmon.

3. Avoid excess red meats, milk, dairy, eggs, margarine, and shortenings.
4. Consume a high-fiber diet, especially if elimination is a problem.

Supplementation

Routine supplementation (page 86) *plus*

Vitamin C: Increase to 8–10 grams daily, preferably in crystal form
Evening primrose oil: Increase to 6–8 capsules daily
MaxEPA: Increase to 6–9 capsules daily
Micellized Vitamin E: 2 ml daily (300 IU)
Micellized Vitamin A: 7 drops daily (20,000 IU)
Chelated zinc: 25–50 mg daily
(children one-third to one-half dose)

See Digestive Support, page 264.

Additional Recommendations

1. Aerobic exercise is important therapy for skin disorders. Exercise aerobically three to four times weekly (see Chapter 18), never to exhaustion. Wear cotton exercise clothes, do not let sweat remain on body, and shower with lukewarm water immediately after. Do not exercise for at least three hours after eating.
2. Make use of stress-management techniques: meditation, yoga, biofeedback, and deep relaxation.
3. Apply evening primrose oil to affected areas twice daily to soften dry, scaly skin.

See also ATOPIC ALLERGIES and ASTHMA.

Fibrillation. See CARDIOVASCULAR DISEASE.
Flatulence. See DIGESTIVE DISORDERS and Digestive Support (page 264).

GALLBLADDER PROBLEMS

A small organ attached to the underside of the liver, the gallbladder collects bile and uses it to help the small intestine with the digestion of fats and cholesterol. It also acts as the passageway for secretory IgA antibodies that trickle into the upper intestines, binding with food allergens, bacteria, and other microorganisms potentially harmful to the body. A malfunctioning gallbladder may indicate trouble with food allergy or with essential-fatty-acid metabolism.

The result of chronic imbalance in bile production and cholesterol levels is gallstones, small fatty "pebble" formations that may cause plenty of trouble for over 16 million people in this country. The symptoms of gallbladder disease can range from mild gastrointestinal upset to devastating upper abdominal pain, and include gas and belching, food intolerance, and sharp pain in the upper right section of the abdominal cavity after eating or during the night.

Food allergy seems to have a profound effect on the entire liver/gallbladder system. The presence of food allergies is somehow associated with a tremendous added burden on the gallbladder, which must manage not only the digestion of dietary fats, but also continually store and release secretory IgA antibodies to coat and neutralize particles of allergic food and bacteria entering the stomach. *A great deal of gallbladder surgery could be avoided if gallbladder sufferers would address their allergy problems.*

Joseph G., a patient, came to us with knifelike pains in his side (symptomatic of cholelithiasis, the presence of gallstones). He was on medication that had disturbing side effects, and he was about to give in and schedule surgery. Instead, we put him on a program of allergy elimination, a low-fat diet, and digestive support. His pains steadily subsided. He never had that operation, and today he is entirely off medication.

Dr. Jonathan Wright, the well-known columnist for *Prevention* magazine, reports he no longer refers gallbladder patients to surgery since he discovered the problem of delayed food allergy in 1979.

Protocol for Gallbladder Problems

Dietary Management

1. Basic Optimum Health Program: elimination of allergic foods, rotation diet. See Part IV.
2. Eliminate saturated and trans fats.
3. Eat plenty of fresh vegetables.
4. Eat slowly and chew food well, to aid in digestion.

Supplementation

Routine supplementation (page 86) *plus*

Evening primrose oil: Increase to 6–8 capsules daily
MaxEPA: Increase to 6–9 capsules daily
Lipotrophic formula (choline/inositol/lecithin/methionine): 2 capsules after each meal (to assist fat metabolism)

See Digestive Support, page 264.

Additional Recommendations

1. Bile salt supplements may be helpful, but they can have side effects and should be taken only under medical supervision.
2. Exercise is particularly helpful for the metabolism of fats. The goal: aerobic exercise in your target heart range for thirty minutes four to five times weekly. See Chapter 18.

Gastrointestinal candidiasis. See CANDIDIASIS.

GLUTEN SENSITIVITY
(Celiac Sprue/Gluten Gastroenteropathy)

Gluten sensitivity is a form of food sensitivity that has far-reaching repercussions, and these are often difficult to pinpoint. It is a reaction in the mucous lining of the intestine to a protein, alpha gliadin, found in wheat, rye, barley, and oats. Acting as an allergen, the gliadin protein combines with IgG antibodies to form immune complexes in the intestinal mucous lining. These immune complexes appear to stimulate the growth of "killer" lymphocytes, leading to immune-system weakness. Common in both children and adults, gluten sensitivity is often associated with pronounced nutritional deficiencies. It is also thought by some medical authorities to be a factor in such diverse illnesses as multiple sclerosis, sarcoidosis, nephrosis, dermatitis herpetiformis, autism, schizophrenia, and rheumatoid arthritis.

The symptoms of gluten sensitivity in adults are often those of secondary nutritional deficiencies: e.g., iron, folic acid and/or B12 deficiency anemia; weight loss, edema, skin problems, and bone pain. In children, symptoms may be iron deficiency anemia, severe abdominal bloating and trouble with bowel movements, or failure to thrive and grow. Because those with gluten sensitivity have impaired digestive systems, they are likely to suffer from other food allergies and malabsorption problems as well. Until the digestive problems are corrected and the mucusal lining healed, dietary changes and supplementation are often only partially effective.

Because a gluten-free diet is so restrictive, a diagnosis of gluten sensitivity should not be made casually. On the other hand, once diagnosis is confirmed, total elimination of all gluten products from the diet indefinitely is an absolute must. This is not easy, because so many commercial products, such as frankfurters, sausage, cold cuts, soups, and baked beans, frequently use wheat flour as a filler. One patient who had responded very quickly to his gluten-free rotation diet was surprised to have his symptoms re-emerge after a few months. When we investigated, it turned out that he was occasionally eating hotdogs and bologna.

When it comes to gluten sensitivity, even a little can be too much. It is very important to familiarize yourself with the ingredients in any prepared and processed foods you eat. And when in doubt, leave it out! A guide to gluten-containing and gluten-free foods can be found in Table 55, pages 376–77.

Protocol for Gluten Sensitivity

Dietary Management

1. Basic Optimum Health Program: elimination of allergic foods, rotation diet. See Part IV.
2. Keep an accurate and detailed food diary (see page 256, plus Table 50 for example, plus diary blank, page 487), so that you can identify problem foods if any symptoms turn up.
3. Beware of all fillers in prepared foods. Read labels carefully.
4. Eliminate cereal and bakery products made from wheat, barley, rye, and oats. (Substitute rice, potato, and soy flours, and cornmeal, for other flours and grains.)
5. Eat foods that are rich in iron and thiamine, since elimination of grains robs you of valuable sources of these nutrients.

Supplementation

Routine supplementation (page 86) *plus*

Evening primrose oil: Increase to 6–8 capsules daily
MaxEPA: Increase to 6–9 capsules daily
Micellized Vitamin A: 10,000 IU daily (2 drops)
B complex: 1 capsule twice daily with breakfast and lunch
Iron: (if serum ferritin tests show depletion 100–200 mg daily)
Zinc chelate: 25–50 mg daily

See Digestive Support, page 264.

Additional Recommendations

Because of the restrictive nature of a gluten-free diet, a diagnosis of gluten sensitivity should only be determined after thorough medical

Table 55 — Gluten-free Diet Guidelines		
Food Category	**Foods Allowed**	**Foods Not Allowed**
Beverages	Milk, milk substitutes, fruit juices, soft drinks, tea, coffee, herbal teas.	Coffee substitutes made with cereal, milk drinks mixed with malt or cereal added, beer, ale.
Eggs	Hard- or soft-cooked, fried, poached, scrambled.	Eggs in sauces containing cereal flours that are not allowed.
Meat, poultry, fish, meat substitutes	Beef, veal, lamb, pork, chicken, turkey, fish, shellfish, glandular meats, cheese, cottage cheese, cream cheese, natural cheese, dried beans and peas, nuts, nut butters.	Any commercially prepared product containing cereals that are not allowed. Luncheon meat, wieners, meat loaf, sausage, meat or fish patties, and gravies usually contain one of the grain products that are not allowed and should be avoided unless made from pure meat. Casserole-type foods made with cereals that are not allowed, canned and frozen foods containing sauces thickened with flour/meal of grains that are not allowed. Cheese spreads containing cereal products that are not allowed as fillers.
Vegetables	Any fresh, frozen, or canned vegetable or vegetable juice.	Vegetables cooked with sauces thickened with grain products (wheat flour, etc.) that are not allowed.
Potatoes and substitutes	White or sweet potatoes, rice, corn, hominy, gluten-free pastas, grits.	Noodles, macaroni, spaghetti.
Fruit	Fresh, canned, frozen, or dried fruits.	Always check the labels of fruit sauces to make sure thickening agents do not contain flours of grains that are not allowed.

Table 55 *(Continued)*		
Food Category	**Foods Allowed**	**Foods Not Allowed**
Fats	Butter, margarine, shortening, oil, salad dressing, made with those cereal flours that are allowed.	Commercial salad dressings made with wheat flour or thickened with other restricted grain flour/meals that are not allowed.
Breads	Breads made from 100% rice flours, cornmeal, soybean flour, gluten-free wheat starch, and potato starch.	Wheat flour bread, oatmeal, rye or barley breads, flour tortillas, commercially prepared biscuits, pancakes, waffles, toaster pastries, crackers made from wheat flour, wheat gluten, and cereal flours that are not allowed.
Cereals	Cereals made from rice or corn, such as cream of rice, boiled rice, corn grits, cornmeal mush, such ready-to-eat cereals as cornflakes, Rice Krispies, puffed rice, rice flakes, etc.	All those containing wheat, wheat gluten, oats, rye, or barley, such as oatmeal, cream of wheat, wheat flakes, Cheerios, shredded wheat. Check the labels for cereal grains that are not allowed.
Soups	Broth, homemade vegetable soups made from foods that are allowed. Creamed soup with cornstarch or potato.	Commercially prepared canned or frozen soups thickened with wheat flour, oats, barley, or rye flour, or those containing whole barley.
Desserts	Fruits, plain or fruited gelatin desserts, tapioca puddings, homemade ice cream.	Commercial cakes, cookies, pastries, pies, puddings, ice cream, etc.

investigation. Don't diagnose yourself. Work with an experienced nutritionist to assure a balanced, optimally nourishing diet.

Gout. See URIC ACID (ELEVATED).
Gouty Arthritis. See ARTHRITIS and URIC ACID (ELEVATED).
Halitosis. See DIGESTIVE DISORDERS and Digestive Support (page 264).
Hardening of the Arteries. See CARDIOVASCULAR DISEASE.
Hay Fever. See ASTHMA.

HEADACHE

"When I had headaches, I only lived half a life. When I had a migraine, everything else was obliterated by the pain—my family, my work, my name. I was living half my life on another planet, a planet of torture and pain."

Devastating, debilitating headaches of various kinds plague 42 million Americans. For some, it's tension headaches, usually characterized by dull, nonthrobbing pain that begins in the back of the neck or head and moves over the head. Cluster headaches, probably the most severely painful of all headaches, are the curse of other lives; usually located behind one eye, they are often described as feeling like a red hot poker being driven into the eye socket; they are often totally incapacitating and can last for hours or even days nonstop, and often occur in batches on a daily basis, followed by periods of calm. Men are the most frequent cluster-headache victims, and for 20 to 25 percent of them, the pain is so severe that they contemplate suicide.

Then there's the migraine headache, the bane of 20 million American lives. Women migraine sufferers outnumber men by nine to one. About 10 percent of migraines are preceded by a classic aura or prodroma, a set of nonpain symptoms that precede the actual onset of the headache, such as flashing lights, upset stomach, or light-headedness, all of which disappear as soon as the pain begins. Triggered by the dilation of arteries in the scalp, the headache is often associated with visual disturbances, nausea, vomiting, sensitivity to light and noise. All of these symptoms are perhaps stimulated by the excruciating pain. Such headaches are exhausting, and the sufferer usually has to sleep it off afterward in order to recover.

Because headaches are the classic intense-pain disorder, a great deal of research has gone into finding out what causes and cures migraine and other headache syndromes. Treatment often starts with drugs, for the relief of pain is the first order of business. But while aspirin and certain painkillers help in some cases, headaches have proved resistant to many drugs, and in most cases they provide only partial or temporary relief anyway. Moreover, drugs are often actually a hindrance to cure. Some are predictably powerful and therefore easily abused by patients desperate to obtain relief at any cost. Nondrug therapies such as acupuncture and biofeedback have helped some sufferers, but again they offer only pain relief (welcome but temporary), not cure.

As to the *cause* of migraine and other headache syndromes (many headache victims suffer from more than one kind of headache), there are lots of theories, few facts. Hormonal imbalances can sometimes be to blame and may explain why some teenagers suffer from migraines that disappear at maturity. Genetic disposition may explain some cases, because headaches do at times run in families. Chronic tension is often blamed for headaches, and some people have successfully reduced the pain and frequency of headaches using relaxation techniques. When all other explanations fail, it is not surprising that the headaches are often decreed to be psychosomatic or the by-product of "emotional problems."

The Food-Allergy Connection

But there are exciting signs of progress. Conventional medicine has finally acknowledged that certain foods, and to a lesser degree additives —particularly certain preservatives and colorings, caffeine, chocolate, certain drugs, cigarette smoke, perfume and other strong odors—may bring on headaches. This gets a bit closer to an explanation, but is still not the whole answer. As long as doctors and pain clinics ignore the possibility of food allergy, they cannot get the whole picture.

The fact is that *over 90 percent of migraines can be traced directly to food allergies.* I say this with complete confidence, based on our own clinical experience at OHL, and on corroborating evidence from published research around the world.

An important placebo-controlled, double-blind study of migraine in adolescents and children, reported in the prestigious British journal *The Lancet,* confirms everything we have witnessed at our clinical laboratories. Here are some of the highlights of the study, which involved eighty-eight subjects, each of whom had suffered migraine headaches (and often their side effects) at least once a week for the past six months to ten years:

- Ninety-three percent of the study subjects experienced dramatic relief when allergenic foods were eliminated from their diet.
- On an allergy-free diet, they experienced relief not only from their headache pain, but from other ailments as well, including epilepsy (twelve of fourteen epileptic children became seizure-free), hyperactivity (thirty-five of forty-one showed dramatic improvement here), and such maladies as "growing pains," abdominal pain, asthma, eczema, rhinitis, etc.
- While it was once believed that a patient would "know" which foods he or she might be allergic to, this study showed that the offending foods were most often unsuspected and often *favorite foods.*
- The double-blind placebo test proved that, with reintroduction of the allergic foods, migraine pain recurred.
- Although seventeen of the eighty-eight test subjects were allergic to only one food, the rest were allergic to a number of foods, and one child had to eliminate twenty-four foods before migraine pain disappeared.
- Skin testing and IgE RAST testing proved to be of little value in determining allergic foods. If the investigators had relied on skin test and IgE results, they would have helped only five of the eighty-eight people.

Not surprisingly, the most commonly allergic foods turned out to be cow's milk, eggs, wheat, orange, benzoic acid (a common food preservative), cheese, rye, tomato, tartrazine (a popular food dye, FD&C Yellow No. 5, found in margarine, orange soda, etc.). It was discovered that in most cases it was not the naturally occurring chemicals in these foods—such as tyramine in chocolate—that caused the reactions, but an allergy to the whole food itself. One interesting side note was that many more reactions were reported to whole wheat than to white flour.

It is also significant that allergic symptoms, including migraines, did not return immediately when the allergic foods were reintroduced into the diet. Instead, it took from one hour to *seven days* before painful symptoms reappeared. Delayed reactions are typical of Type II and Type III IgG-mediated-immune-complex food allergies.

This study has added importance for me because it confirms not only my experience with migraine, but my experience of allergy in general. It is my hope that studies of this kind will be conducted in connection with other allergy-responsive disorders such as rheumatoid arthritis, inflammatory bowel disease, asthma, eczema, hyperactivity, chronic depression, epilepsy, etc. I'm confident the findings will be the same.

I've seen many patients experience substantial relief on our program. One teenage boy who had two to three migraines a week and was fifty pounds overweight was brought in by his mother at the end of a long trek from specialist to specialist. On several drugs and in pain, he had been diagnosed as having chronic learning impairment and emotional disabilities (not such an unlikely consequence of severe chronic pain). The doctors he had seen offered little hope, but his mother remembered him as a bright, happy child and was not ready to condemn him to a stunted existence of pain and underachievement. It turned out that he had numerous severe allergies. This boy not only experienced complete relief from his headaches on our program, he also quickly lost 48 pounds. His mother said that we had given her son back his life.

Another patient, a woman who had pretty much resigned herself to her chronic migraine and tension headaches because her mother and grandmother had suffered the same fate, also got better on our program. And, like so many of our patients, other symptoms improved as well. The bloating, belching, intestinal cramps, and flatulence that she reported at her first consultation had disappeared, as had the hives and rashes that so easily appeared when she used the wrong shampoo or cosmetics. But the most important bonus benefit, as far as she was concerned, was that she was sleeping well for the first time in years.

Headache Treatment

Obviously the first avenue of attack on migraine and other headache syndromes is nothing more than the basic Optimum Health Program —the elimination of allergies and the rotation diet. Three other therapeutic approaches round out our multifactorial approach: essential-fatty-acid and DL-phenylalanine supplements plus exercise.

The PGE1 and PGE3 produced by the conversion of essential fatty acids are anti-inflammatory agents and act as vasodilators, keeping the blood vessels from constricting. DL-phenylalanine (page 00) has proved to be a potent pain reliever when taken regularly. And exercise *between* headache attacks works to increase the production of morphinelike endorphins, to promote oxygenation, and to reduce stress. As usual, the more parts of the therapeutic program you follow, the higher the degree of success you are likely to achieve.

Protocol for Migraine and Other Headache Therapy

Dietary Management

1. Basic Optimum Health Program: elimination of allergic foods, rotation diet. See Part IV.
   Note: At first, the elimination of allergic foods may incur withdrawal headaches. See page 262 for help in minimizing withdrawal problems through the use of Vitamin C therapy.
2. Eliminate all xanthine-containing foods: coffee, tea, cola, chocolate, and medications containing caffeine.
3. Eliminate alcohol.
4. Avoid food colorings, sodium benzoate, and other additives if you are aware of chemical sensitivities. (In the *Lancet* migraine study, two of the top offenders were FD & C Yellow No. 5 and sodium benzoate.)

Supplementation

Routine supplementation (page 86) *plus*

Vitamin C: Increase to 8–10 grams daily
Evening primrose oil: Increase to 6–8 capsules daily
MaxEPA: Increase to 6 capsules daily
Vitamin E: Increase to 400–800 IU daily
Calcium/magnesium: 800 mg calcium/600 mg magnesium
Niacinamide: 500 mg daily
DL-phenylalanine: 2 275-mg capsules three times daily between meals

Additional Recommendations

1. Avoid smoking, cigarette smoke, perfume, and other petrochemical by-products if you are aware of chemical sensitivities.
2. Exercise regularly between headache attacks. Do not exercise during a migraine or when you feel one coming on. Exercise should be moderate, and heart rate should not go above the low end of your optimal aerobic target range. (See Table 51, page 282.)
3. Make a special point to get exercise during stressful periods.
4. Practice meditation, deep relaxation, biofeedback, or yoga to promote vascular and muscle relaxation and to increase endorphin production.
5. Consider undertaking stress- and behavior-evaluation tests to identify possible emotional and life-style headache triggers.

See also PAIN, Chapter 11, and DL-phenylalanine (page 130).

Heartburn. See DIGESTIVE DISORDERS and Digestive Support (page 264).
Heart Disease. See CARDIOVASCULAR DISEASE.

HERPES SIMPLEX, TYPES I AND II

About one dozen of the several dozen varieties of the common herpes virus affect humans. Our concern here is with two of the most common strains. Herpes simplex Type I manifests itself as cold sores or fever blisters, and in rare cases it can affect the eyes or cause serious brain infection. Herpes simplex Type II, or genital herpes, can be dangerous to newborn infants, who are exposed to the virus in their passage through the birth canal; there is also preliminary indication that it may be associated with an increased incidence of cervical cancer.

Genital herpes—thanks to public hysteria and misinformation—has attained the status of a modern-day sexual leprosy. It was not considered a major health hazard until the "sexual revolution." Now some 5 to 10 million Americans are thought to have genital herpes, and it is spreading at a rate of up to half a million new cases a year. However, with the change in sexual climate, the distinction between "above the waist" herpes cold sores and "below the waist" genital herpes has become blurred, and the only way to tell Type I from Type II is through testing.

Herpes has become a shameful disease in the minds of many, in great part because of the stigma attached to having a sexually transmitted disease. Herpes sufferers are often so intimidated by their condition that they seek therapy in groups of like sufferers and socialize only with those who have and understand the problems—physical and social—attached to it. But while herpes is no fun, and severe cases can be painful, the problem is made much worse by shame and stress. For herpes is one of those problems with a high correlation to stress.

The fact is that most of us—probably more than 75 percent of us—are carriers of the herpes virus. Some of us have stronger immune systems than others, and this seems to keep the virus dormant. Although there is as yet no cure for herpes, sufferers can exert considerable control over outbreaks of the virus with a combination of nutritional support and stress management, aimed at strengthening the immune system.

It takes about five to ten days after exposure to the virus for herpes symptoms to appear. In addition to the cold sores on the lips or the rashlike sores on the genitals, symptoms may include fever, swelling, headache, fatigue, and sore throat. This active period (that is, while the lesions are visible) is the danger time—when the disease is communicable. It may last from several days to three weeks. When the sores disappear, the communicable period is over.

Recurrence depends on the severity of the disease and on one's general health and current life stresses. Most herpes victims learn to "read" the signs of an impending attack—often itching or tingling—and are able to exercise caution so as not to spread the disease.

To date, there is no vaccine for herpes, no sure-fire medication. The herpes virus hides out in the nerve endings where the antibodies of the immune system can't reach it, and it comes out only when it's safe—when the patient is weakened by stress, immune-system inhibition, or nutritional deficiencies. Any kind of stress can bring herpes out of hibernation, as can a bad sunburn (this is why herpes simplex Type I is sometimes referred to as sun poisoning or sun blisters) or the hormonal changes at the onset of menstruation. And of course it can be activated by intercourse with someone else with herpes in the active stage.

Herpes Therapy

As the research community continues to look for a comprehensive herpes vaccine, there are some alternative approaches that can have proved successful:

Vitamin C. As might be expected, Vitamin C therapy, because of its ability to stimulate the immune system, can be extremely effective. Vitamin-C-to-90-percent-bowel-tolerance is the usual recommendation, though in severe cases and during outbreaks intravenous C therapy may be warranted. Intravenous Vitamin C can also significantly reduce the time between flare-ups. One patient of ours, who had suffered breakouts almost weekly for a long time, was symptom-free for three months after just three intravenous infusions. More about this therapy on page 00.

Lysine. The amino acid lysine has an antagonistic relationship to arginine, another amino acid that is necessary for reproduction of the herpes virus. Research by Dr. Christopher Kagan indicates that daily doses of 1,200 mg of lysine will overpower the influence of arginine. (Caution: Excess lysine in people prone to hypercholesterolemia will result in higher cholesterol levels.)

Lithium ointments. Topically applied lithium succinate ointments offer substantial symptomatic relief. Applied at the first sign of an outbreak—at the burning or tingling stage—it in many cases prevents blisters from forming; in addition, if blisters are already formed, an application can reduce recovery time significantly. LSO-1 is the name of one such ointment; it is available at health food stores.

Essential fatty acids. The multiplication of the herpes virus may be associated with the release of arachidonic acid from cell membrane stores (where it is normally held in inactive form); it is then converted to inflammatory prostaglandins and prostanoids, causing pain, itching, and irritation. Supplementation with evening primrose oil and MaxEPA helps to block arachidonic acid release and provide anti-inflammatory relief. (Topical application of evening primrose oil alternating with micellized vitamin A application also shows great promise in immediate relief of shingles.)

Herpes, especially genital herpes, is a common problem requiring a calm and reasonable approach to its management and treatment. It is important that herpes sufferers should not despair, or feel embarrassed or "untouchable." Even if the first outbreak of herpes is severe, the disease seems to moderate with time. With a combination of nutritional therapy, supplementation, topical ointments, and stress-reduction techniques, it is entirely possible to live a healthy, normal life.

Protocol for Herpes Simplex, Types I and II

Dietary Management

1. Basic Optimum Health Program: elimination of allergic foods, rotation diet. See Part IV.
2. Eliminate all foods high in arginine such as peanuts and chocolate. (See Table 36, page 186.)
3. Eat more nonallergic foods high in lysine such as eggs, fish, poultry, and brewer's yeast on a rotation basis.
4. Avoid alcohol.

Supplementation

Routine supplementation (page 86) *plus*

Vitamin C: (depending on status of disease) 8–12 grams daily to 90 percent bowel tolerance *or* three consecutive days of intravenous therapy for acute flare-ups (see page 264)
Evening primrose oil: Increase to 6–8 capsules daily
MaxEPA: Increase to 6 capsules daily
Micellized Vitamin E: 1 ml (150 IU) daily
Micellized Vitamin A: 3 drops (10,000 IU) daily
B complex: 1 capsule twice daily with breakfast and lunch

Zinc orotate: 25–50 mg daily
L-lysine: 500 mg daily (routine) *or* 500 mg twice daily between meals (for acute flare-ups) (*Not* recommended in those with elevated serum cholesterol)
Thymus tissue concentrate: (for acute flare-ups) 2 capsules with each meal

Additional Recommendations

1. Apply micellized Vitamin A and evening primrose oil topically to sores twice daily (separately, two hours apart).
2. Apply lithium succinate ointment such as LSO-1 (from health food store) topically, if topical evening primrose oil and micellized vitamin A are not completely effective.
3. Use a sunscreen at all times on target areas, and limit exposure to sun.
4. Use stress-management techniques such as meditation, biofeedback, and yoga to minimize stress-activated outbreaks.

See also STRESS MANAGEMENT, VIRAL INFECTIONS.

High Blood Pressure. See CARDIOVASCULAR DISEASE.

HIVES
(Urticaria, Angioedema)

Hives, or urticaria, is often an immediate Type I reaction to airborne or contact allergens, and sometimes a delayed Type II and III reaction. It causes its sufferers to break out in itchy, raised splotches and may be provoked in one person by food, in another by chemicals or airborne allergens. Or the breakout may be induced by exercise, much as exercise can bring on an asthma attack.

Though hives are notoriously difficult to treat, we have had a better than 50 percent success rate with hives on our program, which, in addition to the elimination of food allergies and a rotation diet, focuses on correcting digestive problems, stress management, and essential-fatty-acid supplements. A protocol for treatment appears below; also refer to the general discussion of ATOPIC ALLERGIES in this section.

Protocol for Hives

Dietary Management

1. Basic Optimum Health Program: elimination of allergic food, rotation diet. See Part IV.

2. Eat small, frequent meals instead of two or three big meals.
3. Eat only a few simple foods at each meal.
4. Increase consumption of cold-seawater fish such as salmon, herring, mackerel.
5. Avoid alcohol.

Supplementation

Routine supplementation (page 86) *plus*

Vitamin C: To 90 percent bowel tolerance (page 114) during flare-ups; otherwise 8–10 grams daily
Evening primrose oil: Increase to 6–8 capsules daily
MaxEPA: Increase to 6–9 capsules daily
Micellized Vitamin E: 1 ml twice daily (300 IU)
Micellized Vitamin A: 8 drops daily (25,000 IU)
Pantothenic acid: 500 mg daily
Magnesium orotate: 600 mg daily
Calcium orotate: 800–1,000 mg daily
Zinc orotate: 50 mg daily
Copper: 1 mg daily

See Digestive Support, page 264.

Additional Recommendations

1. Stress management through the use of biofeedback, deep relaxation, yoga, meditation, and exercise.
2. Exercise-induced hives can be controlled through the elimination of allergic foods, and by taking 1–2 grams of Vitamin C thirty minutes to an hour before exercising (500 mg for children). Exercise should be moderate, not to exhaustion and not undertaken until three to four hours after eating.

See also ATOPIC ALLERGIES.

Hypercholesterolemia. See CARDIOVASCULAR DISEASE.
Hyperlipidemia. See CARDIOVASCULAR DISEASE.
Hypertension. See CARDIOVASCULAR DISEASE.
Hypertriglyceridemia. See CARDIOVASCULAR DISEASE.
Hyperuricemia. See URIC ACID (ELEVATED).
Hypochlorhydria. See DIGESTIVE DISORDERS and Digestive Support (page 264).

HYPOGLYCEMIA
(Low Blood Sugar)

Hypoglycemia has become a commonly diagnosed disease of modern life. Its symptoms can run the gamut of faintness, weakness, palpitations, hunger, nervousness and anxiety, paranoia, crying jags, aches, confusion or fuzziness, visual disturbances, motor weakness, and even personality changes. It is a misunderstood illness, which some authorities feel is grossly overdiagnosed. Long thought to be the result of a weak pancreas and overactive adrenal system, it is now apparent that it is not really a disease in itself, but part of a larger allergy and nutritional problem. Like diabetes mellitus, it develops from long-term allergies, improper diet, and inactivity.

Hypoglycemics, in response to a sugar challenge, produce too much insulin, and this causes blood sugar to drop too rapidly. The result is low blood sugar. But hypoglycemics also tend to be overly sensitive to stress, and when pressured, they produce too much cortisol and adrenaline. The result is a precipitous rise in blood sugar, followed by a sudden fall as the body tries to stabilize itself. The panic and terror that sometimes accompany hypoglycemic attacks are most likely caused by this excess adrenaline. The overwhelming fatigue that follows is associated with the fast-falling blood-sugar level. It is a seesaw that is hard to keep in balance.

Because the frequent association between food allergy and hypoglycemia is often ignored, traditional treatment is usually only partially successful. The standard program of many small, high-protein meals does work to stabilize the blood sugar, but the repetitive diet, in an already weakened system, often leads to the development or intensification of allergies/addictions to the repetitive new battery of foods. Hypoglycemics on such a regimen end up eating frequently not only in an attempt to keep their blood sugar constant, but to mask symptoms of withdrawal from allergic foods. Allergies are often the underlying source of symptoms in the hypoglycemic who needs a "fix" of a favorite food. Conversely, for some people, chronic allergies lead to hypoglycemia.

Merv Griffin was one of those who felt his symptoms getting worse after years on a typical hypoglycemic diet. He turned out to have many allergies, and he had a very difficult time giving up some of his favorite foods. For the first few days, he called us several times, irritable and headachy, dying for just one cup of coffee. But once he made it through those first few days of withdrawal, he felt more stable and vital than he had for years.

Hypoglycemia, when viewed in narrow terms simply as a disorder of low blood sugar and treated in the traditional way, can become more and more serious. The problem of food allergy must be addressed. One of our patients, who had long adhered to a hypoglycemic diet, had nevertheless gotten slowly and steadily worse. When he came in, he'd been having frequent headaches for fifteen years and had gotten to the point of waking during the night, vomiting from the pain. His pain and headaches were gone on the third day of his diet, never to return. Eighteen months later he had lost 80 pounds. He was no longer hypoglycemic and was able to eat, with few exceptions, what he wanted on a rotating basis.

Hypoglycemic Therapy

As with other blood-sugar disorders, therapy must start with regulation of the diet. In addition to the elimination of allergies and a rotation diet, caution must be taken to avoid blood-sugar overload, which leads to plummeting blood-sugar levels. Eating a candy bar is no way to handle a hypoglycemic attack. That temporary rise goeth before a fall.

Exercise is important because of its role in stabilizing the blood sugar: During exercise, insulin is not needed to transport sugar into cells. If no other physical problems are present, the goal should be thirty minutes of aerobic exercise five times weekly.

Protocol for Hypoglycemia

Dietary Management

1. Basic Optimum Health Program: elimination of allergic foods, rotation diet. See Part IV.
2. Eat small meals, including snacks of vegetables and other complex carbohydrates. Be sure to have a small portion—1 to 3 ounces—of a complete protein (page 445) at each meal.
3. Avoid all simple sugars. Eat fresh fruit only after carefully testing to see if you have any reaction.
4. Avoid caffeine and tobacco, both adrenal stimulants.
5. No alcohol. It is not only high in sugar, but most alcoholic beverages are made from highly allergenic foods and contribute to allergy by causing a leaky gut or increased mucosal permeability.

Supplementation

Routine supplementation (page 86) *plus*

Vitamin C: 3 500-mg capsules after each meal (Use buffered calcium ascorbate; do not take to bowel tolerance)
Evening primrose oil: Increase to 6–8 capsules daily
MaxEPA: Increase to 4–6 capsules daily
Micellized Vitamin A: 3 drops twice daily (20,000 IU)
Micellized Vitamin E: 1 ml twice daily (300 IU)
B complex: 1 capsule with breakfast and lunch
B6: 250 mg with breakfast and lunch
Pantothenic acid: 250 mg with each meal
Zinc orotate: 25–50 mg tablet with breakfast and dinner
GTF chromium: 200–400 mcg daily
Calcium: 800–1,000 mg daily
Magnesium: 600–800 mg daily

Additional Recommendation

Aerobic exercise (under a doctor's supervision when warranted), with a goal of thirty minutes five times weekly.

Also see BLOOD-SUGAR DISORDERS.

HYPOTENSION
(Low Blood Pressure)

Here's a potential problem we see more and more often at our clinic, especially in young women. One of our patients is a perfect illustration of the misguided habits that can lead to low blood pressure. She arrives at our office on the run, a bit late: rail thin, beautifully made up, every hair in place—for her exercise class. "It's one of those marathon things," she explains. "You know, four hours of aerobics, and then you collapse. I do it twice a week." She goes on to explain about her daily jump-rope regimen and the four hundred sit-ups she does each morning. She takes out a bottle of pills. Her vitamins? No, she explains, water pills, diuretics. "It's the only way I can keep my weight down. I gain weight so easily —all I have to do is look at food." Chronic crash dieting, too many diuretics, and too much exercise without adequate nutrition—this woman, like so many of her contemporaries, was a prime target for hypotension (and perhaps dangerous cardiac arrhythmias).

Hypotension can be arbitrarily defined as a blood pressure below 100/70, in association with such symptoms as chronic fatigue, light-headedness, and dizziness. This condition is often found in malnourished women and teenage females, in people who are chronically depressed or inactive, or those suffering from allergies, chronic fatigue, intolerance to cold, or malnutrition.

It may also be associated with excess alcohol consumption, iron deficiency anemia, fever (leading to dehydration), anorexia, chronic diarrhea, bulimia or severely restrictive diet, overly strenuous exercise, abuse of diuretics, heart disease, hypothyroidism, hypoadrenalism (underactive adrenals), or the use of antidepressive medication.

Protocol for Hypotension

Dietary Management

1. Basic Optimum Health Program: elimination of allergic foods, rotation diet. See Part IV.
2. Drink plenty of liquids—at least eight glasses of bottled water daily.
3. Adequate quality protein (see page 444).

Supplementation

Routine supplementation (page 86) *plus*

Vitamin C: Increase to 6–8 grams daily
Vitamin B5: 500 mg daily
Vitamin B6: 500 mg daily
Multiple amino acid supplement: 2–4 capsules twice daily between meals

Additional Recommendations

1. Eliminate alcohol.
2. Exercise in moderation (see Chapter 18).
3. A doctor's supervision is required for treatment of possible infections, or heart disease, for thyroid medication if needed, and slow reduction in medications, especially diuretics.

HYPOTHYROIDISM

The thyroid is the central regulatory gland of the metabolism. Hypothyroidism, or underactive thyroid, may underlie a number of conditions, including stubborn obesity, coronary heart disease, elevated cholesterol levels, malabsorption, hypochlorhydria, fatigue, dry skin, intolerance to cold, and a generally lowered immune-system functioning. The cause is often hard to pinpoint. Do thyroid problems trigger metabolic imbalances? Or does it work the other way around, with absorption problems and a weakened immune system causing thyroid problems? But half of those with depressed thyroid function are also hypochlorhydric and have malabsorption and metabolic disorders; these include difficulty with clearing CICs (circulating immune complexes) from the bloodstream and problems with the absorption of many nutrients, especially zinc and the fat-soluble vitamins, plus problems with the conversion of beta carotene to Vitamin A and the utilization of B6 and B12.

Diagnosis of hypothyroidism can be difficult, and many of the standard blood tests are most likely unreliable. A better way to determine hypothyroidism may be to take your basal temperature for five days running, early in the morning, as follows:

- Use an oral thermometer with markings to a tenth of a degree. Shake the thermometer down below 95 degrees F the night before and place it within easy reach of your bedside.
- Upon awakening—before you get out of bed and move around—take your axillary (armpit) temperature; this method is most accurate. Place the thermometer firmly under your armpit and let it remain there for ten minutes.
- Read and record the temperature to the nearest tenth of a degree. Repeat this procedure for five days in a row. A temperature below 97.6 for premenopausal women and 97.4 for men and postmenopausal women, in conjunction with the symptoms mentioned above, indicates probable hypothyroidism.

  Note: Because of temperature fluctuations due to the menstrual cycle, women should begin recordings only on the second or third day of their menstrual flow.

Protocol for Hypothyroidism

Dietary Management

1. Basic Optimum Health Program: elimination of allergic foods, rotation diet. See Part IV.
2. Limit consumption of dairy products, red meat, and eggs.
3. Eat sea vegetables high in iodine and minerals such as kelp, amanori (nori, laver), dulse, and arame. Wash them well to rinse off excess salt.

Supplementation

Routine supplementation (page 86) *plus*

Vitamin C: Increase to 8–10 grams daily
Evening primrose oil: Increase to 6–8 capsules daily
MaxEPA: Increase to 4–6 caps daily
Iodine supplement: Up to 200 mcg daily
Kelp tablets: 2 tablets three times daily with meals

See Digestive Support, page 264.

Additional Recommendations

1. Diagnostic tests: thyroid panel and basal temperature test (explained above). Repeat basal temperature test each month to monitor improvement. Also, serum cholesterol, blood vitamin analysis, blood mineral analysis, the FICA, and serum ferritin.
2. Aerobic exercise four to five times weekly to strengthen immune system and stimulate metabolism. See Chapter 18.

See also IRON DEFICIENCY and Weight Loss, page 198.
Indigestion. See DIGESTIVE DISORDERS and Digestive Support (page 264).

INSOMNIA
(and Other Sleep Disorders)

While some insomniacs adjust to their sleeping problems and even manage to take advantage of their night-owl status, for most sufferers it is a waking nightmare. Long sleepless nights followed by days of exhaustion take their toll on both the physical and mental health of many teenagers and adults.

Conventional therapies for insomnia include the use of sedatives, tranquilizers, and hypnotics such as Valium and chloral hydrate, which can be addictive, have serious side effects, and soon lose their power to do the job. Relaxation techniques and behavioral modification are helpful for some.

But often insomnia and other sleep disorders fall under the heading of BRAIN ALLERGIES (page 341), because of the ability of allergies and nutritional imbalances to affect the sleep center of the brain. Nighttime wakefulness frequently turns out to be nothing more than the body needing a middle-of-the-night fix of an allergic food to keep withdrawal symptoms at bay.

A haggard college senior named Marty came to us after five years of nighttime torture and hundreds of pills—Valium, Dalmane, chloral hydrate. Though these drugs sometimes gave him a welcome night's sleep, he was dragging through his classes with drug hangovers and becoming very worried about his dependence on pills. All it took to get Marty back on track was the elimination of his daily ration of coffee and sweet rolls, along with a couple of allergic foods, plus a nightly dose of L-tryptophan (an amino acid that has proved to be a remarkable natural sleeping pill for many people), and some other nutrients. Three years later, he was still completely off sedatives and only needed his tryptophan sleep aid about once a month.

Protocol for Insomnia and Other Sleep Disorders

Dietary Management

1. Basic Optimum Health Program: elimination of allergic foods, rotation diet. See Part IV.
2. Eat a substantial breakfast and lunch, and a lighter dinner high in complex carbohydrates, low in protein and saturated and trans fats (no eggs, red meat, or dairy products).
3. Eat dinner several hours before bedtime and no late night snacks.
4. Avoid all caffeinated beverages, foods, and medications.
5. Avoid all alcoholic beverages.

Supplementation

Routine supplementation (page 86) *plus*

Niacinamide: 500 mg
B5: Increase to 500 mg daily
GABA (gamma amino butyric acid): 500 mg one hour before bedtime
L-tryptophan: 1–2 grams thirty minutes before bedtime

Add to bedtime supplement if needed

Niacin: 50–100 mg
Calcium: 600–800 mg
Magnesium: 400 mg

Note: Do not take B complex after 4:00 P.M. (midafternoon), especially no B6 and no B12.

Additional Recommendations

Exercise helps dispel tension, makes you comfortably tired, and promotes the metabolism of stress hormones and the production of sleep-enhancing neurotransmitters. A daily thirty-minute aerobic workout should do the trick, but don't exercise right before bedtime.

Do not take naps during the day.

See also BRAIN ALLERGIES, STRESS MANAGEMENT, and L-tryptophan (page 129).

IRON DEFICIENCY AND IRON-DEFICIENCY ANEMIA

Iron deficiency and anemia, extremely common in women of all ages, athletes, pregnant women, and those with malabsorption problems, is discussed in the chapter on minerals (page 118).

Protocol for Iron Deficiency

Dietary Management

1. Basic Optimum Health Program: elimination of allergic foods, rotation diet. See Part IV.
2. Eat organ (liver, kidney) meats once a week.
3. Increase consumption of green, leafy vegetables.
4. Cook in iron pots and skillets.
5. Avoid caffeine.

Supplementation

Routine supplementation (page 86) *plus*

Ferrous fumarate (iron tablets): 50 mg three times daily between meals with nondairy snacks and 500 mg Vitamin C

See Digestive Support, page 264.

Additional Recommendations

1. Diagnostic blood tests: complete blood count (CBC), serum ferritin, TIBC (total iron binding capacity), and percentage of saturation evaluation.
2. Follow-up: repeat serum ferritin after one month. Repeat all other tests every two months until iron level is stabilized.

3. If deficiency has reached anemia stage, have CBC test done each month until condition is eradicated.

Note: Don't overdose on iron. Too much iron in the body (hemochromatosis) is associated with increased incidence of heart disease, diabetes, bacterial infection, and cancer of the liver. This condition is more common in men than in women, but it is possible to *over*compensate for a deficiency.

IRRITABLE BOWEL SYNDROME
(Spastic Colon)

Irritable bowel syndrome is apparently caused by periodic spasm of the colon, producing alternating diarrhea and constipation, abdominal cramping or pain, and perhaps additional symptoms such as gas, flatulence, bloating, bad breath, water retention, and/or visible spasms or twitching in the lower abdominal region. The chronic irritation of the mucosal lining of the intestine may lead to more pronounced inflammation, tearing, and microscopic bleeding.

Triggered in part by severe food allergies, excess dietary fats, and stress, irritable bowel syndrome may lead to serious nutritional deficiencies, absorption problems, lowered immune strength, and other secondary problems. Left untreated, it may be the precursor to more serious intestinal disorders such as ulcerative colitis, Crohn's disease, and diverticulitis.

Irritable bowel problems must be treated as soon as symptoms are recognized, to avoid further complications. Refer to the following protocol and to specific protocols for DIARRHEA and CONSTIPATION, and to Digestive Support, page 264.

Protocol for Irritable Bowel Syndrome

Dietary Management

1. Basic Optimum Health Program: elimination of allergic foods, rotation diet. See Part IV.
2. Increase dietary fiber such as rice bran, soy bran, and fruits and vegetables high in fiber. For a list of high-fiber foods, see page 00.
3. Eliminate all nuts, seeds, and fruits with small seeds such as raspberries and strawberries.
4. Avoid excess saturated fats. Eliminate all trans fats and fried foods.
5. Eliminate dairy products except for yogurt.
6. Avoid caffeine, alcohol, and spices.

7. If IBS persists, drink three to four ounces of aloe vera juice three times a day between meals.

Supplementation

Routine supplementation (page 86) *plus*

Evening primrose oil: Increase to 6–8 capsules daily
MaxEPA: Increase to 9–12 capsules daily
Micellized Vitamin A: 2 drops (10,000 IU) daily
Zinc chelate: 25–50 mg daily

See Digestive Support, page 264.

Additional Recommendations

1. Nutritional deficiencies are often a consequence of irritable bowel syndrome. A blood vitamin analysis and mineral panel is useful to identify any problems.
2. A Hemoccult test (not to be confused with a hemoculture test) to identify blood in the stool is a helpful diagnostic test and can alert you to the possible presence of hidden blood loss, and blood loss anemia. If blood is identified, it is advisable to have an upper and lower gastrointestinal X ray series to rule out more serious inflammatory bowel diseases.
3. Exercise will help restore bowel function to normal. A daily walk after one meal and a program of aerobic exercise gradually building up to thirty minutes a day four to five times weekly should be the goal. See Chapter 18, page 00.

See also DIGESTIVE DISORDERS, CANDIDIASIS, and Chapter 6.

Juvenile Diabetes. See BLOOD-SUGAR DISORDERS, DIABETES, and page 301.

KIDNEY STONES

When the kidneys cannot adequately regulate the levels of calcium, sodium, potassium, phosphate, oxalate, urate, and other substances in the blood, these substances may eventually accumulate in clumps or deposits known as stones. Formed very slowly over time, these stones usually do not make themselves known until they are large enough to obstruct the internal ducts of the kidneys. This obstruction can be very painful, as can the pain that occurs as a stone attempts to move from the kidney into the bladder. Symptoms of kidney stones include the following: extreme pain on either side just above the small of the back, often in waves recurring every few minutes; pain that shifts from the back to the groin area as the stone moves; fever, chills, and nausea; and blood in the urine.

Excess oxalate formation, deficiencies in B6 and magnesium, elevated uric acid, and inadequate consumption of fluids are some of the known conditions that can lead to kidney problems. About 5 percent of the population suffers from kidney stones and more than 200,000 are hospitalized annually for treatment, which can include powerful stone-shrinking drugs and surgery. Because the tendency to kidney stones may be hereditary, those with such a family history should be extra careful about excess milk intake, excessive Vitamin C supplementation, and inadequate Vitamin B6 or magnesium consumption, and should be sure to drink plenty of water every day.

Protocol for Kidney Stones

Dietary Management

1. Basic Optimum Health Program: elimination of allergic foods, rotation diet. See Part IV.
2. Drink *at least* six to eight tall glasses of bottled water a day, the more the better.
3. Restrict intake of milk products.

Supplementation

Routine supplementation (page 86) *plus*

B complex: 2 capsules daily with breakfast and lunch
B6: 250 mg twice daily with meals
Magnesium orotate: 100 mg three times daily after meals

Additional Recommendation

1. For ongoing monitoring of kidney health, have a complete urinalysis, plus a check of serum uric-acid levels, every two to three months.
2. Before beginning additional supplementation, have a lab test to rule out magnesium and B6 deficiencies.
3. If uric acid is elevated, begin supervised program to reduce uric acid, see URIC ACID (ELEVATED).

LEG CRAMPS

Leg cramps are a particular problem for many elderly people. Though not physically damaging, the pain, which often comes on at night, can be quite severe and can make sleeping difficult. Nutritional imbalances, lack of exercise, impaired circulation, and allergies are the usual sources of this common problem.

One patient, who came to us for an entirely unrelated back problem, mentioned in passing that she was accustomed to waking every night with aching legs. Tests showed she was low in folic acid and B12. With these supplements, plus the elimination of allergies and a daily walk, she was able to sleep through the night in just two weeks.

Protocol for Leg Cramps

Dietary Management

1. Basic Optimum Health Program: elimination of allergic foods, rotation diet. See Part IV.
2. Reduce all saturated fats and eliminate all trans fats and fried foods.
3. Make sure the diet is high in fiber, to promote good digestion and elimination.

Supplementation

Routine supplementation (page 86) *plus*

Vitamin C: Increase to 8–10 capsules daily
Evening primrose oil: Increase to 6–8 capsules daily
MaxEPA: Increase to 6 capsules daily
B complex: 1 tablet with each breakfast and lunch
Micellized Vitamin E: 2 ml daily (300 IU)
Calcium: 800 to 1,000 mg daily
Magnesium: 600 to 800 mg daily

Additional Recommendations

1. Have mineral panel for calcium and RBC (red blood cell) magnesium and a blood vitamin analysis for all vitamins. Repeat after one or two months.
2. Aerobic exercise; a good goal is moderate aerobic exertion or brisk walking every other day. See Chapter 18.
3. Elevate the feet above head at least ten to fifteen minutes a day. Simply lie on your back on the floor, and prop your feet up against the wall with legs straight at an angle of at least 45 degrees.

Life Extension. See ANTI-AGING.
Longevity. See ANTI-AGING.
Low Blood Sugar. See BLOOD-SUGAR DISORDERS and HYPOGLYCEMIA.
Maldigestion. See DIGESTIVE DISORDERS and Digestive Support (page 264).
Menstrual Problems. See PREMENSTRUAL SYNDROME.
Migraine. See HEADACHE.

MULTIPLE SCLEROSIS

Multiple sclerosis is a progressive autoimmune disease, characterized by the slow loss of patches of myelin sheaths (coverings) of nerves in the brain and spinal cord. This degenerative process usually strikes its victims between the ages of twenty and forty, causing a wide range of neurological problems. Early symptoms include transient weakness, vertigo, slight stiffness, minor gait-control problems, speech disturbances, and mild emotional disturbances. When the disease is fully established, it causes problems ranging from hysteria, depression, mental apathy, and lack of judgment, to visual and speech disturbances, sensory loss, incontinence, and severe loss of muscle control.

There is no cure for this serious disease, but there are several nutritional and life-style approaches that have proved helpful in managing multiple sclerosis. Allergy elimination often provides immediate relief, especially when gluten sensitivity is a factor (page 374). Aggressive essential-fatty-acid supplementation in conjunction with restriction of saturated and trans fats seems to reduce flare-ups. Regular aerobic exercise is important in minimizing muscle weakness and atrophy. Work and activity levels should be maintained as energetically as possible.

Protocol for Multiple Sclerosis

Dietary Management

1. Basic Optimum Health Program: elimination of allergies, rotation diet. See Part IV.
2. Decrease saturated fats and avoid trans fats and fried foods.
3. Use only small amounts of cold-pressed oils (Table 7, page 144).
4. Eliminate alcohol.

Supplementation

Routine supplementation (page 86) *plus*

Evening primrose oil: Increase to 6–8 capsules daily
MaxEPA: Increase to 6–9 capsules daily
Micellized Vitamin A: 2 drops daily (10,000 IU)
Micellized Vitamin E: 2 drops daily (300 IU)
Octacosonol (wheat germ oil): 2,000 mg twice daily after meals

See Digestive Support, page 264.

Additional Recommendations

1. Progressive exercise program to level of aerobic exertion. See Chapter 18, page 277.
2. Hyperbaric oxygen therapy, though still in the research stage, has shown some promising effects for multiple sclerosis sufferers and may soon be covered under health insurance plans. This administration of 100 percent in an enclosed chamber is similar to therapy that divers use for the bends. Treatment involves one to two hours of pure 100 percent oxygen at two atmospheres of pressure (double the air pressure at sea level) for ten to twenty consecutive days, then follow-up treatments every one to two months indefinitely.

See also GLUTEN SENSITIVITY and Chapter 11 for information on EFAs.

Muscle aches and pains. See ARTHRITIS.
Nontropical sprue. See GLUTEN SENSITIVITY.
Osteoarthritis. See ARTHRITIS.

OSTEOPOROSIS

Osteoporosis is a decrease in bone density and strength that makes the vertebrae, the small bones, and bones of the leg, arm, and hip brittle and prone to cracking. Over 10 million women suffer from this debilitating condition, which usually sets in after menopause. Symptoms include easy bone fracture, receding gums and jaw line, excess loss of calcium from bones into the urine, loss of height, dowager's hump, and shiny skin on the back of the hands.

Exactly why women are so vulnerable to osteoporosis is still being debated. It is clear, however, that osteoporosis develops when the body can no longer regenerate and retain bone mass. This calcium loss may be triggered by any of the following: physical inactivity or excessive activity; nutritional deficiencies that affect bone formation; defective intestinal absorption of calcium, phosphorus, and magnesium, perhaps the result of hypochlorhydria; overconsumption of fluoride; increased sensitivity to endogenous parathyroid hormone; and the hormonal fluctuations of menopause.

Given the tendency for older people to be hypochlorhydric, malnourished, and inactive, it is easy to see why this disease is so prevalent in postmenopausal women. Many medical practitioners ascribe the calcium loss associated with osteoporosis to decreased levels of estrogen and progesterone after menopause and therefore prescribe hormone-replacement therapy for this problem. I disagree with this and feel that osteoporosis can be prevented and treated more successfully with calcium supplementation, direct sunlight, weight-bearing exercise, and the correction of food allergy and absorption problems. Too, studies show that vitamin E (400–800 mg daily) and vitamin A (20,000–50,000 IU daily) can have a positive impact on estrogen and progesterone levels.

Postmenopausal women are not the only ones who are in danger of bone loss these days. A new class of candidates for osteoporosis is young female athletes who have stopped menstruating (amenorrhea) as a result of extensive exercise without adequate nutrition. This artificial menopause, common to female athletes, threatens young bones as much as natural menopause affects older women. Another by-product of extensive exercise (and I stress the word "extensive," for moderate weight-bearing exercise is imperative for bone strength) is a condition in which the pituitary produces large quantities of prolactin. This, in addition to shutting down the pituitaries, seems to interfere with the metabolism of essential fatty acids, and that in turn may lead to bone degeneration as a result of prostaglandin imbalance.

I feel that osteoporosis is almost entirely preventable if allergies are eliminated, hypochlorhydria is corrected, the proper nutrients are provided in the diet, and a moderate level of weight-bearing exercise and activity is maintained throughout life.

Protocol for Osteoporosis

Dietary Management

1. Basic Optimum Health Program: elimination of allergic foods, rotation diet. See Part IV.
2. Reduce consumption of saturated and trans fats.

3. Eat only low-fat dairy foods and particularly yogurt, which is more easily digested.
4. Eat many dark, green, and leafy vegetables, such as broccoli and spinach.
5. Avoid diet drinks containing phosphates.
6. Avoid overconsumption of animal protein (also high in phosphates).

Supplementation

Routine supplementation (page 86) *plus*

Vitamin C (in form of calcium ascorbate): Increase to 6–10 grams daily
Evening primrose oil: Increase to 6–8 capsules daily
MaxEPA: Increase to 4–6 capsules daily
Vitamin E: Increase to 400–800 IU daily
Vitamin A: 20,000–50,000 IU daily
Vitamin D: 400 IU daily
Calcium: 500 mg three times daily with meals
Magnesium: 500 mg twice daily with meals

See Digestive Support, page 264.

Additional Recommendations

1. Diagnostic tests: RBC (red blood cell) magnesium test to determine magnesium level; test for blood levels of Vitamin D and phosphorus.
2. Repeat RBC magnesium test monthly until deficiency is corrected.
3. Weight-bearing exercise is crucial to the maintenance of strong bones. A lifelong commitment to moderate aerobic exercise and strength training will prevent osteoporosis in later life. Runners, walkers, and bodybuilders (weight lifters) have the densest bones. However, premenopausal women should not exercise to the point of amenorrhea. For older women, studies have shown that exercise has a corrective effect for those already experiencing bone loss. Even routine walking, along with some form of strength training, is of great benefit. See Chapter 18, page 277.
4. Expose face and arms to sun, at least twenty to thirty minutes twice weekly, for Vitamin D benefits.

PAIN

Chronic pain is the backdrop to millions of lives. There are 70 million Americans with chronic back pain, 36 million arthritis sufferers, 20 million with migraines. Pain can show up in the nerves, the muscles, or the bones. It can be traced to menstrual problems, injury, disease, or may have no explainable cause. *One out of three people will have to deal with chronic pain in one form or another in his lifetime.*

I can often pick out the pain sufferers who come into our clinic. Their faces are engraved with stress, their brows furrowed, their frowns permanent, their posture defeated. But there is nothing more satisfying to me than seeing the change wrought in them by a few weeks or months of therapy. Relief from pain, often for the first time in years, often after they had given up hope of relief, makes whole new persons of them. For me, the sheer elation, the new-lease-on-life attitude of such patients is a greater reward than that of helping an athlete to improve his performance or seeing a patient shed unwanted pounds.

At OHL, we see patients who have tried just about everything—from the predictable to the dangerous to the worthless—to relieve their pain. Everything, that is, except what could truly make them well: dietary changes, a few supplements that have proved to have potent pain-relieving powers, and in some cases exercise.

Relief often comes very fast. One man who had lived with pain in his arm and shoulder for ten years, who was unable to lift his arm over his head and could hardly sleep at night because of the swelling in his hands, was on his way to complete relief in just seven days.

Sometimes it's hard for people to believe that allergy and diet are such powerful influences on our health. We had a patient, a lawyer, whose years of intense back spasms had just about driven him to suicide before he came to us. Pain-free for the first time in years after starting our program, he couldn't quite believe, even in his euphoria, that such a drastic change could have been brought about without drugs or surgery, in fact with nothing more than our usual pain program. So after about a year and a half free of pain, he drifted back into drinking and being careless about rotating foods. Not surprisingly, he noticed one day that his back pain had turned up again. So he came back to us for a new series of allergy tests and a pep talk, went back on the program, and the pain predictably disappeared.

For some pain sufferers the psychological effects are as devastating as the physical pain. A patient named Jeanette had long suffered debilitating lower back pain, though no doctor could find any apparent trauma. Some doctors had suggested braces; others recommended surgery. All had loaded her up with drugs. "I became convinced that this pain must be in my head," she said. "The guilt and depression became almost as bad as the pain. I started to think that I deserved the pain, that I was bringing it on myself. When I came here, I was elated to learn that my pain came from an identifiable source, that it was my diet causing my pain, and my diet could relieve it. It made a big difference not to feel helpless in the face of such discomfort. The pain lessens every week. And exercise is helping me to overcome the secondary damage I did to my muscles."

The Treatment of Chronic Pain

It is possible to transcend pain in rare instances of nerve-circuit overload or intense distraction. This phenomenon has been observed in wartime when soldiers in the intense noise and chaos of battle don't feel their wounds. It happens when a football player doesn't notice his dislocated shoulder until the game is over. But for most sufferers pain is a constant presence, and its relief or avoidance becomes an understandable obsession.

Chronic pain condemns tens of millions to a lifelong dependency on expensive drugs, and to experimenting with every new pain-relief technique that comes along, from the radical to the rational to the ridiculous.

Drugs do little or nothing to address the causes of pain and often mask the signs that would identify its cause. The side effects of drugs range from the ringing in the ears and digestive-tract bleeding associated with aspirin, to the bleeding ulcers, bone demineralization, and sugar diabetes associated with prednisone and other steroids. Many patients who take painkilling drugs risk kidney damage and nutritional deficiencies. Barbiturates disturb mental acuity. And many drugs lose their effectiveness over time: Dosages have to be increased, side effects escalate, and it often becomes necessary to graduate to stronger drugs in order to get pain relief. Many, of course, like codeine and Demerol, are highly addictive.

Fortunately, effective alternatives to drug therapy exist and are proliferating as the nature of pain becomes more fully understood.

Pain Relief and Cure

Even the nondrug alternatives to pain do not provide cure, for they don't address the causes of pain. At OHL we are often able not only to provide relief from pain, but get rid of it entirely by clearing up the cause of the pain. Our pain-relief program centers on allergy elimination and supplementation with certain nutrients, especially a newly discovered nutrient pain reliever, the amino acid DL-phenylalanine.

The relief from chronic pain is sometimes as simple as eliminating allergic foods from the diet. We know that allergic responses cause irritation to muscles, joints, nerves, and the digestive tract and that the chemical mediators released in allergic reactions can lead to the pain associated with everything from arthritis and migraine to muscle cramps and chronic back pain. At OHL, we have seen time and time again how the elimination of allergic foods works to relieve pain, often in patients who had suffered for years and tried all kinds of drugs and therapies.

The Lancet in a 1978 article, "Food Allergy: Fact or Fiction," reported the case of a thirty-seven-year-old woman who had suffered years of apparent cardiac pain. Diagnosed as having a pulmonary embolism, she had been taking large doses of heparin and warfarin (anticoagulants). Then, when another doctor's X ray didn't reveal any abnormalities, she was diagnosed as suffering from "effort syndrome," a wishy-washy diagnosis later amended to "cardiac neurosis." The woman's symptoms worsened, and soon she was living in fear of a heart attack, subsequently began suffering from agoraphobia, never leaving the safety of her home.

And there she remained until she was referred to Royal Southern Hospital Clinic in Liverpool. Here a dietary history revealed that she was a self-confessed tea fiend, which led to allergy testing and the discovery that she was extremely allergic to coffee, tea, and tomatoes. Her heart pain and other symptoms completely disappeared when she avoided those allergens. Six months later she had conquered her long-festering psychological symptoms and is now leading a perfectly normal life.

Nutrient supplements play a major part in pain therapy. Essential-fatty-acid supplements—evening primrose oil and MaxEPA—encourage production of the anti-inflammatory prostaglandins with the reduction of pain sensitivity.

But the most exciting and important nutrient supplement for pain relief is the amino acid DL-phenylalanine. DLP has proved effective in 70 to 80 percent of the chronic pain patients in stimulating endorphin production and in reducing inflammation associated with chronic pain. Not only is it nonaddictive, it seems to increase in effectiveness over time. Since it is not classified as a drug, it requires no prescription—so far. Studies have turned up no side effects at the therapeutic dose range. DL-phenylalanine does not work like aspirin; you don't take two pills when you feel a headache coming on. It must be taken over time for its effectiveness to take hold in the system. More about DL-phenylalanine and dosages can be found on page 130.

Protocol for Pain Relief

Dietary Management

Basic Optimum Health Program: elimination of allergic foods, rotation diet. See Part IV.

Supplementation

Routine supplementation (page 86) *plus*

Vitamin C: To 90 percent bowel tolerance (see page 114)
Evening primrose oil: Increase to 6–8 capsules daily
MaxEPA: Increase to 6–9 capsules daily
Vitamin E: 400–800 IU daily
Calcium: 1,000 mg a day
Magnesium: 1,000 mg a day
DL-phenylalanine: 2 375-mg capsules twice a day between meals (see page 00 for guidance, restrictions)
L-tryptophan: 2–3 grams before bedtime

Additional Recommendations

1. Exercise is an important factor in the treatment of many pain syndromes. Details can be found under individual pain-disorder headings. Also refer to Chapter 18.
2. Stress-management techniques, including exercise, are often extremely beneficial in pain management.

See also ARTHRITIS, HEADACHE, PREMENSTRUAL SYNDROME, Chapter 11 (page 137), and DL-Phenylalanine (page 130).

Platelet Aggregation. See CARDIOVASCULAR DISEASE.

PREMENSTRUAL SYNDROME (PMS)

Premenstrual syndrome provides a vivid example of how biochemical imbalances affect mood and emotional and physical well-being. Women have always been at the mercy of the physical discomforts and emotional roller coaster of their menstrual cycle. The travails of PMS seemed to come with the territory. Many women have grown up feeling that their monthly cramps and moods were all their fault, all in their heads, the signs of feminine weakness and emotional imbalance. It is only recently that the medical community has realized that PMS is not to be blamed on its victims and that certain therapeutic measures can greatly reduce its effects.

About 40 percent of women suffer from PMS to a noticeable degree. Some are totally immobilized each month with depression and pain; others simply get bloated and cranky. Physical symptoms may include the following: bloating and weight gain as a result of water retention; headache; breast tenderness; pelvic discomfort or pain; a change in bowel habits; increased appetite (particularly sugar cravings); weakness and tiredness or general aches and pains. On a list of psychological symptoms would be these: nervousness or anxiety; irritability; mood swings; loss of concentration; depression; change in sexual desire; insomnia; forgetfulness; crying spells; and mental confusion and fatigue. One month may be bad, another mild.

The good news is that the vast majority of PMS is the result of biochemical imbalances that are manageable through nutritional intervention. PMS appears to be the direct result of prostaglandin imbalances, food allergies, blood-sugar disturbances, and hormonal fluctuations. There are also indications that PMS sufferers have unusually high levels of the hormones estrogen, progesterone, and prolactin, which may account for fluid retention and cause smaller blood vessels to contract and spasm. Moreover, changing hormone levels during the menstrual cycle affects carbohydrate metabolism and the production of corticosteroids by the adrenal glands. The key to controlling PMS is to regulate hormonal balance and restore healthy prostaglandin levels so that PGE2 cannot overwhelm the beneficial effects of PGE1 and PGE3. Researcher Dr. David Horrobin says that PMS is almost always connected to PGE1 deficiency (more about this on page 150).

Unfortunately, conventional therapy for PMS is clearly inadequate. The frequent use of diuretics may deprive the body of potassium and magnesium, which may in turn impair hormonal balance. The use of tranquilizers dulls the wits, does nothing to cure this syndrome, and can lead to abuse of the drugs. And anti-prostaglandin drugs, such as Anaprox, block not only the PGE2 (which causes inflammation and water retention), but the beneficial prostaglandins, and these are major cure factors in PMS.

A shy, angry, antisocial seventeen-year-old came to our office complaining of the acne and obesity that had made her life miserable since she was fourteen. But she didn't see the larger picture until we went carefully through her health history and were able to show her how intimately connected her problems were to her menstrual periods. We put her on the protocol described below and told her to keep a careful diary of her moods, her weight, and her acne breakouts. Her first period went pretty much as we expected: She didn't feel like leaving the house, she gained 4 pounds, failed a history test, fought with her brothers, and described herself as "a waste." By the second month even she couldn't miss the changes. Her weight was down 9 pounds, she hadn't had any new acne flare-ups, and her skin was really clearing up. And her mood? "I feel lighter, not just in my body, but my head too—I'm no longer depressed," she told me.

Protocol for Premenstrual Syndrome

Dietary Management

1. Basic Optimum Health Program: elimination of allergic foods, rotation diet. See Part IV.
2. Eliminate refined sugars.
3. Decrease salt intake.
4. Decrease consumption of caffeine, chocolate, alcohol, and tobacco.
5. Decrease red meat and dairy products.
6. Eliminate fried foods.
7. Increase leafy green vegetables.

Supplementation

Routine supplementation (page 86) *plus*

Vitamin C: Increase to 8–10 grams daily
Evening primrose oil: Increase to 6–8 capsules daily
MaxEPA: Increase to 6 capsules daily
Micellized Vitamin E: 1 ml per day (150 IU)
Micellized Vitamin A: 3 drops per day (10,000 IU)
B complex: 1 capsule after breakfast and lunch
B6: 250 mg daily after breakfast or lunch
Calcium: 600 mg
Magnesium orotate or chelate: 400 mg

Note: Supplementation is especially important in the two to fourteen days before the beginning of your period.

Additional Recommendations

Exercise is important in PMS, because it relieves stress and fluid retention and promotes regulation of adrenal glands, hormone production, and prostaglandin levels in the blood. In addition, deep relaxation techniques can help ease irritability and mood swings. A good goal is thirty minutes of aerobic exercise four to five days a week. It is particularly important to exercise during the symptomatic period. See Chapter 18.

See also BRAIN ALLERGIES, STRESS MANAGEMENT, and Chapter 11.

Psoriasis. See ECZEMA.
Respiratory Problems. See ASTHMA.
Rheumatism. See ARTHRITIS.
Rheumatoid Arthritis. See ARTHRITIS.
Smoking. See ADDICTION.
Spastic Colon. See IRRITABLE BOWEL SYNDROME.
Sprue. See GLUTEN SENSITIVITY.
Stomachache. See DIGESTIVE DISORDERS and Digestive Support (page 264).

STRESS MANAGEMENT

I've emphasized several times in this book that excess stress, whether caused by physical or emotional trauma, plays a big part in both the development and exacerbation of disease and illness. There is a big difference between "eustress," the good kind of stress that charges us up and helps us to move forward through life, and "dis-stress," the kind associated with too many things to do under too much pressure, too often associated with undiagnosed allergies and poor nutrition.

Just about everyone goes through stressful periods at one time or another in life. With luck, those periods are not of long duration, and we have the health and stamina to get through them without permanent damage. But if stress is chronic, and there is no hope of change, we will eventually sacrifice our health on the altar of a high-pressure job, or a low-quality diet and undiagnosed allergies, or alcohol and drugs, or an abrasive relationship, and be too weakened to recover fully.

What are the signs of dis-stress? Many of them are all too familiar: irritability, trouble sleeping, inability to concentrate, feelings of tension and anxiety, headaches, mental and physical fatigue, depression, digestive disorders, back pain and muscle tension, sweating, racing thoughts. Without relief, these stress symptoms will lead to all manner of serious health problems, from diminished immune strength, elevated blood pressure, coronary vasospasm, and atherosclerosis to adrenal and prostaglandin imbalances, perhaps even cancer.

Obviously the first line of defense against stress overload is changes in the way we live—from finding time to relax and sleep restfully, to getting enough exercise, to cutting down on drinking or smoking, to quitting an impossible job. Although nutritional supplementation and the elimination of allergies can't be expected to do the whole job indefinitely, the following stress-management protocol is a basic foundation for reclaiming good health.

Protocol for Stress Management

Dietary Management

1. Basic Optimum Health Program: elimination of allergic foods, rotation diet. See Part IV.
2. Increase consumption of foods high in calcium, magnesium, and potassium. See individual listings in the mineral tables beginning on page 174.
3. Avoid refined, simple sugars.
4. Avoid caffeine and alcohol, both highly stressful to the system.
5. Reduce sodium chloride (table salt) intake to guard against hypertension.

Supplementation

Routine supplementation (page 86) *plus*

Vitamin C: Increase to 8–10 grams
Evening primrose oil: Increase to 6–8 capsules
MaxEPA: Increase to 4–6 capsules
B complex: 1 capsule at breakfast and lunch
B5: 500 mg daily
Niacinamide: 100–500 mg daily
Magnesium: 600 mg daily
Calcium: 800 mg daily
L-tryptophan: 500 mg once to three times daily between meals

In cases where the adrenal system has been severely compromised by stress:

Vitamin C: To 90 percent bowel tolerance or intravenous Vitamin C therapy if needed (pages 114, 264)
Pantothenic acid: 250 mg three times daily after meals
Multiple free-form amino acids: 2–4 capsules twice daily between meals

Additional Recommendations

1. Diagnostic tests: blood pressure check, resting heart rate, lipid profile, FICA, blood vitamin analysis, and blood mineral analysis.
2. Aerobic exercise, four to five times weekly, will help to rebalance adrenal hormone levels, elevate endorphin levels, stimulate a weakened immune system, and relax muscle tension. It is in general an excellent way to burn off stress. See Chapter 18, page 277.
3. Deep-relaxation techniques such as yoga, biofeedback, and meditation are particularly effective in restoring proper adrenal levels, calming internal systems, and relaxing tense mind and muscles. Furthermore, it has been demonstrated that relaxation improves the cardiovascular system.

See also CARDIOVASCULAR DISEASE: Hypertension (page 355), Atherosclerosis (page 350).
Stroke. See CARDIOVASCULAR DISEASE.
Tension. See STRESS.
Tension Headache. See HEADACHE.

TINNITUS

Tinnitus is the perception of sound in the ears in the absence of acoustic stimulation. These phantom noises may take the form of a dull drone, buzzing, a high-pitched whine, or ringing in the ears. The noises may be loud or soft or may vacillate up and down the scale; they may be intermittent or persistent. It may be possible to ignore them, or they can drive you to distraction and impair hearing. It can be hard to hear or even think with the Indianapolis 500 going on in your head.

The origin of tinnitus can be difficult to pin down, for it may be a consequence of such diverse problems as hypertension, arteriosclerosis, anemia, Ménière's syndrome, toxic levels of carbon monoxide or heavy metals, allergies, essential-fatty-acid metabolic disorder, or of the overuse of aspirin, diuretics, quinine, or some antibiotics. The following protocol will reduce symptoms in many cases.

Protocol for Tinnitus

Dietary Management

1. Basic Optimum Health Program: elimination of allergic foods, rotation diet. See Part IV.
2. Restrict sodium chloride (table salt) intake.

3. If indicated, Protocol for Heart Disease, page 00.
4. If anemic due to nutritional problems, see IRON DEFICIENCY AND ANEMIA.

Supplementation

Routine supplementation (page 86) *plus*

Evening primrose oil: Increase to 6–8 capsules daily
MaxEPA: Increase to 6 capsules daily
Niacin: 50 mg daily to begin; over four weeks gradually increase to 200 mg twice daily with meals

Additional Recommendations

1. Have blood pressure checked to rule out hypertension.
2. Have complete blood count to rule out anemia.
3. Have FICA to rule out severe food allergies.
4. Have blood vitamin analysis and blood mineral analysis to rule out vitamin and mineral deficiencies.

See also Chapter 11.

Tobacco. See ADDICTION.
Type I Juvenile Diabetes. See BLOOD-SUGAR DISORDERS, DIABETES, and page 299.
Type II Diabetes. See BLOOD-SUGAR DISORDERS and DIABETES.
Ulcerative Colitis. See IRRITABLE BOWEL SYNDROME.

ULCERS
(Duodenal or Peptic)

Ulcers, long believed to be caused by excess hydrochloric acid, are now being viewed differently—as a possible allergic and nutritional disorder. Research indicates that ulcers develop in the mucosal lining of the stomach and intestinal tract when there are problems with appropriate production of and protection by mucous secretions. Food allergies are associated with this, as are excessive dependency on aspirin, prednisone, or other anti-inflammatory drugs that block prostaglandin production. (Certain prostaglandins function to stimulate production of mucus, the function of which is to protect the gastrointestinal mucosa from the hydrochloric-acid action.)

Sometimes there are no indications that an ulcer is developing until the condition is serious. Only about half of ulcer sufferers have a consistent set of symptoms. Others may have only occasional complaints about upset stomach or stomach pain, burning or gnawing feelings in the stomach, feelings of acute hunger or pain after eating or lying down. A high-stress life, the not-so-great, high-fat, low-fiber American diet, chronic allergies, and essential-fatty-acid deficiencies are the breeding ground for ulcers. No wonder over 8 million people in this country have ulcers of the esophagus, stomach, or intestines.

Protocol for Ulcers

Dietary Management

1. Basic Optimum Health Program: elimination of allergic foods, rotation diet. See Part IV.
2. Cut down on saturated fats and eliminate trans fats.
3. Avoid alcohol and caffeine.
4. Avoid aspirin and other anti-inflammatory, antiprostaglandin medications, especially if hydrochloric-acid production (as determined by a Heidelberg gastrogram) is normal or on the low side.
5. Use 2 tablespoons linseed oil on a salad every day.
6. Drink 3 ounces of aloe vera juice (available at health food stores) twenty minutes before each meal.

Supplementation

Routine supplementation (page 86) *plus*

Evening primrose oil: Increase to 6–8 capsules daily
MaxEPA: Increase to 6–12 capsules daily
Micellized Vitamin A: 3 drops (10,000 IU) daily
B5: 250 mg three times daily after meals
Zinc chelate: 25–50 mg after one meal

See Digestive Support, page 264.

Additional Recommendations

1. Diagnostic test: Heidelberg gastrogram.
2. Avoid milk therapy of any kind. Often an allergic food, it may aggravate ulcers rather than soothe them.
3. Stress-management techniques can help restore HCl and mucus balances and will generally promote healing of the entire gastrointestinal system.

See also STRESS MANAGEMENT, IRRITABLE BOWEL SYNDROME, and Chapter 11.

Upset Stomach. See DIGESTIVE DISORDERS and Digestive Support (page 264).

URIC ACID (ELEVATED)
(Hyperuricemia, Gouty Arthritis)

The inability of the blood, kidneys, and intestinal tract to maintain healthy low levels of uric acid can often be traced to an overly rich high-fat diet, obesity, food allergies, and kidney disease.

Elevated uric-acid levels may lead to gouty arthritis, an inflammation of the joints caused by deposits of uric-acid crystals. This can be disfiguring to joints and can cause extreme pain.

Even when a high uric-acid level hasn't reached the arthritis stage, it is a serious problem and can be difficult to treat unless underlying causes are addressed and eliminated. It's no wonder gout is associated with the high life of the upper classes, with rich, heavy meals and liberal imbibing.

Protocol for Elevated Uric Acid

Dietary Management

1. Basic Optimum Health Program: elimination of allergic foods, rotation diet. See Part IV.
2. Eliminate saturated and trans fats. No red meats, nuts, seeds, or organ meats.
3. Avoid alcohol.
4. Drink at least six to eight tall glasses of water every day; the more the better.
5. Drink four large glasses of cherry juice diluted by half with water every other day.

Supplementation

Routine supplementation (page 86) *plus*

Vitamin C: Increase to 8–10 grams daily, slowly and gradually
Vitamin A: 10,000 IU three times daily
Vitamin E: Increase to 400 IU daily

Additional Recommendations

1. The best diagnostic test is a blood-chemistry panel showing uric-acid levels. This test should be repeated every month or so until uric-acid levels are controlled.
2. Aerobic exercise three to five times weekly. See Chapter 18, page 277.
3. Weight loss, if indicated. See Chapter 18.

See also ARTHRITIS, HYPERTENSION.

Urticaria. See HIVES.
Vaginitis. See CANDIDIASIS.
Vascular Headache. See HEADACHE.

VIRAL INFECTION

The best way to prevent and manage viral infections is to strengthen the immune system. We are all exposed to viruses regularly, but only certain people at certain times are unable to fight them off. Any advantage we can garner through good nutrition and a strong immune defense is to our benefit.

Once a virus hits, though, our best course is to help the body flush out the virus with lots of fluids and that magic virus fighter, Vitamin C. Fever, because it stimulates the immune system, is the body's natural defense against virus. Fever is part of the healing process and should be allowed to run its course unless it is dangerously high or persistent. Exceptions to this would be infants with a fever over 104 degrees, fever associated with seizures or stiff neck, pregnant women, or those with advanced heart disease. Aspirin, which lowers fever and thus interferes with the body's attempt to destroy the virus, should be avoided if the discomfort is bearable.

Protocol for Viral Infection

Dietary Management

1. Basic Optimum Health Program: elimination of allergic foods, rotation diet. See Part IV.
2. Reduce saturated- and trans-fat intake.
3. Avoid excess sugars, which suppress the immune system, fuel the virus, and are taxing on the system.
4. Avoid caffeine and other stimulants that tax the adrenal and immune systems.

5. Drink eight to ten tall glasses of bottled or distilled water every day.

Supplementation

Routine supplementation (page 86) *plus*

Vitamin C: To 90 percent bowel tolerance for three days; reduce to 75 percent for duration of symptoms. See page 114.

If viral infection persists, add

Evening primrose oil: Increase to 6–8 capsules daily
MaxEPA: Increase to 6 capsules daily
Vitamin A: 25,000–100,000 IU daily for five days
Zinc orotate or zinc picolinate: 100 mg daily for five days
Copper: 2 mg daily
Thymus tissue supplement: 2 tablets daily, if viral infection is chronic

Additional Recommendations

Do not take antibiotics indiscriminately. Antibiotics are for *bacterial,* not viral, infections.

Yeast infection. See CANDIDIASIS.

Afterword: A Healthy Future?

Just a few final words about the prospects for medicine, and for your health. I believe that we are on the brink of a renaissance in modern medicine and that the next fifteen to twenty years will be crucial and exciting ones. During this time, there will be a gradual shift in emphasis, away from drugs, surgery, and dealing with disease *after* the fact. We will see the considerable powers of science and technology brought to bear on those health factors that are at the core of the Optimum Health Program—focus on life-style and risk factors, disease prevention, nutritional treatment of disease, self-care, immune function, allergy, supplementation, and exercise. In this ideal medical climate, equal respect and attention will be given to both the prevention and cure of disease. Here are some of the advancements I foresee for medicine in the near future:

- Attention will be focused more on the *existing* scientific information that supports the health theories espoused in this book.
- We will re-evaluate our total reliance on "pure" scientific method, which works for stones and stars but not often for humans, in favor of a view that recognizes the phenomenon of individual idiosyncrasy and the multifactorial nature of health and disease.
- We will discard the misguided and dangerous idea that "normal" can be equated with "healthy." We will get a working definition of good health, based on optimum rather than marginal guidelines, which encompasses the principle of biochemical individuality.
- It will be recognized that the patient possesses the primary responsibility in health maintenance, and the doctor/patient relationship will reflect this view.
- Medical school education will focus *primarily* on nutrition and life-style factors in disease. Physicians will represent the new wave in medical care, acting as role models in changing the course of medicine, especially today's young medical students. For the first time in many years, doctors will outlive their patients.
- Hospitalization will *routinely* include in-depth nutritional,

immunological, and allergy testing, and aggressive supplementation will be a routine component of hospital nutrition.

- There will be a recognition that surgery is a traumatic event that must be compensated for with aggressive oral and intravenous supplementation.
- There will be a focus on immune-system stimulation rather than suppression (i.e., chemotherapy), in treating cancer and other immune-system disorders.
- Infectious diseases will be treated nutritionally in conjunction with antibiotics, the dangers of which (associated with overuse), are now becoming widely recognized.
- Prenatal nutrition will become a prime focus of obstetrics. Blood samples taken from the umbilical cords of infants at birth will provide valuable information on blood levels of nutrients, the presence or absence of a tendency toward allergy and other diseases.
- The importance of breast-feeding will be viewed with a certain urgency, to the point that surrogate nurses for mothers unable to breast-feed will be accepted alternatives.
- Treatment of the elderly, who are frequently malnourished as a consequence of allergy and impaired digestion, will routinely include parenteral (intravenous) nutrient therapy.
- Psychiatric treatment will become a mix of "talk" therapy, nutrition, exercise, and stress management. Serious mental disorders and addiction will increasingly be treated nutritionally, in conjunction with talk therapy and life-style change.
- The underlying nutritional and immunological causes of allergy and autoimmune disease will be recognized. The therapy of choice for these disorders will become exclusively the province of nutritionally oriented physicians.

Now this is, admittedly, an optimist's view, and I am acutely aware that things could turn out differently. For modern medicine stands at an important crossroads. To move forward, we must stem the rising tide of degenerative disease and bring under control the overwhelming costs of medical care. But medicine cannot grow and meet the challenges of the future unless it broadens its scope and as long as it is hamstrung by the powerful vested interests of the FDA, the medical establishment, and the pharmaceutical industry.

Orthodox medicine may well be approaching a dead end. And I believe that the business community, which suffers the effects of poor employee health, and the insurance companies, which in the end have to pay the ever-escalating costs of poor health, will eagerly support change. There are indications of this support already, as corporations establish in-house fitness centers and upgrade the food in the company dining room—measures that universally result in decreased absenteeism and increased productivity. Insurance companies, slowly but surely, are starting to pay claims for non-mainstream therapies and for health care provided by health maintenance organizations—alternative group medical practices that charge all-inclusive annual fees and understandably, therefore, focus on prevention and self-care.

In the end, though, the future of medicine lies with *you.* It is your own actions and not the action of government or the curative powers of physicians and their potions that will keep you healthy. The place to start in your quest for optimum health is with your own nutritional and life-style habits, voting with your dollars by purchasing healthier, less chemicalized foods, with whatever noise you can make in favor of cleaning up the environment and in favor of your right to choose the type of health care you want. If there is to be a healthy future—for you, for your children, and for your loved ones—you, and only you, can make it happen. The potential for change is great. And the time for change is *now.*

Appendices

Glossary

ADDICTION. A maladaptation of the body to chronic STRESS, usually in the form of a drug or food. In order for the body to tolerate the stressful substance, the substance becomes incorporated as a necessary part of the body chemistry, resulting in a continuous need for it; withdrawal symptoms appear if the substance is withheld.

ADRENALINE. A "stress" hormone produced by the ADRENALS.

ADRENALS. Tiny glands, located atop the kidneys, which produce the so-called stress hormones: ADRENALINE, noradrenaline, and CORTISOL.

AMINO ACIDS. The building blocks of PROTEINS. Many are "essential" and must be gotten from protein foods in the diet; others are synthesized in the body from dietary proteins.

ANTIBODY. A PROTEIN, produced by B-lymphocyte plasma cells, which fights off the effects of a specific ANTIGEN, clearing it from circulation. The antibodies primarily involved in food allergy are IgG, IgE, IgA, and IgM.

ANTIGEN. Any substance that stimulates the production of an ANTIBODY when introduced into the system, i.e., dust, pollen, dander, petroleum products, drugs, bacteria, viruses, or an allergic food.

ANTIOXIDANTS. Certain chemicals and nutrients that block the destructive ability of FREE RADICALS, and thus must be present in sufficient quantities to protect vital tissue from damage. They include Vitamins A, C, E, B1, B5, B6, and beta carotene, the minerals zinc and selenium, the amino acid cysteine, and the chemicals BHT and BHA.

ARACHIDONIC ACID. A fatty acid, derived from saturated dietary fats. It is the PRECURSOR of "inflammatory" PROSTAGLANDINS of the 2 series.

ATOPIC ALLERGY. Often an IgE-mediated, Type I immediate reaction. It is involved with the release of HISTAMINE and other CHEMICAL MEDIATORS from the MAST CELLS and basophils, usually in response to airborne or contact irritants, but often to foods. Asthma, hay fever, rhinitis, and hives are the most common atopic allergies.

BASAL METABOLISM. The rate at which the body converts calories to energy when at rest.

BASAL TEMPERATURE. The temperature of the body at rest after a night's sleep.

BILE. An emulsifying substance, essential for the digestion and metabolization of fats. It is produced by the liver from cholesterol and stored and released by the gallbladder.

BLOOD SUGAR. GLUCOSE.

BRADYKININ. A powerful, pain-inducing CHEMICAL MEDIATOR.

BROWN FAT. The high-metabolic-fat tissue that makes up 10 to 15 percent of human body fat, located deep in the body along the ribs, shoulder blades and chest cavity.

CARBOHYDRATES. One of the three essential food groups, consisting of all compounds with carbon, hydrogen, and oxygen. They include starches, sugars, and related substances. Carbohydrates provide the primary energy source for the body.

CHEMICAL MEDIATORS. Chemicals released by certain cells of the immune system. They initiate a chemical chain reaction, usually involving inflammation.

CHOLESTEROL. A steroid alcohol involved in the biosynthesis of bile acids, adrenal hormones, sex hormones, and vitamin D. It is transported in the blood by low-density lipoprotein (LDL) and high-density lipoprotein (HDL).

CIRCULATING IMMUNE COMPLEX (CIC). An IMMUNE COMPLEX in the bloodstream.

CIS FATS. Fatty acids in their natural form, which the body is able to metabolize successfully. (Cf. TRANS FATS.)

CLINICAL ECOLOGY. Study of the impact of environmental conditions on the health of the body, especially the effect on allergy.

COMPLEMENT. A complex group of at least twenty different proteins, which are activated in the final stages of inflammatory allergic reactions, linking the antigen-antibody reaction to the inflammatory response, associated with the recruitment of other PROTEINS and cells involved in inflammation.

CORTISOL. A stress HORMONE derived from CHOLESTEROL and produced by the ADRENALS, in part as a response to stress.

CYTOTOXIC TEST. A food-allergy test that measures the damage done to white blood cells when put in contact with potential allergens. Among other drawbacks, it must be conducted under extremely rigorous and time-consuming laboratory conditions.

DEGENERATIVE DISEASE. Any chronic condition that causes a system or organ to lose function over a period of time. Cardiovascular disease, osteoporosis, and arthritis are prime examples.

DELTA-6-DESATURASE. The enzyme primarily responsible for the conversion of *cis linoleic acid* to GAMMA LINOLENIC ACID on the pathway to PGE1, and of *alpha linolenic acid* to EICOSAPENTAENOIC ACID on the pathway to PGE3.

DIS-STRESS. Harmful STRESS, such as illness, psychological overload, chronic nutritional deficiencies, or excessive exercise.

DOCOSAHEXAENOIC ACID (DHA). An ESSENTIAL FATTY ACID, derived from *alpha linolenic acid.* It is a PRECURSOR to PGE3.

EDEMA. Swelling of tissue as a result of water retention in the cells.

EICOSAPENTAENOIC ACID (EPA). An ESSENTIAL FATTY ACID, derived from *alpha linolenic acid.* It is a PRECURSOR to PGE3.

ENZYME. A PROTEIN catalyst produced by and formed in all cells, responsible for most of the chemical reactions of the body.

ESSENTIAL FATTY ACIDS. Nutrient fats that the body cannot produce on its own and which must therefore be obtained from dietary sources. *Cislinoleic acid* and *alpha linolenic acid* are true essential fats. GAMMA LINOLENIC ACID, EICOSAPENTAENOIC ACID, and DOCOSAHEXAENOIC ACID are often referred to as essential fatty acids, because dietary sources are scarce, and because many diet and life-style factors inhibit their synthesis in the body from cis linoleic and alpha linolenic acids. Essential fatty acids are the PRECURSORS to the PROSTAGLANDINS of the 1, 2, and 3 series.

EU-STRESS. Beneficial STRESS that allows the body to extend its limits and express its stored energy and emotions in a life- and health-promoting manner.

FIBER. The nondigestible cellular matter in vegetables, fruits, and grains, which aids in the absorption and clearance of toxins from the body and is needed for proper elimination.

FICA (Food Immune Complex Assay). The automated test clinically developed by Optimum Health Labs to measure the level of food-specific IgG ANTIBODIES and IMMUNE COMPLEXES in the blood.

FREE RADICALS. Chemically reactive substances produced in normal metabolism. They are highly destructive to tissue and are especially implicated in cancer, inflammatory disease, and cardiovascular disease. Their activity is neutralized by ANTIOXIDANTS.

GAMMA LINOLENIC ACID (GLA). An ESSENTIAL FATTY ACID, derived from *cis linoleic acid.* It is a PRECURSOR to PGE1.

GASTROINTESTINAL MUCOSA. The vital ⅛-inch-thick mucous lining of the gastrointestinal tract. It acts as a barrier against the passage of unwanted substances into the bloodstream and promotes the absorption of desirable substances. The integrity, or impermeability, of the gastric mucosa is vital to good health.

GLUCOSE. Blood sugar, the main unit of fuel used by every cell in the body. Its primary source is CARBOHYDRATES in the diet; excess is stored in the liver and muscle cells. The body synthesizes further glucose from certain AMINO ACIDS and glycogen.

HCl (hydrochloric acid). A gastric juice, produced in the stomach as an essential aid to digestion.

HDL (high-density lipoprotein). A fat protein molecule of CHOLESTEROL transportation that acts beneficially to remove excess cholesterol from circulation. Also see LDL.

HGH (human growth hormone). An important hormone released by the pituitary gland, important in the growth of children, immune function, and METABOLISM in adults.

HISTAMINE. A usually abundant CHEMICAL MEDIATOR, released by the MAST CELLS and basophils, most often in response to the presence of an allergen.

HORMONE. A substance released by one organ to regulate the function of other cells through stimulation or inhibition. Examples of hormones includes thyroid, adrenaline, progesterone, estrogen, insulin, and growth hormone.

HYPOCHLORHYDRIA. Deficiency of hydrochloric-acid secretion in the stomach in response to food. This common digestive disorder, which involves insufficient HCl production, is often found in conjunction with allergies, excessive alcohol consumption, and prostaglandin imbalance.

Ig (immunoglobulin). A chemical substance produced by plasma cells released into the bloodstream and secretions to bind with antigens. There are five major types: IgG, IgA, IgE, IgM, and IgD.

IgA (immunoglobulin A). The major class of ANTIBODY in tears, saliva, and airway and intestinal secretions. The secretory ANTIBODY released by the gallbladder as a first step in food-allergy response.

IgD (immunoglobulin D). The IgD ANTIBODY is present in human blood in very small quantities, presumbly due to its role as a receptor ANTIBODY on the surface of certain white blood cells. It seems to function in triggering the production of other antibodies by these cells.

IgE (immunoglobulin E). The ANTIBODY most commonly involved in Type I, immediate allergic reactions and also parasitic infections. It functions in allergic reactions due to its attachment to the surface of MAST CELLS and basophils. When the IgE antibodies react with allergens, the mast cell and basophil in turn respond with the release of pharmacologically active chemicals, which are responsible for the symptoms of allergy.

IgG (immunoglobulin G). The most important ANTIBODY in delayed food-allergy reactions, also involved in combating microorganisms and their toxins. IgG makes up about 80 percent of all serum antibodies.

IgM (immunoglobulin M). An ANTIBODY that binds with an ANTIGEN as it enters the bloodstream, tagging it for identification by the immune system. The first active defense against blood-borne bacteria. In humans, IgM constitutes about 10 percent of all antibodies.

IMMUNE COMPLEX. A large molecule, or macromolecule, formed by the combination of an ANTIBODY (usually IgG) and an ANTIGEN (often an allergic food, but also drugs, toxins, bacteria, viruses, and parasites).

INSULIN. A hormone produced primarily by the PANCREAS, the function of which is the regulation of blood sugar, or GLUCOSE. A lack of insulin production is associated with Type I juvenile diabetes mellitus.

LDL (low-density lipoprotein). A protein molecule that functions as a transport molecule for cholesterol, generally detrimental in excessive amounts. Also see HDL.

LESION. The diseased area of a tissue or an organ.

LIPID. An organic substance composed of carbon and hydrogen, as well as some oxygen. The main lipids in human blood are CHOLESTEROL, TRIGLYCERIDES, fatty acids, and phospholipids.

LUMEN. The empty space inside a tube; i.e., the lumen of the gastrointestinal tract.

M CELL. A specialized immune cell found in the lining of the digestive tract. Its function is to sample food and other substances eaten and to communicate the presence of ANTIGENS to the immune system, so that antibodies are produced if needed.

MAST CELLS. Guardian cells found in large quantities, primarily in the lining of the air passages and gastrointestinal tract and around small blood vessels, which release HISTAMINE, PROSTAGLANDINS, and other CHEMICAL MEDIATORS in response to allergens.

METABOLISM. The bodily conversion of a substance to its end product or use—e.g., the conversion of calories to heat and energy.

METASULFITES. A class of common chemical additives, widely used as a preservative in processed foods and to keep fresh foods looking fresh. Metasulfites are implicated in a wide varity of allergic reactions.

MICELLIZATION. The suspension of fat-soluble vitamins (specifically A and E) in a water base, to increase absorption and utilization.

MINERAL. An inorganic substance, vital to bodily functions, which must be obtained from dietary sources.

NIGHTSHADES. A plant family, the *Solanaceae,* which includes such popular foods as potato, tomato, pepper, paprika, and eggplant (as well as the drugs atropine and hyoscine). Nightshades are often associated with arthritis, according to some authorities.

OPIOIDS. A group of substances produced by the body that have narcoticlike properties, i.e., endorphins, enkephalins, dynorphins.

PANCREAS. An organ located behind the stomach and connected to the small intestines, which is vital to digestion and the regulation of blood sugar. It functions as an endocrine gland in the regulation of blood sugar, producing and releasing INSULIN and *glucagon* into the bloodstream. It functions as an exocrine gland in the digestive tract, producing and secreting digestive enzymes and bicarbonates.

PGE1. The generally beneficial series of PROSTAGLANDINS produced from cis linoleic acid and GAMMA LINOLENIC ACID.

PGE2. The potentially destructive series of PROSTAGLANDINS produced from ARACHIDONIC ACID (saturated fat).

PGE3. The generally beneficial series of PROSTAGLANDINS produced from *alpha linolenic acid* and EICOSAPENTAENOIC ACID.

pH. A measure of the acid or alkaline level of any substance. On a scale of 1–14, 1 is extremely acid, 7 is neutral, and 14 is extremely alkaline. The pH of the stomach is usually 2.0 or less, the blood 7.3 or so.

PLATELET. The smallest formed element in the blood, instrumental in blood clotting. Because of its clotting function it is perhaps the initiator of such pathologies as atherosclerosis.

PRECURSOR. An intermediary step in a chain of chemical reactions that indicates the approach to—or causes—the formation of an end reaction or condition. For example, GAMMA LINOLENIC ACID is a precursor of PGE1.

PROSTAGLANDINS. Short-lived, hormonelike substances, produced from ESSENTIAL FATTY ACIDS. They are found in virtually all cell membranes and control most metabolic functions. There are three major groups of prostaglandins; their levels must be kept in balance for optimum health.

PROSTANOIDS. A group of inflammatory CHEMICAL MEDIATORS associated with allergic symptoms, derived from ARACHIDONIC ACID. They include PGE2, PGF2 alpha, thromboxane A2, prostacyclin, and leukotrienes.

PROTEIN. A nitrogen-containing organic molecule, formed from AMINO ACIDS, literally speaking the framework and building block of all tissue. Protein is necessary for thousands of intricate biochemical reactions.

PSYCHOSOMATIC. An adjective used to describe a disease condition caused by psychological, as opposed to physiological, factors. The condition itself may cause secondary physical problems that are in and of themselves disease factors.

SENSITIVITY. A term often used (incorrectly) to mean *allergy.* It describes an abnormal response to external (usually chemical) irritants, but it is not a true ANTIBODY/ANTIGEN allergic reaction.

SEROTONIN. A brain neurotransmitter, the product of tryptophan metabolism, that influences mood and sleep, among other things.

STRESS (dis-stress). Any influence that upsets the natural equilibrium of the system.

THYMUS GLAND. The master gland of the immune system, located behind the breastbone, just above the heart.

TRACE MINERAL. An essential mineral, but one that is needed only in a minute amount for the maintenance of health.

TRANS FATS. Fatty acids in a form that the body is not able to metabolize successfully. They result form the alteration of CIS FATS by means of overheating, hydrogenation, and refining. Two common examples are the fats in margarine and shortening.

TRIGLYCERIDES. A type of body fat, formed by the binding of glycerol and fatty acids, obtained from fats in the diet. They are the main storage fats in man, accounting for 95 percent of fat tissue.

VITAMIN. An organic substance, essential to life. Vitamins must be obtained from dietary sources.

Mail-Order Food Sources

Deer Valley Farm
R.D. 1
Guilford, NY 13780
(607) 764–8556
Organic products, mostly grown on their organic farm. For organically raised poultry, beef, pork, and lamb, this is one of the best facilities in the country. Free catalog.

Ener-G Foods, Inc.
6901 Fox Avenue
PO Box 24723
Seattle, WA 98124
(206) 767–6660
Gluten- and wheat-free products, such as white and brown rice breads, rice hamburger buns, and wheat-free pastas. Ener-G also has some gluten-free sweets and an egg replacer for those with an egg allergy.

Walnut Acres
Penns Creek, PA 17862
(717) 837–0601
Canned and fresh vegetables from their own fields, organically grown; also dried fruits, nuts, and fresh preservative-free nut butters. Walnut Acres is one of the few organic farms that sells fresh vegetables in small quantities.

Better Foods, Inc.
251 North Washington St.
Greencastle, PA 17225
(717) 597–3105
A good source of grains, breads, honeys, syrups, cheeses, pastas, and vegetarian entrees, all additive-free. The catalog, available for a dollar, lists all the basic foods they carry, gives their nutritive values, and offers tips on preparing them.

Sources of Common Allergens

FOODS CONTAINING YEAST

Breads and Flours

Breads
Crackers
Pastries
Pretzels
Cake and cake mix
Hamburger and hotdog buns
Cookies
Flour enriched with vitamins from yeast
Rolls, homemade and canned
Milk fortified with vitamins from yeast
Meat fried in cracker crumbs

Other Hidden Sources of Yeast

Mushrooms
Truffles
Cheese of all kinds
Buttermilk
Cottage cheese
Vinegars (apple, gin, pear, grape, distilled)
Catsup
Mayonnaise
Olives
Pickles
Sauerkraut
Condiments
Tomato sauce
Chili peppers
Canned mincemeat
Gerber oatmeal
Barley cereal
Alcoholic beverages (whiskey, wine, brandy, rum, vodka)
Root beer
Malted products (cereals, candy, malted milk drinks)
Citrus fruit juices (frozen or canned)
Horseradish
French dressing
Salad dressing
Barbecue sauce
Many vitamin products are, in fact, derived from yeast or are their sources yeast.

Nutrients

B complex
Multivitamins with B complex
Selenium
Other trace minerals

SUBSTANCES CONTAINING CORN

Adhesives
Envelopes
Stamps
Stickers
Tapes
Ales
Aspirin and other tablets
Bacon
Baking mixes (biscuits, piecrusts, doughnuts, pancake mixes)
Baking powders
Batter for frying
Beers
Beverages (carbonated)
Bleached wheat flour
Bourbon and other whiskies
Breads and pastries
Cakes
Candies
Catsup
Cheeses
Chewing gum
Chili
Chop suey
Instant coffee
Cookies
Cornflakes
Cough syrups
Cream pies
Milk in paper cartons
Oleomargarine
Peanut butters
Canned peas
Powdered sugar
Preserves
Puddings, custards
Rice (coated)
Salad dressings
Sandwich spreads
Sauces for meats and sundaes
Sherbets
Dates (confection)
Deep-fat frying mixtures
French dressing
Fritos
Frostings
Fruits (canned and frozen)
Fruit juices
Frying fats
Gelatin dessert
Glucose products
Graham crackers
Grape juice
Gravies
Grits
Hams (cured/tenderized)
Ice creams
Inhalants (bath and body powders)
Popcorn
Starch
Jams, jellies
Meats (bologna, sausage)
Similac
String beans (canned and frozen)
Soups (creamed and vegetable)
Soybean milks
Sugar, powdered
Syrups: Commercial preparations (cartose, glucose, Karo, Puretose, Sweetose)
Talcums
Teas, instant
Toothpaste
Tortillas
Vegetables (canned, creamed, frozen)
Vanilla
Vinegar, distilled
Wines (some American wines are corn-free)

To the above list, add most available Vitamin C preparations, powder or tablet, which are derived from hydrolyzed cornstarch.

FOODS CONTAINING EGG

Baking powders
Batters for deep-frying
Bavarian cream
Boiled dressings
Bouillons
Breads
Breaded foods
Cakes
Cake flour
Fritters
Frostings
French toast
Griddle cakes
Glazed rolls
Hamburger mix
Hollandaise sauce
Ices
Ice cream
Icings
Macaroons
Malted cocoa drinks (Ovaltine, Ovomalt, and many others)
Macaroni
Meat loaf
Meat jellies
Marshmallows
Meat molds
Meringues (French torte)
Noodles
Pastes
Pancakes
Pancake flours
Patties
Puddings
Pretzels
Salad dressings
Sauces
Sausages
Sherbets
Soufflés
Spaghetti
Spanish creams
Soups (noodle, mock turtle, consommés)
Tartar sauce
Timbales
Waffles
Waffle mixes
Wines (often "cleared" with egg white)

FOODS CONTAINING WHEAT

Beverages

Beer
Cocomalt
Gin (any drink with grain neutral spirits)
Malted milk
Ovaltine
Postum
Whiskies

Breads

Biscuits
Crackers
Matzos
Muffins
Popovers
Pretzels
Rolls

Certain Kinds of Bread

Corn, gluten, graham, pumpernickel, rusk, rye, (rye products are not entirely free of wheat), wheat, soy, zwieback

Cereals

Bran flakes
Cornflakes

Cream of Wheat
Crackels
Farina
Grape-Nuts
Krumbles
Muffets
Pep
Pettijohns
Puffed wheat
Ralstons wheat cereal
Rice Krispies
Shredded Wheat
Triscuits
Wheatena
Other malted cereals

Flours

Buckwheat flour
Corn flour
Gluten flour
Graham flour
Lima bean flour
Patent flour
Pumpernickel flour
Rye flour
White flour
Whole wheat flour

Pastries and Desserts

Cakes
Candy bars
Chocolate candy
Cookies
Doughnuts
Frozen pies
Pies
Puddings

Nonbread Wheat Products

Dumplings
Macaroni
Noodles
Spaghetti

Miscellaneous

Barley malt
Bouillon cubes
Chocolate candy
Chocolate (except bitter cocoa and bitter chocolate)
Cooked mixed meat dishes
Cooked sausages (wiener, bologna, liverwurst, lunch ham)
Fats used for frying foods that are rolled in flour
Gravies
Griddle cakes
Hamburger
Hot cakes
Ice cream cones
Malt products
Mayonnaise
Meat rolled in flour
MSG
Pancake mixtures
Sauces
Soups
Synthetic pepper
Thickening in ice creams
Waffles
Wheat cakes
Wheat germ
Vitamin E from wheat-germ oil
Yeasts (some)

FOODS CONTAINING MILK

Baker's bread
Baking powder biscuits
Bavarian cream
Bisques
Blancmange
Boiled salad dressings
Butter
Buttermilk
Butter sauces
Cakes
Candies
Cheeses

Chocolate
Chowders
Cocoa drinks, mixtures
Cooked sausages
Cookies
Cream
Creamed foods
Cream sauces
Curds
Custards
Doughnuts
Flour mixtures
Food au gratin
Food fried in butter (fish, poultry, beef, pork)
Fritters
Gravies
Hamburgers
Hard sauces
Hash
Hot cakes
Ice creams
Junket
Malted milk
Mashed potatoes
Meat loaf
Oleomargarine
Omelets
Ovaltine
Ovomalt
Piecrust made with milk products
Prepared flour mixtures (biscuits, cake, cookies, doughnuts, muffins, pancakes, piecrust, waffles)
Rarebits
Salad dressings
Scrambled eggs and scalloped dishes
Sherbets
Soda crackers
Soufflés
Soups
Spumoni
Whey
Zwieback

FOODS CONTAINING COTTONSEED

Note: This listing is given to show the many uses to which cottonseed oil is put and the many things to be considered when it is recommended that all contact with cottonseed be avoided.

Cottonseed may be contacted in any of these forms:

Cottonseed Meal Products

Cottonseed cake and meal are used as (1) fertilizer and (2) feed for cattle, poultry, horses, hogs and sheep; (3) the flower is used for human food. It is used sometimes to make gin. It is also used to make xylose or wood sugar. Xylose has a sweet taste and may be used in soft drinks, but to our knowledge, it is not used in the common soft drinks. Be sure to watch for and avoid all these contacts.

Cottonseed Oil

The finest cottonseed oil is used for food. Most salad oils contain this oil, as do most oleomargarines. Mayonnaises and salad dressings are almost always made with cottonseed oil, unless made at home. Lard compound and lard substitutes are made with cottonseed oil. Sardines may be packed in cottonseed oil. Most commercial frying and baking (cakes, breads, fish, popcorn, potato chips, and doughnuts) are done with cottonseed oil. This oil is used almost universally in restaurants.

Cottonseed is used in some cosmetics.

Cottonseed oil is used to polish fruit at fruit stands. Check for this!

Cottonseed is secreted in the milk of animals. Since these seeds are often fed to cattle, you will have to omit milk if you cannot get it from animals not fed cottonseed.

Cottonseed Oil Products*

Shortening

Advance
Bakerite
Mrs. Tucker's
Scoco
Jasimine
Creantex
Humko
Jewel
Snowdrift
Crisco
Flako
Armour's Vegetable

Oleomargarines

Meadowlake
Cotton Blossom
Allsweet
Nucoa
Dixi
Good Luck

Salad oils

Wesson
Winco
Mrs. Tucker's
Contadina
Magnolia
Jewel Oil
Margherita
Crustene
Esskey
Armour's Star

Miscellaneous Cottonseed Oil Products

Barbecue sauce
Popcorn in oil
Dry lemonade mix
Sweet and sour dressing
Tartar sauce
Cheese pizza mix

FOODS CONTAINING THE NIGHTSHADES

The Nightshades

1. White potatoes (includes the red-skin potato; does not include the yellow sweet potato or the yam)
2. Eggplant (includes all sizes, shapes, and kinds)
3. Tomatoes (includes yellow, plum, cherry, and ground cherry tomatoes)
4. Tobacco (includes all sources of tobacco: pipe, cigar, and cigarette tobacco; first- and second-hand smoke)
5. Paprika
6. Chili peppers (includes cherry, red cluster, pimiento, chili, long, red, Tabasco, and cayenne peppers)
7. Garden peppers (includes bell and sweet green garden peppers)
8. Certain drugs (includes all drugs containing atropine, belladonna, and scopolamine; found in most sleeping pills)

*This is only a partial list of shortenings, oleos, and salad oils.

White Potato Is Found In:

Some inexpensive yogurts
Some baby foods
Beef stew (hash)
Some biscuits (from potato flour)
Some breads
Potato chips
Clam chowder
Consommé
Some doughnuts
Some gravies
Yeast (?)
Some fish cakes
Meatballs
Meat loaf
Pirogies
Frozen beef, chicken, turkey pies
Taco sauce
Many dry canned soups (e.g., green pea, split pea)
Mixed vegetables (frozen and canned)
White potato starch

Chili Peppers Are Found In:

Relishes
Stuffed salad olives
Smoked herring
Many frozen pies (chicken, turkey)
Frozen onion rings
Some Italian bread crumbs
Frozen chicken legs
Seasoned cookies
Frozen crabs
Chinese mixed vegetables
Many herb teas (as capsicum)
Other capsicum-containing foods
Pinkish-colored cheeses
Some Vitamin C tabletsSo-called natural flavors (used in sodas, spices, etc.)
Many salad dressings
Foods labelled with the word "spices"
Most Italian foods
Many snack dips (bean, enchilada)
Many mayonnaises
Soy sauce (has red pepper)
Some pickles
Hamburger relish
Some gravies
Some cough lozenges
Some pain ointments
Bologna
Hotdogs
DOES NOT include black and white pepper

Paprika Is Found In:

Some cheeses
Some herb teas
Some so-called natural flavors (used in sodas, spices, etc.)
Some peanut butters
Dry-roasted peanuts
On macaroni salads in restaurants
Most mayonnaises (labelled or not)
Foods labelled with the word 'spices"
Spiced salts
Some salad dressings
Sprinkled over fish dishes and seafoods in restaurants

Tomatoes Are Found In:

Some baby foods
Tomato sauce
Chili sauce
Barbecue sauce
Tomato paste
Some meat sauces
Bloody Mary mix
Many vegetable and meat stews
Tomato juice
Chicken mixes for fried chicken
Most salad dressings (Russian, NL French, Thousand Island)
Tortilla chips
Some herring fillets
Many TV dinners
Canned spaghetti and meatballs
Many delicatessen foods
Many soups
Vegetable juices (e.g., V-8)
Canned baked beans
Canned chow mein
Hamburger Helper
Most Italian food (frozen, canned, and dry)
Meat loaf
Spanish rice (canned)

FOODS CONTAINING SOYBEAN

Bakery Goods

Breads
Rolls
Cakes
Pastries (many)
Several crisp crackers

Sauces

Heinz Worcestershire sauce
La Choy Sauce
Lea & Perrin sauce
Oriental Show You Sauce

Cereals

Buc Wheats
Cellu Soy Flakes
Honey Comb
Sunlets
Super Sugar Crisp

Salad Dressings

E-P-K French dressing
Many brands of oil
Many prepared salad dressings

Meats

Lunch meats
Pork link sausage

Candies

Caramel
Hard candies
Nut candies

Milk Substitutes

Mull-Soy
Sobee

Miscellaneous

Baby foods (some contain soybeans or soy flour. Check all labels.)
Cheese, tofu, natto, and miso (as well as some others)
Coffee substitutes
Crisco, Spry, and other shortenings
Custards
Dry lemonade mix
Ice cream (some brands)
Lecithin (invariably derived from soybean and used in candies to pre-

Miscellaneous *(cont'd)*

vent drying and to emulsify the fats.)
Oleomargarine and butter substitutes
Soybean noodles, macaroni, and spaghetti
Soups (check the labels)
Soybean sprouts (served as vegetables in some Chinese dishes)

Contact Sources

Varnish, paints, enamels, printing ink, candles, celluloid, cloth, massage creams, linoleum, paper sizing, adhesives, fertilizer, nitroglycerine, paper finishes, blankets, grease, Gro-Pup dog food, French's fish food, soap, automobile parts, fodder, glycerine, textile dressings, lubricating oil, and illuminating oil.

New Soybean Contacts

Many new contact sources are to be expected each year with the introduction of new products. If you remember that soybeans are used in flour, oil, milk, and nuts, it will be possible to anticipate most of the new contacts with soybean products.

Substitutes and Alternatives to Allergic Foods

DAIRY ALTERNATIVES

Nondairy Sources of Calcium

When you limit your intake of milk, cheese, and dairy products, take care that you are still getting enough dietary calcium from other sources:

Fish
Salmon
Sardines
Shrimp
Clams
Crabmeat
Oysters
Cod
Haddock

Vegetables
Kelp
Chick-peas
Collard greens
Turnip greens
Broccoli
Cabbage
Carrots
Parsley
Watercress
Romaine
Summer squash
Onions

Grains and Nuts
Pistashios
Sesame seeds
Sesame butter
Soy
Oat flakes
Buckwheat
Cream of wheat
Whole wheat
Brown rice
Carob flavor

Fruit, etc.
Figs
Molasses
Maple syrup
Maple syrup
Eggs

Milk Alternatives

When looking for a milk substitute to use as a beverage or as an addition to cereals, nuts offer a reasonably high calcium source. A heaping teaspoon of carob powder added to 8 ounces of nut milk will provide the calcium equivalent of cow's milk.

Almond Milk

Makes 1 cup

½ cup blanched almonds
water

1. Place blanched almonds in blender.
2. Add enough water to cover blender blades.
3. Blend at high speed until creamy.
4. Add water to get consistency desired.
5 Strain if desired through fine sieve.

Note: Cashew, sunflower, or sesame seeds may be substituted for almonds. Follow same procedure.

Soy Milk

Soy milks are available prepared or in powdered form at health food stores.

Both the above milks can be sweetened with a small amount of malt (if you are not allergic), honey, molasses, or maple syrup. Flavorings such as carob, vanilla, or cinnamon are also good. Fruits such as banana or peaches make a "milkshake."

Butter Alternatives

Butter is very high in saturated fats and cholesterol. Even if you are not allergic to it you may want to cut down or eliminate it from your diet in favor of cold-pressed polyunsaturated vegetable and seed oils that are high in essential fatty acids.

Beware of processed margarines, however, for all are high in trans fats. Furthermore, they often contain highly allergic preservatives, food colorings, and other chemicals; read the labels carefully. Ideally, use only cold-pressed vegetable and seed oils and use nut spreads or other condiments in place of butter on toast.

Lite Better Butter

Makes 1½ cups

4 ounces butter, room temperature
½ cup unrefined cold-pressed oil
⅓–½ cup filtered spring water

1. Add butter and oil to blender.
2. Whip slowly.
3. Gradually add water until mixture is smooth.
4. Transfer to covered container and store in refrigerator.

Whipped Cream Substitute

Makes 1 cup

1 very ripe banana
1 egg white

1. Puree or mash the banana.
2. Beat egg white to soft peaks.
3. Add banana and continue beating until well blended with firm peaks.

The Cheese Alternative

Cheese is also high in saturated fats and cholesterol; even if you are not allergic, you might want to consider alternatives to this common diet staple.

Tofu, or soybean curd, is a useful substitute in cooking, on sandwiches, and in salads. Highly nutritious, it contains as much protein as cheese, has no cholesterol, and has one-third the calories. It can be kept fresh by storing it in water in the refrigerator, slicing as needed.

Marinated in fresh cold-pressed oils and herbs, it takes on a wide variety of flavors and can be served as a side dish to fish and chicken.

It can be used for cooking in place of cheese toppings or mixed in with vegetable casseroles.

Tofu can also be used as a substitute for eggs in some recipes: 2 ounces tofu equal 1 egg.

Tofu Sour Cream Substitute

Makes 1½ cups

8 ounces tofu
1 tablespoon lemon juice

1. Bring 2 cups water to a boil. Add ½ teaspoon salt.
2. Drop in tofu and allow water to return to a boil.
3. As soon as it begins boiling again, remove from heat and allow to sit for 3 minutes.

4. Remove tofu, drain, and place in center of 2 layers of 12-inch × 12-inch cheesecloth. Twist double layers of cloth tightly to drain all excess liquid. Remove cheesecloth.
5. Combine tofu and lemon juice in blender.
6. Puree till smooth.

Tofu Yogurt

Makes 2 cups

12 ounces tofu | *¼ teaspoon salt*
2 tablespoons of honey | *½ teaspoon vanilla*

1. Blend all ingredients together in blender or food processor.
2. Store in refrigerator, covered tightly.

This product may be used in any recipe that calls for yogurt.

And tofu ice cream, Tofutti (nondairy, no cholesterol), is available in most parts of the country. It tastes great, but it is high in simple sugar, so eat it only in moderation.

QUALITY PROTEIN WITHOUT MEAT

Meat, particularly red meat, is the main source of protein in the American diet. While meat provides whole proteins needed for amino-acid balance, it is also high in saturated fats and cholesterol and calories; many people eat meat too often. However, it can be eliminated from many recipes without sacrificing flavor or nutrition.

Vegetables, grains, and seeds, when combined properly, offer the same nutritional balance. The protein from various plant sources complement each other, forming "complete" proteins when eaten together. Because amino acids (the building blocks of proteins) are not stored in the body, you must eat complementary plant sources together to form the complete protein you need.

Complete proteins are formed by eating foods from any two groups in the chart on the following page.

WHOLE GRAIN ALTERNATIVES

Fortunately for those with wheat allergies or gluten intolerance, there are many other grains to choose from. Several nutritious (and often neglected) alternatives to wheat are discussed on the following pages.

Figure 8

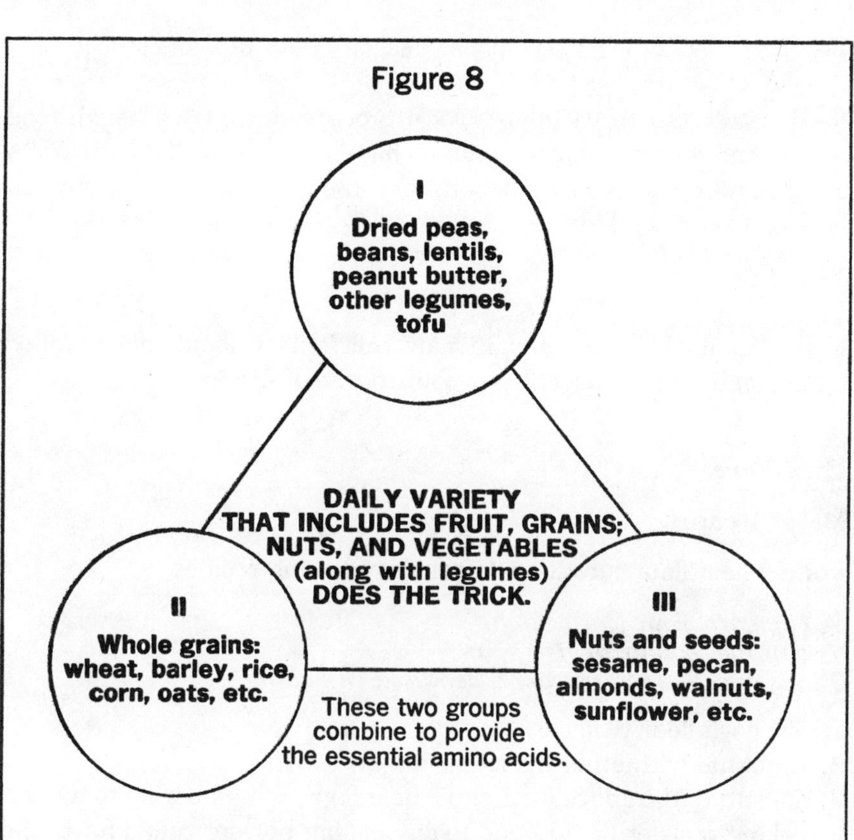

Combine groups I and II in such items as:

1. Corn-soy pones.
2. Rice and "curry" (made with lentils).
3. Bean and pea soups with wheat or whole grain crackers.
4. Rice-bean toppings.
5. Peanut butter sandwiches.
6. Noodle (whole grain)-bean casseroles.

Combine groups I and III in such items as:

1. Use ⅙–⅒ part nuts and seeds in roasts, patties, etc.
2. Garbanzo-sesame dip.
3. Garbanzo-cashew spread.
4. Roasted seeds with meals.
5. Nuts with meals.

Combine groups II and III in such items as:

1. Cereals with nuts or seeds.
2. Whole grain breads with nut and seed spreads.
3. Whole grain cookies and bars with nuts and seeds added.
4. Breads and rolls with added nutmeats.
5. Rice or millet pilaf.

If you can't find them in your local grocery store, try a health food outlet. And remember, grains can be highly allergenic. Rotate them! A list of allowed and prohibited foods for those with gluten sensitivity can be found on page 376.

Corn

Corn is a valuable grain, high in many nutrients. It should not be relied on alone, however, since it is a poor source of niacin.

Corn Flour

Makes 1 cup

For a wheat flour substitute in common baking recipes:

½ cup corn flour (cornstarch)
½ cup rye, potato, or rice flour
2 teaspoons baking powder when used in baking

1. Sift corn flour twice.
2. Combine with other flour.
3. Substitute the above for 1 cup wheat flour, remembering to use the baking powder (in addition to any baking powder called for in the recipe).

Cornmeal

Stone-ground cornmeal has a nutrient-rich germ and a fine flavor. Yellow cornmeal is higher in Vitamin A than white meal. It can be used for toppings, muffins, breads, and cereals. To cook cornmeal cereal:

2 cups water
1 cup cornmeal

1. Bring water to a boil.
2. Add cornmeal and stir well.
3. Reduce heat and simmer for 25 minutes, stirring frequently.

Cornmeal and flour can be used in the following foods:

Tacos	Breads	Chips
Tortillas	Cereals	Snack sticks
Fritters	Pastas	Polenta

Whole Grain Rice

Whole grain brown rice offers both nutrition and variety to any diet. Avoid white or polished rice, since it is stripped of most nutrients.

Whole grain rice can be served in combination with almost any food, added to a wide variety of casseroles, or toasted in a hot skillet to give a nutlike flavor to toppings on vegetables and soups.

Makes 2 cups

2 cups water
1 cup rice

1. Bring water to a boil. Add rice and stir several times.
2. Cover and lower heat to gentle simmer.
3. Simmer without removing the cover for 45 minutes.
4. Remove from heat and let sit, covered, for 5 minutes.

Rice Flour

Rice flour can be used in baking in place of wheat. Substitute 7/8 cup rice flour for 1 cup wheat flour. For baking, do *not* use "sweet" rice flour. It is too sticky. Save it for use in sauces and gravies.

Rice flour and whole rice can be used in the following foods:

Crackers
Cakes
Casseroles
Cereals
Snack bars (granola, etc)
Complement to beans and vegetables

Puffed Rice

Puffed rice makes great cereal. It can also be heated in the oven and seasoned with oil, curry, and ginger for snacks.

Rye

Rye can be used in baking, but may be too heavy for use alone in leavened doughs. Substitute 1¼ cups rye for 1 cup wheat flour. Sourdough starter is often used in all-rye breads.

Rye Meal

Rye meal is simply coarse-ground rye flour. Substitute 1 cup of rye meal for 1 cup of wheat flour.

Rye meal, whole rye, and rye flour can be used in the following foods:

Cream of rye cereal
Crackers
Breads (Essene brand)

Barley

Barley is another valuable grain, easy to use in soups, as a side dish, or as a complement to vegetable casseroles. When substituting barley flour for wheat flour, use ⅔ cup barley for each cup of wheat. Barley flakes can be used as a hot cereal or a substitute for oatmeal in baking.

Whole Barley

Makes 3 cups

To serve as a side dish:

1½ cup water
½ cup whole barley

1. Bring water to a boil and add barley.
2. Cover and simmer for 30 to 40 minutes.

Whole barley and barley flakes can be used in the following foods:

Cereal
Soups
Breads and muffins
Complement to beans and vegetables

Oats

Oats are higher in protein than any other grain and are quickest to prepare. Be sure to use unprocessed rolled or steel-cut oats.

Oat Flour

Can be used in combination with other flours for baking in a mixture that is ⅓ oat flour to ⅔ other flour. Results are best when the oat flour is soaked in enough boiling water to moisten and then the shortening is added to that mixture. When it is cooled, add the other flour and leavening.

Oatmeal

Makes 2 cups

Oatmeal can be used as a filler in casseroles or to replace wheat flour in some recipes. Use 1½ cup rolled oats for each cup of wheat flour. Oatmeal cereal is an old favorite:

2 cups water
1 cup oats
dash salt
cinnamon
raisins if desired

1. Bring water to a boil. Stir in oats and salt.
2. Cover and simmer for 15 minutes.
3. Uncover and add cinnamon and raisins. Cook for 5 minutes more.
4. Serve with milk or yogurt.

Oatmeal and oat flour can be used in the following foods:

Cereals
Breads and muffins
Toppings

Millet

Millet is a small golden pearl, highly alkaline and filled with vitamins and minerals. Though an uncommon grain in Western countries (for human diets), it can be used in many common recipes, as well as exotic cookery. Millet flour is available, although recipes calling for it are hard to find.

Whole Millet

Makes 2 cups

When cooked as a side dish:

2½ cups water
1 cup millet

1. Bring water to a boil.
2. Add millet and stir several times.
3. Cover and lower heat to simmer. Cook for 30 to 40 minutes.
4. Let stand, covered, away from heat, for 5 minutes before serving.

Once you have cooked the millet, it can be used for millet cereals as well. Another interesting variation is a millet burger.

Millet Burgers

Makes 6 servings

4 cups cooked millet
2 eggs, beaten
⅓ cup toasted sesame seeds or sunflower seeds
seasoning as desired

1. Mix ingredients. Chill for 10 minutes.
2. Form patties.
3. Dredge in a sprinkling of flour.
4. Heat ¼ cup oil in skillet.
5. Brown patties on both sides, about 10 minutes altogether.

Cooked soybeans, rice, or kidney beans may be used in place of the millet. Grated cheese may be added, as may Tomato Sauce Substitute (see page 459) for a topping.

Millet can be used in the following foods:

Puffed cereal
Hot cooked cereal
Millet flour (if available) for muffins and breads

Buckwheat or Kasha

Buckwheat is not a grain at all, but the seed of an herb that somewhat resembles rice. As a flour it makes good griddle cakes and muffins. The Japanese make a noodle from 100 percent buckwheat flour marketed under the name "Soba." The coarse-ground version of this grain is known as groats.

Buckwheat Groats

Makes 2 cups

To prepare as a cereal:

2½ cups water
1 cup buckwheat (kasha: can be purchased already toasted)

1. Bring water to a boil.
2. Add buckwheat and stir briefly.
3. Cover and lower heat.
4. Simmer for 15 minutes.
5 Remove from heat and let stand for 5 minutes.

OTHER FLOUR SUBSTITUTES

Carob

Not strictly speaking a grain, carob powder is ground from the pod of a leguminous evergreen tree of the Mediterranean area. When used to replace wheat flour, it must be combined with another flour: 1/8 to 1/4 cup carob flour to 7/8 cup of the other. Do not bake at temperatures over 300 degrees F since it scorches very easily.

Carob can serve as a satisfying substitute for chocolate. Here is a simple carob "chocolate sauce."

Makes 1½ cups

1 cup sifted carob powder
1 cup water
1/4–1/2 cup honey
2 tablespoons oil

1. Blend all ingredients in blender or mixer.
2. Pour into pan and bring to a boil.
3. Keep heat very low and stir constantly.
4. Simmer for 8 to 10 minutes, being careful not to burn.
5. Store in covered jar in the refrigerator.

Soy Flour

Soy contains twice the protein and half the starch of whole wheat flour. Although it cannot be substituted in most recipes for wheat flour, it can be added to other flours to increase the nutritional value of foods.

Potato Flour (Starch)

Potatoes are a wonderful food—if the nightshades (see page 437) are not a problem for you. You can use potato flour as a wheat substitute in sauces, gravies, and cakes, especially when combined with another flour.

As a thickener, use 1½ teaspoons potato flour for 1 teaspoon wheat flour. In baking use 5/8 cup potato flour for 1 cup wheat flour.

Fiber Foods: Sources of Nongrain Dietary Fiber

An optimal diet is high in fiber, which is essential to good digestion, regulation of cholesterol, and intestinal health. Whole grains are an excellent source, but grains present the problem of allergy when eaten too frequently. To get enough fiber in your diet without eating members of the cereal grain family, we suggest that you substitute vegetables, legumes, and fruits high in fiber.

TIPS FOR INCREASING DIETARY FIBER

- Don't peel fruits and vegetables before eating.
- Increase consumption of beans and other legumes.
- Eat fresh fruit for dessert instead of sweets.
- Eat at least one serving of raw vegetable each day.
- Eat your potato skins.
- Use chopped fruit as a topping for yogurt and cereals.

Table 56 — Nongrain Sources of Dietary Fiber

Fiber Content of Vegetables	Grams of Fiber per Average Serving	Fiber Content of Fruit	Grams of Fiber per Average Serving
Artichokes (French)	.96	Apples (all varieties)	1.0
Beans		Blackberries	4.1
Lima (fresh)	.90	Blueberries	1.2
Snap (string)	1.05	Figs	
Beet greens	1.05	Fresh	1.7
Broccoli	1.30	Dried	1.8
Brussel sprouts	1.30	Huckleberries	1.2
Parsnips	1.65	Pears	1.4
Peas (green, shelled)	1.65	Raspberries	
		Black	3.5
		Red	2.8
Squash (winter)	1.40	Strawberries	1.2
		Tangerines	1.0
Sweet potatoes	1.00	Watermelon	.9

Sugar Alternatives

For allergy as well as nutritional reasons you should be cutting back or eliminating your consumption of sugars, especially refined ones. At the very least you should avoid white table sugar (sucrose) when possible in favor of sugars with some nutritional value, and you should rotate the sugars you do use. Below is a list of commonly used sugars, names you are likely to discover on the manufacturer's labels of processed supermarket foods.

SUCROSE

A sugar obtained from beets and sugar cane. Sucrose is the source of refined white table sugar. It has no fiber, no vitamins, no protein, no minerals—only "empty" calories. It is highly allergenic and addictive. Sucrose is broken down in the digestive track into glucose and fructose.

RAW SUGAR

A sugar obtained from the evaporation of sugar cane juice. Raw sugar is coarser than sucrose and tan in color, and it does retain some of the nutrients found in raw cane.

TURBINADO

A refined "raw" sugar with the impurities and molasses removed. Since it's molasses that contains the nutrients found in unrefined sugar, turbinado has fewer nutrients and more empty calories than raw sugar.

BROWN SUGAR

Refined soft sugar crystals coated in molasses syrup give brown sugar a heartier flavor and color. It is 91–96 percent sucrose.

TOTAL INVERT SUGAR

A liquid sweetener, sweeter than white table sugar. It is formed by chemically and enzymatically splitting sucrose into glucose and fructose.

HONEY

A combination of simple sugars: glucose, fructose, maltose, and sucrose.

CORN SYRUPS

Sweet syrups produced by the action of enzymes or acids on cornstarch and composed of the simple sugars fructose and dextrose. Highly addictive and allergenic, corn syrup is found in many commercially prepared foods. Dextrose from corn is often blended with sucrose to make refined table sugar.

FRUCTOSE (or levulose)

Fruit sugar. It appears naturally in fruits, though it may be derived from corn products. Fructose is considerably sweeter than sucrose.

DEXTROSE (or glucose)

A crystalline sugar occurring widely in nature. Also called corn sugar, it is often sold blended with white sugar, and is extensively used in bakery products, soft drinks, and processed foods.

LACTOSE

Natural milk sugar. Prepared lactose is used mostly by the drug industry.

SORBITOL, MANNITOL, MALITOL, AND XYLITOL

Sugar alcohols. They all occur naturally in fruits but are also commercially produced from dextrose (a corn derivative) and other plant sources. Often used as sugar substitutes.

Recipes

BAKING AND COOKING SUBSTITUTIONS

It's the little incidental ingredients that can pose a big problem when you are working out a diet that avoids allergenic foods. Here are some simple tricks:

Thickener for Sauces and Gravies

For 1 tablespoon wheat flour, substitute

½ tablespoon arrowroot powder, or
½ tablespoon rice flour, or
2 teaspoons tapioca flour, or
½ tablespoon cornstarch, or
1 tablespoon buckwheat flour, or
½ tablespoon potato flour (starch)

Salt

For salt, substitute the equivalent quantity of

- kelp powder
- lemon juice
- tamari soy sauce
- miso (if not allergic to yeast and soy)
- Morton's Lite Salt
- all-purpose seasoning mix (recipe follows)

All-Purpose Seasoning Mix

2 teaspoons onion powder
¼ teaspoon pepper
¼ teaspoon garlic powder
1 teaspoon dry mustard
1 teaspoon paprika
½ teaspoon dried thyme
½ teaspoon celery seeds
2 teaspoons dried basil flakes
½ teaspoon dried parsley flakes
½ teaspoon dried marjoram

1. Mix together any or all of the above.
2. Use as seasoning on fish, chicken, eggs, and stews.

Eggs

In cooking, 1 egg can be replaced by

½ teaspoon baking powder
2 tablespoons lemon juice or water

1. Blend well and add to recipe.

or

2 ounces drained fresh tofu (soybean curd)

1. Remove as much liquid as possible.
2. Beat till smooth and creamy and add to recipe.

or

Egg replacer, available at the health food store.

Milk

In baking, 1 cup of milk can be replaced by

1 cup water
½ teaspoon baking soda
1 teaspoon lemon juice or vinegar

Blend well and add to recipe. Substitute any juice for water if you desire.

Honey

Honey may be used in place of refined sugar in most recipes. It is sweeter than sugar however: ½ to ¾ cup honey equals 1 cup sugar. Remember to remove 1 to 2 tablespoons liquid from recipe for each cup of honey you use to replace refined sugar.

BASIC CONDIMENTS AND SAUCES

Many of those convenient condiments and flavorings we have come to depend on from the jar and bottle—everything from catsup to mayonnaise to tomato sauce—contain numerous chemicals and highly allergenic ingredients and sugars that are undesirable. The following recipes are included to help you prepare easy substitutes. Look in your favorite whole-food cookbook for even more suggestions.

Sauces

Cashew Spread

Makes ½ cup

If you are allergic to eggs you may want to use commercially available soy mayonnaise. But if soy allergy is also a problem, consider this alternative:

1 cup raw, unsalted cashews
1 teaspoon dry mustard
½ cup cold-pressed safflower oil
2 tablespoons lemon juice

Optional:

½ teaspoon celery salt
1 clove garlic, minced

1. Place cashews and mustard in food processor or blender.
2. Puree till smooth.
3. Slowly add oil, continuing to blend.
4. Add lemon juice very slowly. Season to taste.

Substitutions

- Use almonds or tahini (sesame butter) for cashews.
- Use ½ teaspoon minced ginger in place of mustard.
- Use white distilled vinegar for lemon juice.
- Use sea salt for celery salt.

Additional Sauces Made with Mayonnaise

Once you have found a mayonnaise substitute, you can make any or all of the other sauces that generally call for a mayonnaise base. For example:

- tartar sauce
- aioli sauce
- horseradish sauce
- curry mayonnaise
- fruit salad mayonnaise
- sauce verte for fish
- remoulade
- Russian dressing
- Thousand Island dressing

Another variation possible in many recipes, although it does alter taste and texture slightly, is to use yogurt in place of all or part of the mayonnaise.

Tomato Sauce Substitute

Makes 3 cups

A staple for almost every cuisine from Italian to American, basic tomato sauce can be a problem if you must eliminate nightshades from your diet. But the following are very palatable alternatives.

2 pounds carrots
1 large beet
juice of 1 lemon

1. Scrape the carrots and beet and cut into chunks.
2. Place in boiling water. Cook for 10 minutes.
3. Drain and place in food processor or blender. Add lemon juice and blend till creamy, adding just enough water to facilitate blending. Season if desired with flavoring agents such as celery seed, dill, salt, or basil. If food processor or blender is not available, mash with fork in a bowl.

Substitute for equal quantities of tomato sauce in any recipe.

Additional Sauces Made with Tomato Sauce Substitute

Once you've mastered the simple basic sauce above, you can add a wide variety of seasonings, to adapt it for many types of dishes.

- barbecue sauce
- tomato-cheese sauce
- shrimp cocktail sauce
- Mexican sauce
- spaghetti sauce—with or without meat
- creole sauce

Catsup

Makes 1½ cups

2 pounds tomatoes
1 medium onion
4 tablespoons honey
½ cup cider vinegar
½ teaspoon celery salt
1 teaspooon salt
½ teaspoon pepper

1. Quarter tomatoes and mince onion.
2. Place all ingredients in a heavy saucepan.
3. Simmer until tomatoes are soft.
4. Put through food mill or strainer.
5. Return to pan. Simmer, stirring often, until sauce is desired consistency.

Substitutions

- Vinegar may be reduced to ¼ cup. Add ½ cup tomato juice if desired.
- Green pepper may be used in place of onion.
- Lemon juice may be substituted for vinegar.
- Horseradish may be added to make a shrimp cocktail sauce.
- Chili powder may be added to make a Mexican sauce.

Tomato Paste

Makes 2 cups

2 tablespoons oil or butter or combination of both
1 medium onion
2 teaspoons flour
3 pounds ripe tomatoes, chopped
1 teaspoon honey (optional)
2 cloves garlic, minced
1 tablespoon chopped parsley
1 bay leaf
salt to taste

1. Heat oil in large saucepan
2. Mince onion and add to pan. Sauté until tender.
3. Slowly stir in flour to make roux.
4. Cook for 3 minutes to remove raw taste.
5. Add tomatoes, honey, garlic, parsley, bay leaf, and salt.
6. Cover pan and cook slowly for 10 minutes.
7. Uncover, stir and simmer for 1 hour until rich and thick.
8. Remove bay leaf.
9. Store in refrigerator or freezer until needed.

Substitutions

Any seasoning may be used in place of those specified. Suggestions: basil, tarragon, rosemary.

Salsa

Makes ½ cup

1 clove garlic, minced
½ cup chopped onion
1 tablespoon oil
4 large fresh tomatoes, chopped
Green chili peppers to taste
¼ teaspoon salt

1. Sauté garlic and onion in oil.
2. Add tomatoes, chili peppers, and salt.
3. Simmer uncovered for 7 to 8 minutes.
4. Chill. Serve with Mexican food, vegetables, or corn chips.

Nut Sauces and Spreads

Oriental dishes, dips with fresh vegetables, sandwiches, and dessert toppings can all be made with nut sauces and spreads.

Nut Butter Deluxe

Makes 1½ cups

1 cup nut butter
1 cup toasted sunflower seeds
½ cup raisins
2 tablespoons honey

1. Put all ingredients into blender.
2. Blend until smooth and store in refrigerator.

Substitutions

- Any nut butter may be used. Health food stores normally carry sesame, sunflower, almond, peanut, and cashew butter.
- Sesame seeds can be used in place of sunflower seeds.
- Dates or any dried fruit may be used in place of raisins.
- Unsweetened apple sauce may be used in place of honey.

Spicy Nut Sauce

Makes 1 cup

2 tablespoons chopped green pepper
1 small onion, minced
1 tablespoon oil
1 cup chopped tomato
¼ teaspoon salt
½ teaspoon chopped jalapeño pepper or ¼ teaspoon cayenne pepper
⅓ cup nut meal (walnuts, pecans, or sunflower seeds, ground into a meal)
¼ cup water

1. Sauté green pepper and onion in oil until tender.
2. Add tomato and cook for 5 minutes or until soft.
3. Stir in salt, pepper, and nut meal.
4. Gradually add water, stirring to make a creamy sauce.
5. Heat through and adjust spices to taste.

Peanut Sauce for Vegetables, Rice, or Noodles

Makes ½ cup

½ cup yogurt
2 tablespoons peanut or other nut butter
2 teaspoons prepared mustard
dash fresh lemon juice

1. Blend yogurt into peanut butter.
2. Add remaining ingredients.
3. Serve with hot or cold vegetables.

BREADS, MUFFINS, PANCAKES, AND CRACKERS

There are many alternatives to using wheat flour in baking breads, crackers, muffins, and biscuits. Yeast-free doughs are also available and easy to make. If you rely on these recipes and read through your favorite cookbook, you'll have many tasty choices.

The Universal Cracker Recipe

Makes 6 servings

Many health food stores offer specialty flours: corn, barley, millet, buckwheat, oat, lima bean, garbanzo bean, tapioca, potato flour, rice, and so on. You can also make your own using a hand mill or a small electric nut and seed grinder, available at health food stores. To make crackers, experiment with the following recipe until you get the consistency and taste you want. You'll be surprised how *easy* it is, and you avoid the problems of yeast, sugar, additives, preservatives, etc.

1 cup flour
½ teaspoon baking soda (optional)
¾ cup liquid (water, soup, or milk
2 teaspoons oil
seasoning as you wish: garlic, herbs, seeds, nuts, or grated vegetables

1. Combine flour and baking soda
2. Blend in liquid.
3. Add oil and seasonings.
4. Pour onto lightly oiled cookie sheet.
5. Bake at 375 degrees for 5 to 10 minutes. Flip and bake 3 more minutes.

Substitutions

- For the flour you may use any grain.
- For the liquid: milk, soy milk, nut milk, vegetable broth or puree, vegetable soup.

Basic Pancake Recipe

Makes 3 to 4 servings

½ cup unbleached white flour
½ cup whole wheat flour
2 teaspoons baking powder
1 teaspoon sea salt
1 cup milk
2 eggs
2 tablespoons oil
2 tablespoons honey (optional)

1. Combine dry ingredients.
2. Slowly add milk.
3. Stir in eggs, oil, and honey.
4. Drop by tablespoonfuls onto hot griddle.
5. Turn when bubbles appear.

Substitutions

- Rice, oat, corn, rye, barley, or a combination of any flours may be used in place of wheat.
- Soy or nut milk, or unfiltered fruit juices, may be substituted for cow's milk.
- One teaspoon baking powder and 2 tablespoons liquid may be used to replace the eggs.
- Maple syrup may be substituted for the honey.

Basic Crepes

Makes 15 to 20 crepes

½ cup milk
¼ cup water
2 large eggs
½ teaspoon sea salt
2 tablespoons oil
⅓ cup unbleached white flour
⅓ cup whole wheat flour

1. Place milk, water, eggs, salt, and oil in blender or mixing bowl and blend till smooth.
2. Slowly add flours, stirring in evenly.
3. Refrigerate for at least 2 hours, preferably overnight.
4. Place a 6-inch crepe pan or skillet over moderate heat.
5. Brush lightly with oil.
6. Stir batter before spooning out each crepe.
7. Pour ¼ cup batter into pan; swirl and tip pan until batter coats the bottom evenly. Do this quickly.
8. Cook for 1 minute or until you can easily slide crepe and flip it over. Cook for 30 seconds more.
9. Stack crepes on ovenproof platter and keep warm in low oven until ready to fill.

Substitutions

One cup potato flour (starch) may be used to replace both unbleached white and whole wheat flour.

Basic Waffle Batter

Makes 8–10 waffles

1½ cups rolled grain flakes
2¼ cups water
⅓ cup nuts or seeds
1 tablespoon oil
½ teaspoon salt (optional)

1. Blend all ingredients in blender at high speed until light and foamy.
2. Let stand while waffle iron is heating. Reblend to thin mixture if necessary.
3. Pour into waffle iron and bake for 8 minutes or until golden brown.

Substitutions

- Flakes may be oat, barley, wheat, or rye.
- Nuts may include one or several of the following: peanuts, cashews, filberts, almonds, sunflower seeds, or pecans.

Barley Drop Biscuits

Makes 16 biscuits

2 cups barley flour
4 teaspoons low-sodium baking powder
½ teaspoon sea salt
4 teaspoons oil
1 large egg, or 2 teaspoons Ener-g Egg Replacer, or ¼ cup plain low-fat yogurt, diluted with ¼ cup water*
½–1 cup water

1. Preheat oven to 425 degrees.
2. Mix dry ingredients.
3. Stir in oil with fork.
4. Add egg, egg replacer, or yogurt. If using egg, beat thoroughly first. Stir well.
5. Slowly add water until mixture is moist but thick.
6. Drop large heaping spoonfuls onto oiled cookie sheet.
7. For 2½-inch biscuits bake for 20 to 30 minutes; bake less time for smaller biscuits.

Rye Flatbread

Makes 4–6 servings

Rye flatbread is both dietetic and flavorful. It can be made easily:

2 cups rye flour
½ teaspoon salt
2 teaspoons baking powder
¼ cup nonfat dry milk powder (optional)
2 tablespoons cold pressed oil
⅔ cup water

1. Mix all dry ingredients.
2. Add oil and water and stir till stiff dough is formed.
3. Knead dough on floured surface (use rye flour) about 4 to 6 minutes.
4. Roll, in sections, till thin and flat. Cut into size you desire.
5. Oil and flour a cookie sheet.
6. Bake at 400 degrees for 10 to 12 minutes or until a light golden color.

Variations

Sprinkle ¼ cup finely grated cheese over the dough 5 minutes before done.

*See Mail-Order Food Sources, page 431.

Buckwheat Sunflower Bread

Makes 8–10 servings

½ cup sunflower seeds
2 cups buckwheat flour
1 teaspoon baking soda
½ teaspoon baking powder
⅛ teaspoon nutmeg or cinnamon
1¾ cups nut milk or soy milk
¼ cup honey
1 teaspoon tamari soy sauce

1. Grind sunflower seeds in blender, using short bursts of high speed.
2. Combine sunflower seeds with other dry ingredients in bowl.
3. Separately mix nut or soy milk, honey, and tamari.
4. Add liquid mixture to the dry ingredients and stir until combined.
5. Place in lightly oiled 8½-inch × 4½-inch bread pan and bake at 350 degrees for 50 minutes.

Corn Bread

Makes 6–8 servings

2 cups yellow cornmeal
3 teaspoons aluminum-free baking powder
½ teaspoon sea salt
1 cup soy milk
2 ounces tofu, crumbled
3 tablespoons honey

1. Combine cornmeal, baking powder, and salt.
2. Mix soy milk, tofu, and honey together until smooth.
3. Stir into dry ingredients until just well blended.
4. Pour into a buttered or lightly oiled 8-inch square pan.
5. Bake at 350 degrees for 20 minutes. Serve hot.

Substitutions

Baking powder may be replaced by ¼ teaspoon of baking soda dissolved in ½ teaspoon of any acid such as lemon or lime juice or vinegar, or by cream of tartar.

Barley Muffins

Makes 6 muffins

2 cups barley flour
1 teaspoon baking powder
¼ teaspoon sea salt
½ teaspoon cinnamon
¼ teaspoon nutmeg
¼ cup chopped prunes
½ cup mashed cooked sweet potato
1 cup apple juice
2 tablespoons oil

1. Combine dry ingredients.
2. Add prunes, sweet potato, juice, and oil. Mix well.
3. Lightly oil muffin tin and fill ⅔ full.
4. Bake at 400 degrees for 12 to 15 minutes.

Substitutions

- One small ripe banana may replace sweet potato.
- One cup coconut pineapple juice may replace the apple juice.

Buckwheat Muffins

Makes 6 muffins

2 cups buckwheat flour
1 teaspoon low-sodium baking powder
½ teaspoon salt
⅔ cup apple juice
1 tablespoon oil

1. Mix dry ingredients.
2. Add juice and oil. Stir well.
3. Bake in lightly oiled muffin tin at 350 degrees for 10 to 15 minutes.

Substitutions

Any juice may replace the apple juice.

Millet-Bean-Peach Muffins

Makes 6 muffins

1 cup lima bean flour
⅔ cup finely ground millet meal
1 teaspoon low sodium baking powder
¼ teaspoon salt
½ teaspoon cinnamon
6-ounce jar peach puree (or fresh peaches, pureed in blender or food processor)
1 tablespoon oil
2 ounces pecans (optional)

1. Combine dry ingredients.
2. Blend peaches and oil in blender or mixing bowl.
3. Place peach mixture in bowl. Slowly add dry ingredients, stirring continually.
4. Add nuts if desired.
5. Fill oiled muffin tin ⅔ full.
6. Bake at 400 degrees for 15 minutes or until done.

Substitutions

- 1/4 teaspoon cloves may replace 1/2 teaspoon cinnamon.
- Apricot or pear puree may replace peaches.

Banana-Oat Muffins

Makes 6 muffins

1⅔ cups oat flour
1 teaspoon baking powder
1/4 teaspoon salt
1/2 teaspoon cinnamon
3/4 cup mashed banana
1 tablespoon oil
1/4 cup chopped filbert or other nuts

1. Combine all dry ingredients.
2. Stir in banana, oil, and nuts. Mix well.
3. Fill lightly oiled muffin tin ⅔ full. Bake at 400 degrees for approximately 15 minutes.

Rye Muffins

Makes 6 muffins

1 1/2 cups rye flour
1/2 teaspoon salt
1 teaspoon baking powder
1/2 teaspoon anise or fennel seeds (optional)
1/3 cup raisins
1/4 cup chopped pecans
1/2 teaspoon grated orange rind
1 pureed orange plus enough juice to make 3/4 cup
1 tablespoon oil
1/2 teaspoon vanilla

1. Combine dry ingredients.
2. Add orange mixture, oil, and vanilla.
3. Stir well.
4. Fill lightly oiled muffin tin ⅔ full. Bake in 375 degree oven for 12 to 15 minutes.

Substitutions

- Dates or other dried fruit may be used in place of raisins.
- Walnuts or almonds can replace pecans.

Rice-Soy Bread

Makes 1 loaf

2 cups brown rice flour
½ cup soy flour
1 teaspoon baking soda
2 teaspoons baking powder
1 teaspoon salt
6 teaspoons sesame oil
¾ cup coconut or soy milk
¼ cup honey

1. Sift together dry ingredients.
2. Blend liquid ingredients.
3. Add liquid to dry mixture and stir well.
4. Pour into oiled 9-inch×5-inch loaf pan.
5. Bake at 350 degrees for 35 minutes.

Soy-Blueberry Muffins

Makes 6 muffins

1 cup soy flour
½ cup rice flour
1 teaspoon low-sodium baking powder
⅛ teaspoon salt
1 egg
¾ cup soy milk
1 tablespoon honey
1 tablespoon oil
¾ cup fresh blueberries

1. Sift together dry ingredients.
2. Beat together egg and soy milk.
3. Add honey and oil to liquid. Blend well.
4. Stir liquid mixture into dry mixture.
5. Add blueberries.
6. Drop by spoonfuls into oiled muffin tin.
7. Bake at 350 degrees for 20 to 25 minutes.

Substitutions

- Two ounces tofu can replace egg. Mash or puree well.
- Egg replacer (from health food store).

MEAT AND FISH

Sesame-Honey Chicken

Makes 4 servings

½ cup tahini
4 tablespoons honey (optional)
2 tablespoons lemon juice
2 tablespoons water
cup yeast-free cracker crumbs
1 pound skinless chicken breasts (with or without bones)
1 teaspoon dried tarragon
½ teaspoon onion powder
salt to taste

1. Blend tahini, honey, lemon juice, and water.
2. Place cracker crumbs in shallow dish.
3. Add tarragon, onion powder, and salt to crumbs. Stir to blend in.
4. Dip chicken pieces in tahini mixture.
5. Roll in cracker crumbs.
6. Bake in shallow dish at 350 degrees for 45 minutes or until done.

Substitutions

- Soy milk or nut milk may be used in place of water.
- Yeast-free bread crumbs may be used in place of cracker crumbs. Toast bread first, then roll into fine crumbs.
- Any unsweetened fruit puree may be used in place of honey.
- Herbs such as rosemary or thyme may replace tarragon.

Turkey Patties

Makes 4 servings

¼ cup chopped onions
dash onion powder
dash fresh or dried thyme
1 pound freshly ground turkey meat

1. Add onions, onion powder, and thyme to ground turkey, and knead to mix.
2. Form chopped turkey into 4 patties.
3. Broil for 5 minutes on one side. Turn and broil till done.
4. Serve like hamburgers.

Poached Salmon

Makes 2 servings

1 medium onion
1 stalk celery
1 carrot
½ cup chopped fennel leaf (optional)
2 tablespoons oil or butter
1 quart water
½ cup white wine or ¼ cup lemon juice
1 large salmon steak, about 2 pounds
hollandaise sauce or mayonnaise
drained capers

1. Chop vegetables.
2. Sauté in oil in skillet for 5 minutes.
2. Pour in liquids and simmer for 5 minutes.
3. Place salmon carefully in boiling liquid.
4. Lower heat to gentle simmer. Cover tightly.
5. Cook approximately 8 minutes per pound.
6. Remove salmon very carefully so it doesn't break.
7. Serve hot with hollandaise sauce or cold with mayonnaise and capers.

Substitutions

Any fish may be poached in a similar fashion. Swordfish, halibut, and tuna are thick, steaklike fish. For whole fish such as snapper or bass consult your favorite cookbook for cooking times. Since fish tends to break when cooked, you may want to use a fish poacher or wrap the fish in cheesecloth squares while poaching.

SOUPS

A soup may consist of just about anything you want plus some liquid. There is no vegetable or bean or even fruit that hasn't been turned into a soup by some inventive cook. Here we offer a few basic recipes: bean soup, potato soup, and gazpacho, a "soup" in salad form.

Any Bean Soup

Makes 4–6 servings

½ small onion
1½ carrots
1 stalk celery
1 tablespoon oil
1½ quarts water
⅓ cup barley
1 cup cooked beans (navy, garbanzo, lentil, black or other beans, or black-eyed peas)
½ teaspoon soy sauce
¼ teaspoon dried marjoram
¼ teaspoon dried thyme
pepper to taste
parsley for garnish

1. Chop onion, carrots, and celery.
2. Sauté vegetables in oil for 5 minutes.
3. Bring water to a boil and add the sautéed vegetables.
4. Add barley and cover. Simmer at low heat for 45 minutes.
5. Add cooked beans and seasonings. Simmer for 30 more minutes.
6. Serve with parsley garnish.

Substitutions

- Rye, millet, whole oats, or rice can be used in place of barley.
- To add beef: Brown meat cubes in oil and seasonings. Cut into bite-sized, well-trimmed chunks. Cook with barley till tender. Degrease liquid. Complete soup as above.
- For chicken soup, add chicken chunks to barley with or without bones. Cook till tender. Remove bones, chop chicken, and replace in pot. Add beans and prepare as above.

Basic Potato Soup

Makes 4–6 servings

2–4 tablespoons oil or butter
3 cups diced potatoes
3 cups diced leeks
2 quarts water
salt and pepper to taste

1. Heat oil in skillet and sauté potatoes and leeks until tender but not browned.
2. Bring water to a boil and add vegetables.
3. Simmer for 30 minutes.
4. Remove vegetables from stock and puree in food mill or blender. Add salt and pepper to taste.
5. Slowly add to hot broth, stirring constantly, until you have desired consistency.

Substitutions

- Vegetable, beef, or chicken stock may be used in place of water.
- Milk or cream can be added as the last step, for added richness.
- Any spices can be added for extra flavor.
- This soup, when kept a thick puree, provides an ideal gravy and sauce thickener, free of dairy or grain.

Gazpacho Salad Soup

Makes 4–6 servings

3 diced fresh tomatoes
1 clove garlic
1 medium cucumber, diced and seeded
1 medium onion, diced
1 green pepper, seeded
cayenne or chili pepper
1/4 cup olive oil
1/4 cup lemon juice
3/4 cup tomato juice

1. Blend tomatoes, garlic, cucumber, onion, and green pepper at high speed in food processor or blender until well mixed.
2. Add seasonings, oil, and lemon juice. Blend again.
3. Pour in tomato juice.
4. Chill. Serve cold and garnished with a slice of cucumber or chopped onion.

Substitutions

- Watercress can be used in place of the cucumber.
- You may add 2 slices of diced bread as a thickener if you wish; or croutons may be added as a garnish.
- Experiment with other vegetables such as steamed asparagus, broccoli, or zucchini. All should be well peeled after cooking and cooled before being added to blender.

SALADS AND DRESSINGS

Gone, thank goodness, are the days when a salad meant a plate of forlorn and wilting iceberg lettuce. Salads are an interesting and complex part of modern American cookery. A salad can even serve as a whole meal. Don't hesitate to use cold grains such as rice or lentils as a salad base, or to serve "hot" salads with gently warmed greens or rounds of exotic broiled goat cheese.

Seaweed Salad

Makes 4 servings

1 package dried arame seaweed
1/4 cup vinegar
1 tablespoon grated fresh ginger
1/2 cup chopped onion

1. Soak seaweed in water for 5 minutes. Drain and pat dry.
2. Toss in bowl with remaining ingredients.
3. Chill for 1 hour to allow flavors to blend.

Substitutions

Soy sauce or carrot juice may be used in place of vinegar.

Vegetable Noodle Salad Orientale

Makes 6 servings

1 package oriental rice noodles
1/2 head red cabbage
2 cups chopped spinach
1 medium zucchini
1 medium crooked neck squash
1/4 cup scallions

1. Boil noodles, drain, and chill.
2. Shred cabbage. Chop spinach.
3. Slice zucchini and squash into paper-thin rounds.
4. Slice scallions.
5. Combine ingredients.

Lentil Salad

Makes 4 servings

2 stalks celery
1 medium onion
2 cloves garlic
2 tablespoons oil
1 cup dried lentils
1 quart water

1. Chop celery, onion, and garlic.
2. Heat oil in saucepan and sauté vegetables.
3. Add lentils and water.
4. Bring to boil.
5. Lower heat and simmer covered for 30 minutes; do not let lentils get mushy.
6. Drain and cool.
7. Dress with one of dressing recipes that follow.

Tabouleh Salad

Makes 4 servings

1½ cups water
1 cup dry bulgar wheat
3 scallions, diced
1 tomato, chopped
½ cup Oil and Vinegar Dressing dressing (see below)
6 fresh mint leaves, minced

1. Bring water to a boil and pour over bulgar wheat. Let sit in pan till all liquid is absorbed and wheat is fluffy.
2. Mix in vegetables and dressing and chill.
3. Before serving, sprinkle minced mint leaves over top.

Substitutions

- Use onions, peppers, or garlic for scallions.
- Use chopped cucumber for tomato.
- Use parsley or basil for mint.

Spanish Bean Salad

Makes 6 servings

1 cup cooked kidney beans
1 cup cooked navy beans
½ pound cooked string beans
1 medium onion, chopped
⅓ cup Chili-Cumin Dressing (recipe follows)

1. Place all ingredients in mixing bowl, draining beans first.
2. Toss and add dressing.
3. Chill for several hours, stirring occasionally.

Substitutions

- Any cooked bean may be used in this recipe.
- Cooked brown rice may be used in place of one of the beans.

Basic Oil and Vinegar Dressing

Makes ⅓ cup

6 tablespoons oil
2 tablespoons vinegar
1½ teaspoons prepared mustard
¼ teaspoon onion powder
⅛ teaspoon salt and pepper
herbs

Mix all ingredients well, making sure they are blended.

Substitutions

- Any oil may be used.
- Lemon or lime juice or a special flavored vinegar may be used.
- 1 clove pressed garlic may be added in place of onion powder.
- Chopped basil, tarragon, mint, turmeric, and coriander all are good additions.

Chili-Cumin Dressing

Makes ⅓ cup

¼ cup oil
2 tablespoons vinegar
1 clove garlic, minced
1 teaspoon chili powder
½ teaspon ground cumin
½ teaspoon salt
¼ teaspoon pepper

1. Combine all ingredients in a jar and shake well.
2. Chill.

Substitutions

- Lemon or lime juice or rice vinegar may be used in place of vinegar.
- Onions or chives may be used in place of garlic.

ASSORTED DIPS

For use with crackers, vegetable sticks, or sandwiches, these versatile dips are delicious.

Avocado Spread

Makes ¾ cup

1 ripe avocado
2 teaspoons lemon or lime juice
2–3 tablespoons diced green pepper
2 tablespoons minced onion
2 tablespoons chopped coriander

1. Cube avocado and place in bowl. Mash avocado to thick paste.
2. Add remaining ingredients.
3. Stir till blended but not too mushy.

Substitutions

- Alfalfa sprouts may be used in place of coriander.
- Green pepper may be omitted.

- 1/4 cup diced tomato may be used.
- Chili powder, garlic, or black pepper may be added.

Eggplant Spread

Makes 2 cups

1 medium eggplant
10 cherry tomatoes
1 clove garlic
1/4 cup onion
sprinkle of parsley
1/2 cup pine nuts
2 tablespoons oil
lemon juice to taste

1. Bake whole eggplant at 375 degrees for 45 minutes or until very soft and tender.
2. Peel and mash.
3. Chop cherry tomatoes.
4. Cut up garlic, onion, and parsley.
5. Chop pine nuts.
6. Add remaining ingredients to eggplant and mix well.
7. Adjust seasoning as desired.

Substitutions

- Any nut may be used in place of pine nuts.
- Tahini may be added.

Garbanzo Bean (Chick-Pea) Hummus

Makes 2 1/2 cups

2 cups cooked, drained chick-peas
1/4 cup liquid from peas
3 tablespoons tahini
1/4 cup lemon juice
1 clove garlic, minced

1. Blend chick-peas with liquid at high speed.
2. Add tahini, lemon juice, and garlic clove.
3. Chill in refrigerator. Before serving, garnish with chopped parsley or paprika if desired.

Tofu Dip

Makes 2 cups

12 ounces tofu
3/4 cup soy mayonnaise
1/2 cup chopped ripe olives
1/2 cup chopped toasted sunflower seeds
2 tablespoons chopped chives
2 tablespoons chopped pimientos
2 tablespoons dried dill
1/2 teaspoons herb salt

1. Drain and mash tofu. Add mayonnaise.
2. Add remaining ingredients.
3. Stir. Refrigerate until ready to serve.

COOKIES, CAKES, AND HEALTHFUL SWEETS

Butternut Squash Flan

Makes 4 servings

1 1/4 cups mashed cooked butternut squash
1/4 teaspoon cloves
1/4 teaspoon cinnamon
3 tablespoons honey
1 1/4 cups low-fat milk or apple juice
2 eggs at room temperature
2 egg whites at room temperature
orange slices

1. Preheat oven to 325 degrees.
2. Blend squash, cloves, cinnamon, and honey to a puree.
3. Scald milk (or heat apple juice).
4. Beat eggs and egg whites together until frothy.
5. Slowly add milk or juice to eggs, whisking well.
6. Add egg mixture to squash mixture in blender.
7. Combine well.
8. Pour into four 1-cup dishes or 1 large dish.
9. Place dishes in a pan of hot water.
10. Bake for 1 hour or until toothpick comes out clean.
11. Remove from oven. Place custard dishes on rack. Place plastic wrap or wax paper over top of custards to retain moisture while cooling.
12. Serve with orange slices at room temperature or chilled.

Carob Custard

Makes 4 servings

2 tablespoons carob powder
2 cups milk
4 tablespoons maple sugar
2 eggs
1/2 teaspoon salt

1. Preheat oven to 325 degrees.
2. Blend all ingredients together.
3. Pour into custard cups and place cups in a pan of hot water.
4. Bake for 20 to 30 minutes or until set.

Substitutions

- Soy or nut milk may be used in place of cow's milk.
- Honey may be used in place of maple syrup.
- Egg substitute or baking soda formula (page 457) may be used in place of eggs.
- You may add raisins or chopped dried fruit if you wish.

Cornmeal Pudding

Makes 4 to 6 servings

3 cups water
½ teaspoon salt
1 cup cornmeal (with germ)
1 cup unfiltered apple juice
½ teaspoon cinnamon
¼ cup raisins

1. Bring water to a boil. Add salt.
2. Combine cornmeal, apple juice, and cinnamon.
3. Stir slowly into boiling water.
4. Simmer on low heat for 10 minutes, stirring occasionally.
5. Add raisins and simmer 5 more minutes or until mixture reaches desired thickness.

Substitutions

- Any dried fruit may be used in place of raisins.
- Any fruit juice may be used in place of apple juice.

No-Flour Oatmeal Cookies

Makes 3 dozen cookies

2 eggs
1 cup maple sugar
2 tablespoons oil or melted butter
1 teaspoon vanilla
1 teaspoon salt
1 cup shredded coconut
1 cup raw rolled oats

1. Preheat oven to 350 degrees.
2. Beat eggs and sugar together.
3. Stir in oil. Add vanilla and salt.
4. Add coconut and oats and mix well.
5. Drop by half teaspoonfuls onto buttered cookie sheet.
6. Bake for 10 minutes or until until golden brown.

Substitutions

- Barley flakes may be used in place of oat flakes.
- Honey may replace the maple syrup.

- Raisins may be used in place of coconut.
- Almond extract may be used in place of vanilla.

Cashew Butter Oat Cookies

Makes 18 to 24 cookies

6 tablespoons cashew butter
3/4 cup honey
1 tablespoon cinnamon
1/2 cup chopped walnuts
1 1/2 cups rolled oats

1. Blend cashew butter and honey well.
2. Blend cinnamon and nuts. Add to honey mixture.
3. Mix in rolled oats.
4. Drop by small spoonfuls onto buttered cookie sheet.
5. Bake at 350 degrees for 12 to 15 minutes.

Substitutions

- Any nut butter may be used.
- Any chopped nut may be used.

Oat Museli

Makes 4 servings

2/3 cup rolled oats
8 dates, chopped
1/4 teaspoon cinnamon
2/3 cup water
1/2 apple
1 banana
1/4 cup nuts
1 cup plain yogurt

1. Combine oats, dates, and cinnamon.
2. Cover with water and let soak overnight.
3. Slice all fruit. Add nuts, fruit, and yogurt to oats.
4. Serve cold.

Apple Crisp

Makes 3–4 servings

Filling:
2 large apples
1/2 cup honey
1 teaspoon cinnamon
1 teaspoon cinnamon

Topping:
1/4 cup rolled oats
1 tablespoon butter
1/4 teaspoon nutmeg

1. Preheat oven to 350 degrees.
2. Peel and thinly slice the apples.

3. Combine all filling ingredients in mixing bowl.
4. Pour into lightly oiled baking dish.
5. Combine all ingredients for topping.
6. Spread over filling.
7. Bake for 1 hour.

Baked Apple

Makes 1 serving

1 large apple
3 tablespoons honey
1/8 teaspoon nutmeg
1/2 teaspoon cinnamon
1 tablespoon butter

1. Preheat oven to 350 degrees.
2. Core apple. Cut 1/2-inch plug from bottom of core and reinsert in bottom of apple.
3. Place in baking dish.
4. Put honey, spices, and butter into hole.
5. Bake for 15 to 30 minutes or until bubbly and tender.

Pumpkin-Date Torte

Makes 4–6 servings

1/2 cup chopped dates
1/2 cup chopped walnuts
2 tablespoons oat flour
1/4 cup sweet butter
dash salt
1/3 cup maple sugar
2/3 cup cooked pumpkin
1 teaspoon vanilla
2 eggs
1/2 cup oat flour
1 teaspoon baking powder
dash nutmeg, ginger, cinnamon, salt

1. Mix together chopped dates and chopped walnuts.
2. Sprinkle with 2 tablespoons oat flour. Set aside.
3. Over low heat melt butter with salt and maple sugar.
4. Blend and remove from heat.
5. Stir in pumpkin and vanilla.
6. Beat and add eggs to pumpkin mixture.
7. In separate bowl sift together oat flour, baking powder, and spices.
8. Add flour mixture to pumpkin mixture. Mix completely. Add date-and-walnut mixture.
9. Pour into 9-inch round pan or 8-inch square pan.
10. Bake at 350 degrees for 20 to 25 minutes.

Wheat-Free Piecrust for All Occasions

Makes 1 crust

1½ cups barley flakes
3 tablespoons honey
6 tablespoons almond butter

1. Preheat oven to 300 degrees.
2. Blend all ingredients together, in food processor or mixer.
3. Press into 9-inch pie plate and refrigerate for 30 minutes.
4. Bake for 15 minutes.
5. Fill with apples, cherries, pumpkin, lemon meringue, etc.

Substitutions

Any flour may be used in place of barley flakes.

BEVERAGES

Apple-Lime Frost

Makes 4 servings

4 cups unfiltered apple juice
juice of two limes
sparkling spring water or club soda

Combine in blender until smooth. Garnish with lime wedge.

Pineapple Chill

Makes 4 servings

2 cups fresh cubed pineapple
1 cup apple juice
½ cup pineapple juice
1½ cups grated ice

Combine in blender until frothy and smooth.

Cranberry Cooler

Makes 8 servings

3 cups cranberry juice
4 tablespoons lime juice or lemon juice
2 tablespoons honey
2 cups orange juice
2 cups club soda

Combine in iced pitcher.

Melon Highball

Makes 4 servings

2 cups diced cantaloupe
2 cups fresh orange juice
1 teaspoon honey
1½ cups crushed ice

Mix all ingredients in blender till frothy.

Blueberry Hill Chill

Makes 2 servings

1 cup fresh blueberries
1 cup pineapple juice
1 cup crushed ice

Blend till frothy.

Yogurt Smoothie

Makes 2 servings

1 ripe banana
1 large peach
1 cup yogurt
1 teaspoon vanilla

Dice fruit and combine all ingredients in blender.

Substitutions

- You may substitute any fruit juice for the yogurt.
- Any fruit may be substituted for the peach. Combinations are also good.
- Vanilla may be omitted.
- Crushed ice will make it a frozen yogurt smoothie.

SNACKS AND SWEET STUFF

Here are a few welcome substitutes for junk food and candy. Also refer to the suggestions for children on page 298.

Munchy Nut, Seed, and Popcorn Snacks

½ cup sunflower, safflower, or sesame oil
½ teaspoon curry powder, or ¼ teaspoon powdered ginger
⅛ teaspoon powdered turmeric
⅛ teaspoon salt
combination of nuts and seeds

1. In a saucepan, combine oil with choice of seasoning.
2. *Briefly* heat mixture on *low* flame till thoroughly heated.
   NOTE: Do not allow the oil to smoke or boil. The object is only to heat the oil enough to release flavors of the spices.
3. Remove from heat, and let sit until oil mixture is warm to the touch but not too hot. Pour into a clean spray bottle.
4. Roast nuts and seeds. Preheat oven to 400 degrees. Place any mixture of raw, unsalted nuts and/or sunflower or pumpkin seeds in a single layer on a cookie sheet. Bake for 5 to 7 minutes or until light golden brown.
5. Remove from oven and spray lightly with oil/spice mixture (use fine setting of spray bottle).
6. Replace in oven for 1 minute to crisp. Remove from oven, and allow to cool. Store in an airtight container.

Low-Calorie Substitutions

Use puffed oats, millet, rice, wheat, corn cereal, or popped corn. Place on cookie sheet, and toast in 400 degree oven for 1 to 2 minutes only. Spray with oil/spice mixture, replace in oven to crisp (approximately 1 minute), cool, and store.

Oil-free Roasted Nuts

1. Spread raw unroasted nuts over bottom of heavy skillet.
2. Place over moderate heat.
3. Shake and stir until well-browned.
4. Store cooled nuts in airtight containers.

Variations

- Add 2 tablespoons soy sauce to pan, stir well.
- Coat with honey for sweet treats.

Fruit Mix

Have a good supply of dried fruits and nuts and seeds in the house. Combine as desired and keep in easy reach.

Frozen Fruit

Frozen bananas, pears, grapes, and oranges make great summertime treats. Just keep fresh fruit handy in freezer. Puree in blender for creamy "sherbet."

Chips

Want salt-free low-fat chips to munch? Buy fresh tortillas and cut into quarters. Sprinkle with curry or garlic powder for extra flavor. Bake on an ungreased cookie sheet at 250 degrees for 20 minutes or until crispy and brown.

Rotation Diet Planning Form

	Day 1	Day 2	Day 3	Day 4
BREAKFAST				
SNACK				
LUNCH				
SNACK				
DINNER				

Date:

Sample Diet Diary Form

Weight:
Hours Slept:

Time	Food and Drink	Supplements	Time	Symptoms	Severity (1–4+)
T:	Early Morning		T:		
T:	Breakfast		T:		
T:	Midmorning		T:		
T:	Lunch		T:		
T:	Midafternoon		T:		
T:	Dinner		T:		
T:	Evening		T:		

Bibliography

GENERAL REFERENCE

Bland, Jeffrey, Ph.D. *Your Health Under Siege.* Brattleboro, Vt. The Stephen Greene Press, 1981.

Brown, Barbara B. *Between Health & Illness.* Boston: Houghton Mifflin, 1984.

Cheraskin, E., M.D., D.M.D., *et al. Diet and Disease.* New Canaan, Conn.: Keats Publishing, 1977.

Friedman, JoAnn. *The Complete Book of Home Health Care: A Guide for Patients and Their Families.* New York: W. W. Norton, 1985.

Kaslow, Arthur L., M.D. *Freedom from Chronic Disease.* Los Angeles: J. P. Tarcher, Inc., 1979.

Lister, J., M.D. "Current Controversy on Alternative Medicine," *New England Journal of Medicine,* 309:24 (December 15, 1983).

Mendelsohn, Robert, M.D. *Confessions of a Medical Heretic.* New York: Warner Books, 1979.

The Merck Manual, 14th ed. Rahway, N.J.: Merck, Sharpe & Dohme Research Labs, 1982.

Reiser, David E., M.D., and David H. Rosen, M.D. *Medicine as a Human Experience.* Baltimore: University Park Press, 1984.

Tortora, Gerard J., and Nicholas P. Anagnostakos. *Principles of Anatomy and Physiology,* 2nd ed. New York: Harper & Row, 1978.

Weil, Andrew, M.D. *Health and Healing: Understanding Conventional and Alternative Medicine.* Boston: Houghton Mifflin, 1984.

ALLERGY

Black, Arthur P., M.D. "A New Diagnostic Method in Allergic Disease," *Pediatrics,* May 1956, pp. 171–176.

Boyles, John H., Jr., M.D. "The Validity of Using the Cytotoxic Food Test in Clinical Allergy," *Ear, Nose & Throat Journal,* April 1977.

Brody, Jane. "Sulfite Food Additives, Used as Preservatives, Are Viewed as Growing Health Problem," *The New York Times,* June 27, 1984, Sec. C, p. 10.

Bryan, W. T. K., and M. P. Bryan. "Cytotoxic Reactions in the Diagnosis of Food Allergy," *Allergy Otolaryngology Proceedings* (1971): 523–34.

Buisseret, P. "Allergy," *Scientific American,* 247: 2 (1982), 86–95.

Coca, A. F. *The Pulse Test.* New York: Arc Books, 1956.

Finn, Ronald, and H. Newman Cohen. "Food Allergy: Fact or Fiction," *The Lancet,* February 25, 1978.

Forman, Robert, Ph.D. *How to Control Your Allergies.* New York: Larchmont Books, 1979.

Hunter, Beatrice Trum. *Fact Book on Food Additives and Your Health.* New Canaan, Conn.: Keats Publishing, 1972.

Randolph, T. G. "The Descriptive Features of Food Addiction: Addictive Eating and Drinking," *Quarterly Journal for the Study of Alcoholism* 17 (1956): 198–224.

———. *Human Ecology and Susceptibility to the Chemical Environment.* Springfield, Ill.: Thomas, 1972.

Rinkel, H. J. "Food Allergy: The Role of Food Allergy in Internal Medicine," *Annals Allergy* 2 (1944): 115–124.

Rowe, A. H., and A. H. Rowe, Jr. "Diagnosis of Allergy" in *Food Allergy: Its Manifestations and Control and the Elimination Diets: A Compendium.* Springfield, Ill.: Thomas, 1972.

———. *Food Allergy, Its Manifestations, Diagnosis and Treatment.* Philadelphia: 1983.

DIGESTION/IMMUNITY

Beisel, W. "Single Nutrients and Immunity," *American Journal of Clinical Nutrition* 35 (2-Supplement) (1982): 417–68.

Bland, Jeffrey, Ph.D. *Digestive Enzymes.* New Canaan, Conn.: Keats Publishing, 1983.

Goldstein, Allan L., M.D. "On Thymosins . . . the Remarkable Hormones of the Thymus Gland that Control Our Immunity and Our Health," *Executive Health,* 18:10 (July 1982).

Hamburger, R. N. "Allergy and the Immune System," *American Scientist* 64 (1976): 157.

Hammerschmidt, Dale, M.D. "On Trigger-Happy Blood Platelets as a Cause of Heart Attacks, Stroke and Other Disease," *Executive Health,* 19:11 (August 1983).

Hayflick, Leonard, Ph.D. "What We are Discovering About Your Body's Amazing Immune System," *Executive Health,* 15:2 (November 1978).

Kluger, Matthew J., Ph.D. "On Fever, Does It Really Harm or Help?" *Executive Health,* 20:6 (March 1984).

Mayron, L. W., M.D. "Portals of Entry—a Review," *Annals of Allergy,* 40:6 (June 1978).

SUPPLEMENTATION—GENERAL

Bland, Jeffrey, Ph.D. *The Justification for Vitamin Supplementation.* Bellevue, Wash.: Northwest Diagnostic Services, 1981.

Passwater, Richard A. *Supernutrition Megavitamin Revolution.* New York: Pocket Books, 1979.

Pfeiffer, Carl C., Ph.D., M.D. *Mental and Elemental Nutrients.* New Canaan, Conn.: Keats Publishing, 1975.

Recommended Dietary Allowances. 8th ed. Washington D.C.: National Academy of Sciences, 1980.

SUPPLEMENTATION—VITAMINS

Braly, James, M.D. *Vitamin Self-Help Guide.* Encino, Calif.: Optimum Health Labs, 1983.

Cameron, Ewan, M.D., and Linus Pauling, Ph.D. *Cancer and Vitamin C.* New York: W. W. Norton, 1979.

Challem, Jack Joseph. *Vitamin C Update.* New Canaan, Conn.: Keats Publishing 1983.

Cheraskin, Emanuel, M.D. *The Vitamin C Connection.* New York: Harper & Row, 1983.

Colgan, Michael, M.D. *Your Personal Vitamin Profile.* New York: William Morrow & Co., 1982.

SUPPLEMENTATION—MINERALS

Bland, Jeffrey, Ph.D. *Trace Elements in Human Health and Disease.* Bellevue, Wash.: Northwest Diagnostic Services, 1979.

SUPPLEMENTATION—AMINO ACIDS

Braly, James, M.D. "The New, Safe, Drug-Free Pain Therapy Alternative—DL-Phenylalanine," *Optimum Health Labs,* 2:2.

Ehrenpreis, S., *et al.* "Further Studies on the Analgesic Activity of D-Phenylalanine in Mice and Humans," *Proceedings of the International Narcotics Research Club Convention, 1979,* 379–82.

Garrison, Robert, Jr. *Lysine, Ttyptophan and Other Amino Acids, Foods for Our Brains, Maintenance for Our Bodies.* New Canaan, Conn.: Keats Publishing, 1982.

SUPPLEMENTATION—ESSENTIAL FATTY ACIDS

Hayflick, Leonard, Ph.D. "On Those Magical Prostaglandins . . .," *Executive Health,* 16:8 (May 1980).

Horrobin, David, M.D., Ph.D. *Clinical Uses of Essential Fatty Acids.* Montreal-London: Eden Press, 1982.

———. *Essential Fatty Acids: A Review.* Kentville, N. S., Canada: Efamol Research Institute.

"It's Not Fishy: Fruit of the Sea May Foil Cardiovascular Disease," *Journal of the American Medical Association,* 247:6 (February 12, 1982).

Passwater, Richard, Ph.D. *Evening Primrose Oil.* New Canaan, Conn.: Keats Publishing, 1981.

NUTRITION/FOOD PREPARATION

Ballentine, Rudolph, M.D. *Diet and Nutrition.* Honesdale, Pa.: The Himalayan International Institute, 1978.

Goldbeck, Nikki, and David Goldbeck. *Nikki and David Goldbeck's American Wholefoods Cuisine.* New York: NAL Books, 1983.

Hardigree, Peggy. *The Mail Order Gourmet.* New York: St. Martin's Press, 1983.

Krause, Marie V., B.S., M.S., RD., and L. Kathleen Mahan, M.S., RD. *Food Nutrition and Diet Therapy.* Philadelphia: W. B. Saunders Co., 1979.

Mandell, Fran Gare, M.S. *Dr. Mandell's Allergy-Free Cookbook.* New York: Pocket Books, 1981.

Reimann, Linda. *The Allergy Snack Book.* Denver: Aurora Books, N.D.

Wright, Jonathan V. *Dr. Wright's Guide to Healing with Nutrition.* Erasmus, Pa.: Rodale Press, 1984.

EXERCISE

Barnes, Lan. "Exercise Is Crucial to New Weight-Loss Theory," *The Physician and Sports Medicine,* 12:2 (February 1984).

Cooper, Kenneth H., M.D., M.P.H. *The Aerobics Way.* New York: Bantam, 1977.

"On Walking: Nature's True—and Painless—Elixir," *Executive Health,* 20:9 (June 1984).

Massimino, Ferdy, M.D. "Aerobics and Fitness," *Triathlon,* April/May 1984, p. 26.

"Is Running Beside a Highway Worse Than not Running at All?" *Prevention,* October 1983.

PARENTS AND CHILDREN

Bahna, S. L., M.D., Furukawa. "Infant Food Allergy Prevention," *Annals of Allergy* 51 (December 1983).

"Clinical Importance of Lactose Deficiency," *New England Journal of Medicine,* January 5, 1984.

Gottlieb, Bill. "Bad Child or Bad Diet?" *Prevention Magazine,* July 1978, pp. 65–71.

Kaiser. *The Feingold Diet Handbook.* San Francisco: Permanente Medical Center.

Oski, Frank A., M.D. *Don't Drink Your Milk.* Syracuse, N.Y.: Mollica Press, Ltd., 1983.

Randolph, T. G. "Allergy as a Causative Factor of Fatigue, Irritability and Behavior Problems of Children," *Journal of Pediatrics* 31 (1947): 560–72.

Rapp, Doris, M.D. *Allergies and the Hyperactive Child.* New York: Simon & Schuster, 1979.

Reed, Barbara, Ph.D. *Food, Teens and Behavior.* Manitowoc, Wis.: Natural Press, 1983.

Rinzler, Carol Ann. *The Children's Medicine Chest.* New York: Berkeley Books, 1984.

Ryan, Allan J. "Do Children Need Physical Education?" *The Physician and Sports Medicine,* 12:4 (April 1984).

Sloan, Sara. *Nutritional Parenting.* New Canaan, Conn.: Keats Publishing, 1982.

Smith, Lendon, M.D. *Knowing Your Child's Behavior.* New York: Pocket Books, 1976.

Swanson, J. M., and M. Kinsbourne. "Food Dyes Impair Performance of Hyperactive Children on a Laboratory Learning Test," *Science* 207 (1970): 1485–87.

THERAPEUTIC APPLICATIONS—ADDICTION/ALCOHOL

Bjarnason, I., *et al.* "The Leaky Gut of Alcoholism: Possible Route of Entry for Toxic Compounds, *The Lancet,* January 28, 1984.
Blakeslee, Sandra. "Scientists Find Biological Causes of Alcoholism," *The New York Times,* August 14, 1984, Sec. C, p. 1.
Horrobin, D. F. "A Biochemical Basis for Alcoholism and Alcohol-Induced Damage, Including the Fetal Alcohol Syndrome and Cirrhosis: Interferences with Essential Fatty Acid and Prostaglandin Metabolism," *Medical Hypotheses* 6 (1980): 929–42.
Randolph, T. G. "Food Addiction and Alcoholism," *Journal of Laboratory and Clinical Medicine* 50 (1957): 940–41.
———. "Specific Food Allergens in Alcoholic Beverages," *Journal of Laboratory Clinical Medicine,* 36 (1950): 976–77.

THERAPEUTIC APPLICATIONS—ANTI-AGING

Batten, Mary. "Life Spans," *Science Digest,* February 1984.
Pearson, Durk, and Sandy Shaw. *Life Extension: A Practical Scientific Approach Adding Years to Your Life and Life to Your Years.* New York: Warner Books, 1982.
Walford, Roy L., M.D. *Maximum Life Span.* New York: W. W. Norton & Co., 1983.

THERAPEUTIC APPLICATIONS—ASTHMA/ATOPIC ALLERGIES

Atherton, *et al.* "A Double-Blind Controlled Crossover Trial of an Antigen-Avoidance Diet in Atopic Eczema," *The Lancet,* February 25, 1978.
"Exercise and Asthma," *The Physician and Sports Medicine,* 12:1 (January 1984).
Fireman, P., *et al.* "Teaching Self-Management Skills to Asthmatic Children and Their Parents in an Ambulatory Care Setting," *Pediatrics* (1981): 341–48.
Lovell, C. R., and J. L. Burton. "Treatment of Atopic Eczema with Evening Primrose Oil," *The Lancet* 278 (1981).
Morton, Alan, R., Ed. D. "Physical Activity and the Asthmatic," *The Physician and Sports Medicine,* 9:3 (March 1981).

THERAPEUTIC APPLICATIONS—BRAIN ALLERGIES

Dohan, F. C., *et al.* "Relapsed Schizophrenics: More Rapid Improvement on a Milk- and Cereal-free Diet," *British Journal of Psychiatry* 115 (1969): 595–96.

Lauersen, Niels, M.D. *Premenstrual Syndrome and You.* New York: Simon & Schuster, 1983.
Ossofsky, H. J. "Endogenous Depression in Infancy and Childhood," *Comprehensive Psychiatry* 15 (1974): 19–25.
Philpott, William H., M.D., and Dwight K. Kalita, Ph.D. *Brain Allergies, The Psychonutrient Connection.* New Canaan, Conn.: Keats Publishing, 1980.
Schwab, Lawrence. "Suicide and Nutrition . . . Can Poor Nutrition Lead to Suicide?" *Let's LIVE,* January 1984.
Shore, R. E., and D. C. Williams. "Reported Psychological and Physiological Symptoms of Tobacco Smoke Pollution in Non-Smoking College Students," *Journal of Psychology* 101 (1979): 203–18.
Snider, L. B., and D. F. Deiteman. "Teenage Girl's Premenstrual Ache Flare Cut with Vitamin B6," *Obstetrics-Gynecology News,* May 1, 1974, p. 5.
Wurtman, Richard J., M.D., and Wurtman, Judith, Ph.D., eds. *Toxic Effects of Food Constituents on the Brain. Nutrition and the Brain,* vol. 4. New York: Raven Press, 1979.

THERAPEUTIC APPLICATIONS—CARDIOVASCULAR DISEASE

Amsterdam, Ezra, M.D., *et al.,* eds. *Exercise in Cardiovascular Health and Disease.* New York: Yorke Medical Books, 1977.
Friedman, Meyer. *Treating Type A Behavior and Your Heart.* New York: Alfred A. Knopf, 1984.
"Hold the Eggs and Butter," *Time,* March 26, 1984.
Kattus, Albert A., M.D. "On Exercise and Cardiovascular Health," *Executive Health,* 20:7 (April 1984).
Kavanagh, Terence, M.D. *Heart Attack, Counterattack!* Toronto: Van Nostrand Reinhold Ltd., 1976.
———. "Magnesium Deficiency and Hypertension: Correlation Between Magnesium Deficient Diets and Microcirculatory Changes in Situ," *Science,* March 23, 1984.
Michener, James A. "Living with an Ailing Heart," *The New York Times Magazine,* August 25, 1984.
"Study Warns Surgeons to Wait on Bypasses," *The New York Times,* October 3, 1984.

THERAPEUTIC APPLICATIONS—PAIN/ARTHRITIS/MIGRAINE

Balagot, R. C., *et al. Advances in Pain Research and Therapy,* vol. 5. New York: Raven Press, 1983.
Bresler, David, M.D. *Free Yourself from Pain.* New York: Simon & Schuster, 1979.
Buist, R., Ph.D. "Migraine and Food Intolerance," *International Clinical Nutrition Review,* April 1984.
Cantterall, W. E. "Rheumatoid Arthritis Is an Allergy," *Arthritis News Today,* 1980.

Egger, J. *et al.* "Is Migraine Food Allergy?" *The Lancet,* October 15, 1983.
Mandell, Marshall, M.D. *Dr. Mandell's Lifetime Arthritis Relief System.* New York: Coward-McCann, 1983.

THERAPEUTIC APPLICATIONS—WEIGHT LOSS

Scanlon, Lynne Waller. *The 21st Century Diet.* New York: St. Martin's Press, 1984.
Schwartz, Bob. *Diets Don't Work.* Galveston, Tex.: Breakthrough Publishing, 1982.
Vaddadi, K. S., and D. F. Horrobin. "Weight Loss Produced by Evening Primrose Oil Administration in Normal and Schizophrenic Individuals," *IRCS Medical Science* (1979): 52.
Vasselli, Joseph, Ph.D., *et al.* "Modern Concepts of Obesity," *Nutrition Review,* 41:12, December 1983.

THERAPEUTIC APPLICATIONS—MISCELLANEOUS

Bates, D., Faucett, *et al.* "Polyunsaturated Fatty Acids in Treatment of Acute Remitting Multiple Sclerosis," *British Medical Journal* 2, (1978): 1390–91.
Brody, Jane. "Study of Various Treatments for Vaginal Yeast Infections Raises Questions About Many," *The New York Times,* June 6, 1984.
Fredricks, Carlton. *Breast Cancer: A Nutritional Approach.* New York: Grosset & Dunlap, 1977.
———. "Multiple Sclerosis: The Rational Basis for Treatment with Colchicine and Evening Primrose Oil," *Medical Hypotheses* 5 (1979): 365–68.
"New Comforts for Old Bones," *Newsweek,* September 17, 1984.
Philpott, William H., M.D. *Victory Over Diabetes.* New Canaan, Conn.: Keats Publishing, 1983.

Index

achiness, 33
acne, 94, 99, 151
addiction, 316–23
  to exercise, 288–89
  therapy for, 321–23
  see also alcoholism; allergy/addiction syndrome
adrenal glands, 47, 68–69, 279, 340
aerobic exercise, 207, 280–83, 285
  stretching before and after, 287
  target pulse rates for, 281–83
aging, 48, 145, 277
  anti-, regimen, 238, 323–26
  degenerative processes in, 323
AIDS (Acquired Immune Deficiency Syndrome), 68
alanine, 127
alcohol, 154–55, 242–43, 255, 350
  dangers of, 240, 241, 346
  leaky-gut syndrome and, 47, 48, 318–19
alcoholism, 317–21
  depression associated with, 320–21
  food allergies and, 318–20
  malnutrition associated with, 320
  therapy for, 99, 130, 135, 153, 321–23
Alka-Seltzer Gold, 74, 265
allergens, *see* food allergens
allergies, 83, 386
  airborne, 69
  atopic, 336–39
  brain, 341–44
  exercise's effects on, 280, 289–90
  overstimulation of adrenals and, 68–69
  supplementation and, 89
  Type I, 37, 54, 55
  vitamin therapy for, 95, 103–4, 108, 113
  see also food allergies
allergy/addiction syndrome, 48, 49, 55–61
  dieting and, 60–61
  food cravings and, 55–58, 60
  masking phenomenon of, 60
  mechanism of, 58–59
  withdrawal from, 55–58, 60, 261–64, 300
allopathic medicine, 18
all-purpose seasoning mix, 456
almond milk, 441–44
aloe vera juice, 265
alpha linolenic acid (ALA), 139, 141, 143, 145, 148, 155

alternative medicine, 16, 22
  disease and medication in, 18–19
  doctor/patient relationship in, 20
  information bias against, 16–17
  nutrition and exercise in, 21
amenorrhea, 402
American Medical Association (AMA), 21, 22
amino acids, 126–36
  dietary and supplementary sources of, 127–29
  essential vs. nonessential, 127
  functions of, 126–27
  supplementation of, 128–29
  therapeutic uses of, 128–29
anaerobic exercise, 281
anaphylaxis, 289–90, 333
ancestors, diet of, 235
anemia, iron-deficiency, 109, 120, 121, 395–96
angina pectoris, 149
anti-aging regimen, 323–26
  Optimum Health Program in, 324
  undereating in, 238, 324–25
antibiotics, 346
antibodies, 58–59, 67, 69–70, 71
anxiety, vitamin therapy for, 109
any bean soup, 472
apple:
  baked, 481
  crisp, 480–81
  -lime frost, 482
arachidonic acid (AA), 139, 142, 148, 150, 154, 293, 328
arginine, 127, 133–34, 135
arthritis, 101, 326–32
  gouty, 105, 326, 415–16
  osteo-, 326
  see also rheumatoid arthritis
aspartic acid, 127
aspirin, 78, 80, 124, 245–46, 328, 334
asthma, 290, 333–36
  allergic responses in, 333–34
  in children, 301, 333, 335
  therapy and protocol for, 95, 334–36
atherosclerosis, 295, 350–55, 357
  cholesterol levels and, 147–48, 351–54
  development of, 350–51
  diet factor in, 138, 147–48, 349
  platelet aggregation in, 350–51, 354–55
  therapy and protocol for, 99, 116, 358–60
athletes, supplements used by, 133, 134
athletic endurance, 99
atopic allergies, 336–39
attention deficit syndrome, *see* hyperactivity
Australia, primitive cultures in, 26
"average" person, as nonexistent, 28–29, 84
avocado spread, 476–77

baked apple, 481
baking, substitutions for, 456–57
banana-oat muffins, 468
barley, 448
  drop biscuits, 465
  flour, 448
  muffins, 466–67
  whole, as side dish, 448
bean:
  -millet-peach muffins, 467–68
  salad, Spanish, 475
  soup, 472
bed-wetting, 299
bell-shaped-curve phenomenon, 31–33
bends, the, 116
beta carotene (provitamin A), 93, 96–97
beverages, 482–83
  apple-lime frost, 482
  blueberry hill chill, 483
  cranberry cooler, 482
  melon highball, 483
  pineapple chill, 482
  yogurt smoothie, 483
bicarbonates, 65–66, 70, 73–74, 265
biotin, 108, 109–10, 346
birth control pills, 346
birth defects, 94, 109
biscuits, barley drop, 465
bloating, 42, 199–200
blood clotting, 116, 148
blood glucose, 148, 349
blood mineral analysis (BMA), 88, 119

blood pressure, 83, 149, 279, 321, 355
  high, *see* hypertension
  low, 390–91
blood sugar, 74, 279, 343
blood-sugar disorders, 106, 340–41
  see also diabetes; diabetes mellitus; hypoglycemia
blood vitamin analysis (BVA), 88
blueberry:
  hill chill, 483
  -soy muffins, 469
B-lymphocytes, 67, 130
body fat percentage, 209–11, 350
bones, 280
  osteoporosis and, 122, 401–3
brain, 279
  disorders of, 153–54
brain allergies, 341–44
breads:
  buckwheat sunflower, 466
  corn, 466
  rice-soy, 469
  see also muffins
breakfast, 237
breast-feeding, 151, 293
brown fat, 149, 203–4, 206
brown sugar, 455
buckwheat, 450–51
  groats, 450–51
  muffins, 467
  sunflower bread, 466
butternut squash flan, 478

caffeine, 240, 255, 290
calcium, 80, 118, 122–23, 356
  breast-feeding and, 293
  deficiencies in, 82, 119, 122
  food sources of, 122–23
  nondairy sources of, 441
calcium oxalate kidney stones, 106, 114, 123
cancer, 68, 353
  beta carotene and, 96
  diet and, 9, 26, 48, 138
  EFA therapy for, 151–52
  Vitamin A and, 94–95
  Vitamin C and, 113
candidiasis, 320, 344–47
  causes of, 345–46
  food-allergy testing and, 225–28
  symptoms of, 345
  treatment and protocol for, 346–47
candy bars, substitutes for, 298
carbohydrates, 236
  complex, 236, 237, 366–67
  digestion of, 65
cardiovascular disease, 348–60
  risk factors in, 349–50
  therapy and protocol for, 358–60
  see also atherosclerosis; heart attacks; heart disease; hypertension
carob, 451
  "chocolate sauce," 451
  custard, 478–79
cashew:
  butter oat cookies, 480
  spread, 458
catsup, 459–60
cellulite, 211
chemical additives, 46, 47, 51, 238–39, 270
chemical hypersensitivity, 338
chewing, 65, 237
chicken, sesame-honey, 470
chick-pea (garbanzo bean) hummus, 477
children, 291–308, 313
  allergy-related diseases in, 301–8; *see also* hyperactivity
  aspirin as risk for, 246
  asthma among, 301, 333, 335
  cow's milk harmful for, 294–95
  exercise for, 297
  food allergies among, 299–301
  healthy, how to bring up, 295–97
  during infancy, 293–94
  menu suggestions for, 298–99
  obesity among, 212
  parents' responsibility to, 291–92
  physical fitness among, 291
  prenatal care and, 292–93
  school lunches for, 296, 299, 343
  snacks for, 296–97, 298–99
  supplementation for, 294, 297
chili-cumin dressing, 476
chips, 298, 485
chloride, 118, 119
chlorine, 81, 244
chocolate, 255, 451
cholesterol, 83, 147–48, 279, 349, 351–54
  correcting imbalances of, 353–54

cholesterol *(cont.)*
desirable level of, 32, 352–53
dietary sources of, 352
functions of, 351
good and bad, 148, 352–53
vitamins for control of, 99, 100, 113
choline, 108, 110–11
chromium, 118
circulating immune complexes (CICs), 71–72
cis-linoleic acid (cLA; cis-LA), 139, 141, 143, 145, 148, 155
therapeutic applications of, 151, 152
Clark, Barney, 22
cobalamin (Vitamin B12), 107–8
cobalt, 118
Coburn, James, 4
Coca, Arthur F., 40–41
coffee, 47, 155, 240–41, 242–43
cola drinks, 255
cold-pressed oils, 144, 270
colds, 45, 113, 124
collagen, 351
Comaneci, Nadia, 210
complement, 71
complex carbohydrates, 236, 237, 366–67
condiments, *see* sauces and condiments
constipation, 360–62
cookies:
cashew butter oat, 480
no-flour oatmeal, 479–80
cooking:
recipes for, 275–76, 456–85
substitutions for, 456–57
tips for, 272–73
copper, 118
corn, 446
bread, 466
flour, 446
substances containing, 433
cornmeal, 446
pudding, 479
corn syrups, 455
cottonseed, foods containing, 436–37
cracker recipe, universal, 462–63
"cradle cap," 151, 370
cranberry cooler, 482
crash diets, 29–30, 201–5
LPL increased by, 204
metabolism slowed by, 29–30, 201–3
overall health harmed by, 204–5
crepes, basic, 464
crime, 343
cumin-chili dressing, 476
custard, carob, 478–79
cyclic AMP (cAMP), 150
cysteine, 127
cystic breast disease, 116, 152
cystine, 127
cytotoxic test, 62, 223–24, 225

date-pumpkin torte, 481
decaffeinated coffee, 241
delta-6-desaturase (DDS), 141, 151
inhibitors of, 145, 152, 153, 154, 155, 206
depression, 33, 362–64
alcoholism and, 320–21
nutritional factors in, 342
treatment of, 106, 130, 280, 363–64
desserts, 478–82
apple crisp, 480–81
baked apple, 481
butternut squash flan, 478
carob custard, 478–79
cashew butter oat cookies, 480
cornmeal pudding, 479
no-flour oatmeal cookies, 479–80
oat museli, 480
pumpkin-date torte, 481
wheat-free piecrust for all occasions, 482
see also snacks
dextrose, 455
DHGLA, 153, 155
diabetes, 74, 106, 152
juvenile, 301–2, 365
diabetes mellitus, 340–41, 364–68
causes of, 365–66
symptoms of, 366
therapy and protocol for, 366–68
diarrhea, 368–69
diets:
crash, 29–30, 201–5
health vs. beauty factor in, 198
national obsession with, 8

undermined by food allergies, 60–61, 199–200
see also overweight; weight loss
digestion, 27–28, 280, 324
of allergens, 38, 50, 58, 69–72
gastrointestinal tract in, 63–66
digestive disorders, 66, 79, 249, 369–70
as allergy symptom, 45, 73–74
constipation, 360–62
diarrhea, 368–69
hypochlorhydria, 73–74, 345, 346, 371
irritable bowel syndrome, 396–97
treatment of, 74, 99, 264–66
dining out, 273–75
dinner, 237
dips, 476–78
avocado spread, 476–77
eggplant spread, 477
garbanzo bean (chick-pea) hummus, 477
tofu, 477–78
disease:
nutritional needs affected by, 80–81
in traditional vs. alternative medicine, 17–18, 19
diuretics, 83
DL-phenylalanine (DLP), 83, 128, 130–32, 363, 381, 406
DMSO test, 222
docosahexaenoic acid (DHA), 139, 145, 147, 155
doctor/patient relationship, 19–20
D-phenylalanine, 131
duodenum, 63, 65–66, 70
dwarfism, 133–34

eating slowly, 237–38
eczema, 151, 370–72
edema (water retention), 42, 199–200
eggplant spread, 477
eggs:
foods containing, 434
substitute for, 457
eicosapentaenoic acid (EPA), 139, 143, 145, 148
supplementation of, 145–47, 155
elderly, mental impairment in, 343
endorphins, 131
entertaining, 274–75
environmental hazards, 50–52, 81
Eskimos, diet of, 26, 147, 148
essential fatty acids (EFAs), 26, 47, 74, 77, 83, 137–57, 355–56
arthritis and immune-related disorders treated with, 150–52
brain-related disorders treated with, 153–54
brown fat metabolism stimulated by, 206
classification of, 139
coronary disorders and, 147–49
deficiencies in, 139–40
diabetes treated with, 152
female problems treated with, 152
food sources of, 141–44, 154
in herpes therapy, 385
hyperactivity and, 153–54, 303
importance of, 139–41
males' vs. females' need for, 154
in obesity therapy, 149–50
in Optimum Health Program, 154–57
problems related to deficiency in, 137
prostaglandins made from, 140, 141, 145
supplementation of, 145–47, 155, 156–57, 328
evening primrose oil, 147, 148, 155, 156
rubbed into babies' skin, 294
side effects of, 156–57
therapeutic applications of, 149–50, 151, 152, 153, 385
exercise, 7, 30–31, 50, 277–90, 349
addiction to, 288–89
aerobic, 207, 280–83, 285, 287
anaerobic, 281
anaphylaxis induced by, 289–90
in arthritis therapy, 331
for asthmatics, 334
for children, 297
crash programs of, 287–88
disregarded by orthodox medicine, 20
equipment and attire for, 288
flexibility, 281
getting started, 287

exercise *(cont.)*
health benefits of, 277, 278–80
along highways or on city streets, 289
metabolism stimulated by, 30, 207–8, 278
nutrient needs increased by, 81, 287
optimal amount of, 33, 282, 286
personal program of, 284–87
during pregnancy, 293
risk factors in, 283–84
set point raised by, 207–8
"staircase" or "plateau" approach to, 288
tips and cautions for, 287–90
eyes, allergy symptoms and, 42

fast-food restaurants, 274
fasting, water, 231–32, 246, 325, 342
fasting and challenge test, 299–30, 231–32
fat(s), 236–37, 270
body, percentage of, 209–11, 350
brown, 149, 203–4, 206
dietary, balance needed in, 138
digestion of, 65
monounsaturated, 138
partially hydrogenated, 138
polyunsaturated, 138, 150
saturated, 47, 138, 139, 147, 154
trans, 143–44, 154
white, 149, 203, 204, 208
see also essential fatty acids
fatigue, 33, 42, 99, 108
Feingold, Benjamin, 304, 341
ferritin, 122
fertility, 103
fever, 246, 416
fiber, dietary, 239
nongrain sources of, 452
FICA (Food Immune Complex Assay), 224–25, 301
fish, cooking, 272, 273
flan, butternut squash, 478
flatbread, rye, 465
flexibility exercises, 281
flours:
barley, 448
carob as substitute for, 451
corn, 446
oat, 448–49
potato, 451
rice, 447
soy, 451
fluoride, 32–33, 118, 240, 244
foam cells, 351
folic acid, 108–9, 110
food allergens:
avoided before exercise, 289
common, sources of, 432–40
cow's milk as, 294–95
cravings for, 55–58, 60
eliminating, for three months, 6
reintroducing, 266–67
substitutes for, 272, 441–51
food allergies, 6, 27, 37–62
alcoholism and, 318–20
atopic allergies related to, 337–38
bloating caused by, 200
breast-feeding and, 293
causes of, 39, 46–53
childhood diseases related to, 301–8
in children, 299–301
chronic pain and, 43, 405–6
damage caused by, 72–74
delayed response to, 38, 39, 54–55
dismissed by traditional medicine, 21, 37, 39–40
eliminating, through rotation alone, 249–50
environmental pollution and, 50–52
exercise and, 50
facts about, 38–39
food variety and, 48
headaches caused by, 379–81
leaky-gut syndrome and, 47–48
liver/gallbladder system affected by, 373
malnutrition caused by, 49–50
mechanism of, 69–72
mental well-being affected by, 341–44
metabolism slowed by, 200
overeating and, 48, 61, 200
pioneering studies on, 40–41
pregnancy and, 292–93
prevalence of, 38
prevented by rotation diet, 248
refined foods and, 46–47

in rheumatoid arthritis, 327–28
self-testing for, 228–33
skin disorders caused by, 370, 371
stress factor in, 52–53
symptoms of, 38, 41–46, 299–300
testing for, 39, 61–62, 221–33, 300–301
weight problems due to, 30, 60–61, 199–200
food-allergy withdrawal, 55–58
in children, 300
coping with, 261–64
symptoms of, 60
Food and Drug Administration (FDA), 83, 132
food and symptom journals, 256–61
food elimination and challenge test, 229–31
Food Immune Complex Assay (FICA), 62, 224–25, 301
free radicals, 71, 81
vitamins for control of, 96, 98, 103, 328
fried foods, 272–73
frozen fruit, 485
fructose, 455
fruit:
frozen, 485
mix, 484
salad, 298

gallbladder, 65, 70
malfunctioning of, 372–74
gamma linolenic acid (GLA), 139, 141, 143, 145, 148, 151
brown fat cells stimulated by, 149–50
mother's milk as source of, 293
supplementation of, 145–47, 155
garbanzo bean (chick-pea) hummus, 477
gastroenteritis, 294
gastrointestinal tract, 63–66
gazpacho salad soup, 473
glutamine, 127, 128
gluten sensitivity, 374–78
glycine, 127
gouty arthritis, 103, 105, 326, 415–16
grains, whole, alternatives to, 444–51
gravies, thickener for, 456
Greenland Eskimos, diet of, 26, 147
Griffin, Merv, 3, 262, 388
groats, buckwheat, 450
growth hormones, 128, 133–34, 279

hangovers, 153
hay fever, 301, 333
headaches, 45, 378–83
food allergies and, 379–81
treatment of, 381–83
health:
average vs. optimum, 10–12, 29
good, principles of, 7
good, thirteen commonsense truths about, 25–34
nation-wide deterioration of, 8–9
responsibility for, 25
Health and Human Services Agency, 9
health food restaurants, 274
health food stores, 271–72, 298
health questionnaire, 215, 216–19
heart, 134, 279
heart attacks, 148–49, 348, 349, 350, 353
repeat, exercise and, 279–80
vitamin therapy after, 113
heart disease, 324, 348–60
diet and, 26, 147, 348
EFAs and, 147–49
therapy and protocol for, 358–60
vitamin therapy for, 105–6
see also atherosclerosis; cardiovascular disease; hypertension
Heidelberg gastrogram, 266
hemoglobin, 120
hemosiderosis, 121–22
herbal teas, 255
herpes, 134, 383–86
therapy and protocol for, 384–86
high-density lipoprotein (HDL), 148, 352–54
histamines, 100, 112
histidine, 127
hives, 386–87
honey, 455
-sesame chicken, 470
substitute for, 457

hormonal imbalances, 94
Horrobin, David, 139–40, 153, 408
human growth hormone (HGH), 133–34, 279
hummus, garbanzo bean (chick-pea), 477
Humperdinck, Engelbert, 5
hydrochloric acid (HCl), 104, 241
  in capsule form, 264–65
  deficiency of (hypochlorhydria), 73–74, 345, 346
  digestion process and, 56–66
  food allergies and, 70, 73–74
hydrogenation, 143–44
hydrostatic weighing, 210
hydroxyproline, 127
hyperactivity (attention deficit syndrome), 14, 302–8, 343
  dietary causes of, 26, 302–3
  EFA therapy for, 153–54
  juvenile delinquency and, 304–5
  nutritional therapies for, 304, 341
  Optimum Health Program as treatment for, 305–8
  parents' questionnaire for, 305, 306–7
  recent increase in, 302–3
  Ritalin therapy for, 304
  symptoms of, 303
  vitamin therapy for, 101
hypertension (high blood pressure), 200, 349, 355–58
  causes of, 47, 355–57
  drug therapy for, 357–58
  therapy and protocol for, 358–60
hypochlorhydria, 73–74, 345, 346, 371
hypoglycemia, 74, 340–41, 343, 388–90
  food allergies and, 388–89
  therapy and protocol for, 389–90
hypotension, 390–91
hypothyroidism, 212, 391–93

IgE RAST (radioallergosorbent test), 39, 62, 222
illness, nutritional needs affected by, 80–81
immune system, 63, 65, 66–69, 83, 108, 324
  adrenals in, 68–69
  in allergy/addiction syndrome, 58–59
  amino acids in, 126–27
  EFAs' effects on, 150–52
  exercise's effects on, 279
  fever in, 246
  in food-allergy reaction, 69–72
  impaired by food allergies, 38, 58
  mechanics of, 67
  strengthened by Vitamin B5, 102–3
  thymus in, 68
  Vitamin C's effects on, 112
  Vitamin E's role in, 115–16
  zinc as stimulant for, 124
immunoglobulin E (IgE), 39, 69, 222, 224
  see also IgE RAST
immunoglobulin G (IgG), 39, 71, 222, 224, 225
infancy, 293–94
infections, 45, 113, 416–17
ingredient labels, 269–70
inositol, 108, 111
insomnia, 280, 393–95
insulin, 74, 152, 279, 301–2, 343, 349, 364–65
insurance, medical, 22, 329
interferon, 67, 151
intestines, 63, 65–66, 74
  food-allergy reaction in, 69–70
intradermal skin test, 222
iodine, 118
IQ (intelligence quotient), 343
iron, 118, 120–22, 123
iron deficiency, 119, 121, 122, 240
  prevalence of, 82, 120
  protocol for, 395–96
irritable bowel syndrome, 396–97
isoleucine, 127

Japanese, diet of, 26, 147
jogging along highways or on city streets, 289
journals of foods and symptoms, 256–61
juvenile delinquency, 26, 304–5
juvenile diabetes, 301–2, 365

Kaposi's sarcoma, 68
kasha, 450–51
Katz, Aubrey, 73
Kavanagh, Terence, 279–80
kidney failure, 350
kidneys, 356–57
kidney stones, 106, 114, 397–98

label reading, 269–70
lactose, 455
lactose intolerance, 123, 295
laxatives, 83, 361
L-carnitine, 134, 293
leaky-gut syndrome, 47–48, 70–71, 241
  alcohol consumption and, 47, 48, 318–19
learning impairments, vitamin therapy for, 101, 109
least common foods test, 229–30, 232–33
leg cramps, 399–400
lentil salad, 474
leucine, 127
Lewin, Joel, 4
L-glutamine, 135–36
life expectancy, diet and, 26, 238, 324–25
lime-apple frost, 482
lipoprotein lipase (LPL), 204
lithium ointments, 384–85
liver, 352, 373
  iron toxicity and, 121–22
L-lysine, 134–35
London, Robert, 116
low density lipoprotein (LDL), 148, 351, 352
L-phenylalanine, 130–31, 132
lunch, 237
  at school, 296, 299, 343
lung cancer, 96
lysine, 127, 128, 134–35
  in herpes therapy, 135, 384

macrophages, 351
magnesium, 80, 82, 118, 123–24, 147
  deficiency in, 119, 356
mail-order food sources, 431
malitol, 455
malnutrition, 27–28, 30, 66, 79
  alcoholism and, 320
  food allergies and, 38, 49–50, 72–73
manganese, 118
mannitol, 455
margarine, 138, 143, 144
Marino, John, 5
Massimino, Ferdie, 5
mast cells, 69, 70, 72, 74, 112, 263
MaxEPA, 89–90, 147, 148, 155, 156
  therapeutic applications of, 151, 152, 385
mayonnaise, sauces made with, 458–59
meat:
  cooking, 272, 273
  substitutes for, 444
medical insurance, 22, 329
medications, 244–46
  caffeine in, 240
  nutrients as, 83
  in traditional vs. alternative medicine, 18
  vitamin absorption affected by, 80–81
medicine, medical profession, 16–23
  costs of, 22
  disease and medication as viewed by, 17–19
  doctor/patient relationship in, 19–20
  future of, 22–23
  information bias in, 16–17
  modern, failure of, 21–22
  nutrition, allergy, and exercise disregarded by, 20–21, 37, 39–40, 77–78
  traditional vs. alternative, 16
melon highball, 483
membranes, 139–40
memory, enhancement of, 103
menstrual bleeding, excess, 94
mental disorders:
  nutritional factors in, 341–44
  vitamin therapy for, 101, 106, 107–8
menu planning, 250–55
metabolic acidosis, 74
metabolic rate:
  crash diets and, 29–30, 201–3
  exercise factor in, 30, 207–8, 278

metabolic rate *(cont.)*
  raising, 205–8
  slowed by food allergies, 200
  time of day and, 206
  white vs. brown fat and, 203–4
metasulfites and metabisulfites, 338
methionine, 127, 134
micellized form, 90, 93, 314–15
middle-ear infections, 294
migraines, 43, 130, 378–83
  food allergies and, 379–81
  treatment of, 381–83
milk, milk products, 122–23, 292
  cow's vs. mother's, 293
  foods containing, 435–36
  harmful effects of, 243–44, 294–95
  lactose intolerance and, 123, 295
  raw, 272
  substitutes for, 441–44, 457
millet, 449–50
  -bean-peach muffins, 467–68
  burgers, 450
  whole, as side dish, 449–50
minerals, 118–25
  blood levels of, 88, 119
  bulk vs. trace, 118
  deficiencies in, 118–19
  food sources of, 118
  hypertension and, 356
  optimum dosages of, 119
  vitamins packaged with, 89, 119–20
  see also specific minerals
mitochondria, 149, 206
molybdenum, 118
Moment, Gardiner B., 327
monounsaturated fats, 138
mood, diet's effect on, 26
MSG (monosodium glutamate), 338
mucus, 45, 70
muffins:
  banana-oat, 468
  barley, 466–67
  buckwheat, 467
  millet-bean-peach, 467–68
  rye, 468–69
  soy-blueberry, 469
  see also breads
multiple sclerosis (MS), 151, 400–401
multivitamin/multimineral capsules, 89, 119–20
munchy nut, seed, and popcorn snacks, 484
muscles, 208, 281
museli, oat, 480

NAD, 100
nails, brittle, 152
narcotic addictions, 316
nervous system, 126, 153, 357
New York, N.Y., jogging in, 289
niacin (Vitamin B3), 100–102, 130
niacinamide, 100, 102
"niacin flush," 100, 102
nicotinamide, 100
nicotinic acid, 100, 102
nightshades:
  arthritis and, 330–31
  foods containing, 437–39
no-flour oatmeal cookies, 479–80
noodle vegetable salad Orientale, 474
noradrenaline, 207, 278
norepinephrine, 132
nut(s):
  oil-free roasted, 484
  seed and popcorn snacks, munchy, 483–84
  see also nut sauces and spreads
nutrient deficiencies, 77–82, 83, 118–19
  ailments caused by, 82
  causes of, 78–81
nutrients, 7
  individual differences in need for, 84
  RDAs as poor guide to, 84–85
  see also minerals; supplements, supplementation; vitamins; *specific vitamins and minerals*
nutrition:
  disregarded in orthodox medicine, 20, 77–78
  educating oneself about, 234–35
  importance of, 25–27
  thirteen basic guidelines for, 234–47
nut sauces and spreads, 461–62
  cashew spread, 458
  nut butter deluxe, 461
  peanut sauce for vegetables, rice, or noodles, 462
  spicy nut sauce, 461–62

oat(s), 448–49
banana muffins, 468
cashew butter cookies, 480
flour, 448–49
museli, 480
oatmeal, 449
cookies, no-flour, 479–80
obesity, 209, 212, 356
EFA therapy for, 149–50
see also overweight
oil(s), 270
-free roasted nuts, 484
vegetable and seed, 142–44, 270
and vinegar dressing, basic, 475–76
opiates, 60
opioids, 59
Optimum Health Labs (OHL), 23–24, 51–52
Optimum Health Program, 195–308
benefits of, 12–13
case histories of, 3–6
for children, 291–308, 313
cooking tips for, 272–73
coping with withdrawal symptoms in, 261–64
digestive support in, 264–66
dining out on, 273–75
exercise in, 277–90
food and symptom journal in, 256–61
goal of, 10–11
learning about your health in, 215–20
nutrition guidelines for, 234–47
recipes for, 275–76, 456–85
reintroducing allergic foods in, 266–67
rotation diet in, 248–56
shopping for, 269–72
summarized, 6–7
supplementation in, 85–90, 261
therapeutic applications of, 311–15; *see also specific ailments*
weight loss as by-product of, 197–214
Optimum Health Weight-Loss Program, 213–14
ornithine, 133–34
osteoarthritis, 326
osteoporosis, 122, 401–3
overeating, 48, 61
overweight:
causes of, 30, 60–61, 211–12
white vs. brown fat in, 203–4
see also diets; obesity; weight loss
oxygenation, 279

pain, chronic, 403–7
food allergies and, 45, 405–6
treatment of, 83, 128, 131–32, 405–7
pancake recipe, basic, 463
pancreas, 47, 65–66, 70, 73–74, 320, 340
pancreatic digestive tablets, 74, 265
pantothenic acid (Vitamin B5), 102–4
para-aminobenzoic acid (PABA), 108, 110
partially hydrogenated fats, 138
parties, eating at, 274–75
patient/doctor relationship, 19–20
Pauling, Linus, 15, 91, 112, 113, 341
peach-millet-bean muffins, 467–68
peanut sauce for vegetables, rice, or noodles, 462
pellagra, 100
pepsin, 65
periodontal disease, 113
personality, diet's effect on, 26
phagocytes, 67
phenethylamine (PEA), 132
phenylalanine, 127, 130–32
DL- form of (DLP), 83, 128, 130–32, 363, 381, 406
dosages of, 132
functions of, 130–31
therapeutic applications of, 131–32
Philpott, William, 41, 301–2
phobias, 343–44
phosphorus, 118, 119
phosphorylation, 97
piecrust, wheat-free, for all occasions, 482
pineapple chill, 482
pituitary dwarfism, 133–34
pituitary gland, 340
platelet aggregation, 83, 141, 148, 280, 302, 354–55
in atherosclerosis, 350–51

poached salmon, 471
pollution, 81
  allergy incidence and, 50–52
polyunsaturated fats, 138, 150
popcorn, nut, and seed snacks, munchy, 483–84
potassium, 118, 119, 356
potassium bicarbonate, 265
potato:
  chips, substitutes for, 298
  flour, 451
  soup, basic, 472–73
  white, foods containing, 438
Powell, John, 5, 133
preeclampsia, 123
pregnancy, 94, 109, 123, 292–93
premenstrual syndrome (PMS), 43, 407–10
  causes of, 408
  symptoms of, 408
  treatment of, 105, 116, 152, 408–10
prenatal care, 292–93
Pritikin, Nathan, 61, 199
Prokop, Dave, 5
proline, 127
prostacyclin (PG12), 150, 302
prostaglandins (PGs), 140–47, 246, 262, 320, 355–56, 408
  balance between 1, 2, and 3 series of, 140–41, 154
  EFAs transformed into, 140, 141–47
  functions of, 140
  PGD2, 149
  PGE1, 140–41, 148, 149, 150, 151–52, 153, 154, 155, 206, 328, 381
  PGE2, 140–41, 142, 148, 149, 150, 151, 328
  PGE3, 140–41, 148, 149, 150, 151–52, 154, 206, 328, 381
  PG12 (prostacyclin), 150, 302
prostanoids, 140, 245
protein, 126, 127–28, 236
  digestion of, 65, 70
  nonmeat sources of, 444
  see also amino acids
psoriasis, 151, 371
psychological disorders, *see* mental disorders
psychosomatic ailments, 33
pudding, cornmeal, 479
puffed rice, 447
pulse tests, 232, 267, 283
pumpkin-date torte, 481
pyridoxine, *see* Vitamin B6

Randolph, Theron, 15, 40, 41, 231, 318
raw foods, 238, 272
raw sugar, 454
recipes, 275–76, 456–85
Recommended Daily Allowances (RDAs), 84–85
  for minerals, 119, 124, 125
  for vitamins, 29, 77, 79, 106, 115, 117
Reed, Barbara, 304–5
refined foods, 46–47, 238–40, 248–49
restaurants, dining in, 273, 274
retinol, *see* Vitamin A
Reyes syndrome, 246
Rhea, William, 231
rheumatoid arthritis, 151, 326–32
  causes of, 327–28
  dietary management for, 330–31
  effects of, 326–27
  exercise as therapy for, 331
  protocol for, 332
  vitamin therapy for, 103, 105, 328
rhinitis, 333
riboflavin (Vitamin B2), 82, 98–100
rice:
  flour, 447
  puffed, 447
  -soy bread, 469
  whole grain, 447
Rinkel, Herbert, 15, 40, 41
Ritalin, 303–4
rotation diet, 6–7, 235–36, 248–56
  allergy elimination and, 249–50
  benefits of, 248–49
  planning, 250–55
  reintroducing allergic foods into, 266–67
  tips for following, 255–56
Rowe, William, 15
Rudin, Donald O., 137
rye, 447–48
  flatbread, 465
  meal, 447–48
  muffins, 468–69

salad dressings, 475–76
basic oil and vinegar, 475–76
chili-cumin, 476
salads, 255, 473–75
gazpacho, soup, 473
lentil, 474
seaweed, 474
Spanish bean, 475
tabouleh, 475
vegetable noodle, Orientale, 474
salivation, 65
salmon, poached, 471
salsa, 461
salt, 47, 243, 270, 356–57
substitutes for, 456
sandwich ideas for lunch boxes, 299
saturated fats, 47, 138, 139, 147, 154
sauces and condiments, 457–62
carob "chocolate," 451
cashew spread, 458
catsup, 459–60
made with mayonnaise, 458–59
made with tomato sauce substitute, 459
salsa, 461
thickener for, 456
tomato, substitute, 459
tomato paste, 460
see also nut sauces and spreads
schizophrenia, 342
EFA therapy for, 153, 154
vitamin therapy for, 101, 106
school lunches, 296, 299, 343
seasoning mix, all-purpose, 456
seaweed salad, 474
secretory IgA, 69–70
seed, nut, and popcorn snacks, munchy, 483–84
seed oils, 142–44
hydrogenation of, 143–44
selenium, 118, 125
Selye, Hans, 52, 68
senility, 101
serine, 127
serotonin, 102, 106, 129–30
sesame-honey chicken, 470
set point, 202, 204, 205
raised by exercise, 207–8
Seventh Day Adventists, 26
Shils, Maurice, 21–22
shopping, 269–72
label reading in, 269–70
mail-order, 431
silicon, 118
Sjögren's syndrome, 151
skin disorders:
acne, 94, 99, 151
eczema, 151, 370–72
skin-fold tests (body fat percentages), 210–11
skin tests (allergies), 39, 61, 221–22
sleep, tryptophan's and serotonin's effects on, 129–30
sleep disorders, 280, 393–95
treatment of, 102, 394–95
small intestine, 63, 65–66, 70, 74
smoking, 47, 154–55, 241, 343, 349, 356
allergy/addiction syndrome and, 59–60
snacks, 483–85
for children, 296–97, 298–99
chips, 298, 485
frozen fruit, 485
fruit mix, 485
munchy nut, seed, and popcorn, 484
oil-free roasted nuts, 484
see also desserts
"soda" substitute, 298
sodium, 118, 119, 243, 270, 356
sodium benzoate, 338
sodium bicarbonate, 265
sorbitol, 455
soups, 471–73
any bean, 472
basic potato, 472–73
gazpacho salad, 473
soy:
-blueberry muffins, 469
flour, 451
-rice bread, 469
soybean, foods containing, 439–40
Spanish bean salad, 475
spicy nut sauce, 461–62
spreads, *see* dips; nut sauces and spreads; sauces and condiments
squash, butternut flan, 478
steaming, 273
stir-frying, 273
stomach, 63, 65, 70, 73–74
stool analysis, 266

stress, 52–53, 206, 357
  management of, 410–12
  nutrient needs increased by, 80
  and overstimulation of adrenals, 68–69
stress hormones, 59, 60, 68
strokes, 349, 350, 353
sucrose, 454
sugars, 47, 240, 241–43, 255, 269, 346
  types of, 454–55
sunflower buckwheat bread, 466
supplements, supplementation, 31, 77–90, 314–15
  amino acids, 128–29
  beta carotene, 96–97
  choline, 111
  cobalamin (Vitamin B12), 108
  essential fatty acids, 145–47, 155, 156–57, 328
  folic acid, 109
  guidelines for personal program of, 85–90
  how much is needed, 84–85
  hypoallergenic, 89
  for infants and children, 294, 297
  inositol, 111
  for juvenile diabetics, 302
  natural vs. synthetic, 89
  niacin (Vitamin B3), 102
  optimal, case for, 83
  for Optimum Health Weight-Loss Program, 213–14
  in orthodox medicine, 20–21, 77–78
  PABA, 110
  pantothenic acid (Vitamin B5), 104
  during pregnancy, 292
  pyridoxine (Vitamin B6), 106–7
  reasons for, 78–84
  riboflavin (Vitamin B2), 100
  storing, 89
  therapeutic use of, 83, 91, 406
  timed-release, 90
  Vitamin A, 90, 95
  Vitamin C, 114
  Vitamin E, 90, 117
  what to take, 85–88
  when and how to take, 88–90, 238, 261
  see also specific vitamins and minerals
sweets, *see* desserts; snacks
sympathetic nervous system, 357

tabouleh salad, 475
tartrazine, 338
teas, 240, 255
tension headaches, 378
thiamine (Vitamin B1), 97–98
thickener for sauces and gravies, 456
thirst, excessive or inappropriate, 42
threonine, 127
thrombophlebitis, 116
thymus, 68, 83, 279
thyroid, underactive (hypothyroidism), 212, 391–93
tinnitus, 412–13
T-lymphocytes, 67, 151
tobacco, 240, 241, 255
  see also smoking
tocopherol, *see* Vitamin E
Tofranil, 130
tofu:
  dip, 477–78
  yogurt, 444
tomato(es):
  catsup, 459–60
  foods containing, 439
  paste, 460
  sauce substitute, 459
tooth decay, 106
torte, pumpkin-date, 481
total invert sugar, 455
trans fats, 143–44, 154
traveling, 273
triglycerides, 83, 148, 279
tryptophan, 80, 127, 129–30
turbinado, 454
turkey patties, 470
tyrosine, 127, 132

ulcers, 245, 413–15
undereating, longevity and, 238, 324–25
universal cracker recipe, 462–63
uric acid, 103, 326
  elevated, 349–50, 415–16

valine, 127
vanadium, 118

vascular disease, 101
  see also atherosclerosis;
    cardiovascular disease;
    hypertension
vasospasm, 148–49, 349
vegetable(s):
  buying, 271
  cooking, 272, 273
  crudités, 298
vegetable noodle salad Orientale,
    474
vegetable oils, 142–44, 270
  hydrogenation of, 143–44
vegetarians, 108, 135
very-low-density lipoprotein
    (VLDL), 352
viral infection, 416–17
Vitamin A (retinol), 77, 80, 82, 92,
    93–95
  beta carotene as precursor of,
    93, 96–97
  food sources of, 93
  functions of, 93–94
  in micellized form, 90, 93,
    314–15
  supplementation of, 90, 95
  therapeutic applications of, 74,
    83, 94–95
  toxicity from overdoses of, 93, 95
Vitamin B1 (thiamine), 97–98
Vitamin B2 (riboflavin), 82, 98–100
  functions of, 98–99
  supplementation of, 100
  therapeutic applications of, 99
Vitamin B3 (niacin), 100–2, 130
  functions of, 100
  therapeutic applications of,
    101–2
Vitamin B5 (pantothenic acid),
    102–4
  functions of, 102–3
  therapeutic applications of, 103–4
Vitamin B6 (pyridoxine), 82, 104–7,
    147
  functions of, 104–5
  supplementation of, 106–7
  therapeutic applications of,
    105–6
  toxicity from overdoses of, 106–7
Vitamin B12 (cobalamin), 107–8
Vitamin C, 74, 77, 79, 80, 92,
    111–14
  anaphylaxis prevented by,
    289–90
  functions of, 112
  supplementation of, 114
  therapeutic applications of, 83,
    91, 113, 384
  withdrawal symptoms alleviated
    by, 262–64
Vitamin D, 91–93
vitamin deficiencies, *see* nutrient
    deficiencies
Vitamin E (tocopherol), 80, 92,
    114–17, 147
  EFA supplementation and,
    156
  functions of, 115–16
  in micellized form, 90, 93,
    314–15
  selenium and, 125
  supplementation of, 90, 117
  therapeutic applications of,
    116–17, 302
Vitamin K, 92
vitamins, 91–117
  B-complex, 74, 80, 92, 97–111
  blood levels of, 88
  discovery of, 91
  dosage units of, 92
  fat-soluble vs. water-soluble,
    92–93
  functions of, 92
  minerals packaged with, 89,
    119–20
  naming and numbering of,
    92
  overdoses of, 78, 92–93
  see also specific vitamins

waffle batter, basic, 464
Walford, Roy, 324–25
water, drinking, 244, 255
water fasting, 231–32, 246, 325,
    342
water retention (edema), 42,
    199–200
weaning, 151
weight, optimum, 208–11
  percentage of body fat and,
    209–11
weight loss, 29–30, 197–214
  allergy factor in, 60–61, 199–200
  "calories in" factor vs. "calories
    out" factor in, 201–5
  health vs. beauty as factor in,
    198

weight loss *(cont.)*
individual set points and, 202, 204, 205, 207–8
metabolic rate and, 201–3, 205–8
Optimum Health Program for, 213–14
right way of, 205–8
on rotation diet, 249
wrong way of, 198–205
see also diets; overweight
wheat:
alternatives to, 444–51
foods containing, 434–35
-free piecrust for all occasions, 482
white blood cells, 67, 71, 242
white fat, 149, 203, 204, 208
Williams, Roger, 102
withdrawal, 316, 317, 321
see also food-allergy withdrawal
Wright, Jonathan, 373

xylitol, 455

yeast:
-base vitamins, 97
foods containing, 432
yogurt:
smoothie, 483
tofu, 444

Zeller, Michael, 40, 328
zinc, 74, 83, 84, 118, 124–25